The
HEALTH AND BEAUTY BOOK

The
HEALTH AND BEAUTY BOOK

Edited by Gillian Cooke

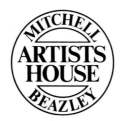

Published in 1979 by Artists House,
Mitchell Beazley Marketing Limited,
Artists House, 14-15 Manette Street,
London W1V 5LB.

Designed and produced for Artists
House by Roxby Press Productions
Limited, 98 Clapham Common
Northside, London SW4 9SG.

ISBN 0 86134 007 8

D. L.: S. S. 539 - 79

Printed in Spain by TONSA,
San Sebastian.

Production: Reynolds Clark
Associates Limited

Contents

Acknowledgements

*The editor and publishers would like to express their gratitude
to the many people who have contributed to this book.*

In particular, the writers of the various chapters:
Anne Boston: Eye Care
Carol Dix and Judy Froshaug: who both provided material for A Healthy Body and A Supple Body
Carolyn Faulder: A Woman's Body, Puberty, Menstruation, Enjoying Sex, Breasts, Birth Control and Menopause
Lesley Garner: Pregnancy and Childbirth
Jean Hutchison: Hair Care and Hair Styling
Brigid Keenan: Body Hair, Skin, Make-up, Hands and Feet, and Margaret McCartney who assisted on the Make-up chapter
Mary Kenny: The Inner Woman and Plastic Surgery
Laura Pank: Clean Outside and In and Dental Care
Catherine Storr: How well do you know yourself?

Appreciation must be expressed especially to Judy Froshaug and Jean Hutchison for compiling most of the Information A to Z and supplying a wide variety of extra material during the final stages of the make-up of the book.

Our thanks go also to those who contributed their expertise to certain chapters:
Lotte Berk for the exercise programme
Kirsty Climo for the make-up of our models and Yvonne Gold who did additional make-up work
Leonard of Mayfair for all the hairstyles
Clare Maxwell-Hudson for massage technique and recipes for natural skin care

The editor and publishers also wish to acknowledge the help of the following people, who painstakingly advised us, read and checked copy, and made suggestions for improvements:
Dr Elizabeth Evans, Department of Nutrition, Queen Elizabeth College, London
Dr M.G. Brush BSc MA PhD
Janice Bumstead SRN MEd
Dr Katharina Dalton MRCS LRCP Gynaecological Endocrinologist
Elizabeth Fern SRN MTD
Dr Jean Infield MRCS LRCP
Professor John Marshall MD FRCP(Lond) FRCP(Ed) DpM of the Natural Family Planning Service
Dr Prudence Tunnadine, Member of the Institute of Psychosexual Medicine
Maurice B. Rothschild BDS LDS RCS, who advised on the dental section and supplied clinical photography for Orthodontics
John Atkins and Jennifer Beeby, Members of the Institute of Trichologists
David Capaldo
Caroline Laing, Wella (Great Britain) Ltd
David Sandler

We also wish to acknowledge the important contribution made by the artists and photographers whose work has helped to give the book its exceptionally high visual standard:
Illustrators:
John Bavosi
Mick Brownfield
Julie Depledge
Jean Maxime Perramon
Photographers:
Terence Donovan
Harry Peccinotti
Robin Saidman
Roger Stowell
Retouching:
Valerie Bennett
Maurice Tait
Redken Laboratories, who supplied the photomicrographs of hair on page 176
The Trustees of the British Museum (Natural History) for permission to reproduce the illustration on page 113

Finally, sincere thanks to all those who assisted in the complicated work of putting the book together:
Ramona Darvas
Kim Evans
Zoë Richmond-Watson
Franny Singer

Introduction

Since the first herbal medicines were accidentally discovered and the first beauty aids employed, there has been a market for information about the way our bodies work, or fail to work, and about techniques for making them more attractive. Many books have been written about health and as many, if not more, about beauty. This one was conceived to meet the need for one encyclopedic book, for and about women, which dealt with two aspects of life that are essentially interlinked: health and beauty.

It would be unfair to claim that THE HEALTH AND BEAUTY BOOK contains everything a woman wants to know about herself; such a book, as far as we know, has not yet been written, nor in practical terms is it likely to be. However, we have attempted to cover as many aspects of being female as possible: from conception and birth to our feelings about sex; the food we eat and its effects on us; how our bodies change over the years and what we can do to slow down the ageing process; and how we can make the most of ourselves and therefore our lives.

From the moment we are born we are given the label 'female', but no two of us are alike – mentally, physically or emotionally – although obviously we share many similar features and physical characteristics. However, once labelled 'female', certain patterns of development and behaviour are expected of us, whether we fulfil these or not. Long-established notions of femininity will be cast upon us. We will be told that little girls do or don't do certain things; and we will read books, be told stories and watch our elders behaving in ways which confirm this. Some of the propaganda will be useful, some of it we may reject as irrelevant to women today. But that we are female remains an unalterable fact.

At puberty, whether we like it or not (and many girls don't), our bodies start to change perceptibly, externally and internally as well. Physically we become capable of having and enjoying sex, and of bearing children, although emotionally and psychologically we are not yet prepared for marriage and motherhood nor, except in rare instances, will we have to accept these roles.

The transition from girl to young woman and from young woman to mature woman takes time and, as in everything else, the processes will be shorter, longer, easier or more complicated depending on a number of factors. The most important of these include genetic inheritance and the environment in which we grow up and live. Our genetic inheritance will to some extent dictate our general health – our potential size and strength, predisposition to certain diseases or physical peculiarities, the basic shape of our bodies, the colour of our eyes, skin and hair. For the rest, the environment in which we are reared – the food we are given, exercise we take, people we grow up with, schools we attend, circumstances in which we live – has an important bearing on the kind of women we ultimately become.

We cannot alter the genetic factor: if we are born beautiful, for instance, we are blessed; if we are born strong and healthy, we are doubly so. But, thereafter, our parents or guardians and later we ourselves are largely responsible for moulding the finished product. The body is sometimes referred to in this book as a machine, because that is in effect what it is. If the machine runs well, it is likely that its components, both internal and external, will also function well. Having a healthy, beautiful body-machine may not guarantee a peaceful mind and a happy soul, but these are more easily achieved through keeping healthy and beautiful than through neglect. And never before have women had so many chances to be both healthy and beautiful. We have all the essential requirements: food in abundance and a wide choice of food at that; medical services that enable us to monitor our health and seek help if we are less than fit, and which in most cases offer us ways of rectifying the situation; the opportunity to keep fit through forms of exercise which are actually enjoyable; thousands of beauty aids, from cosmetics to heated rollers; and access to a mass of information and advice through literature and the media. And yet, the fact remains that many of us are far less fit and healthy than we could or should be.

Physicians, psychologists and sociologists will argue that this is often because we also live with many counter-acting factors. The stresses of life today are numerous: we may try to combine the activities of housewife, mother, working woman and lover; work in polluted atmospheres, often under great pressure; live in over-crowded conditions; over-eat and under-exercise. And, against all this, we are perhaps more aware than ever of trying to beat the time-clock – in the words of the Thirties' song, we are constantly admonished 'to keep young and beautiful . . . if you want to be loved'. Because of the pressures of our modern, industrialized societies, because we are so far removed from the slower, more 'natural' lives of our ancestors, many experts are amazed that our bodies function at maintenance, let alone high-performance, levels – particularly when they are additionally abused by drugs such as alcohol, nicotine, stimulants and tranquillizers. We may even realize that we are behaving unwisely, but seem to be caught on a treadmill of necessary activity or compulsive behaviour, and it takes strength of purpose and a definite goal to be able to slow down and get off.

We hope that THE HEALTH AND BEAUTY BOOK will provide information and guidance to all women, no matter what their age or circumstance. The book describes the essentials for basic healthy living – food, exercise and hygiene – through to more elaborate programmes aimed at developing and maintaining our bodies at a high level of fitness. It explains how our bodies work and the various processes they undergo from birth, through puberty, to the menopause and after. It includes numerous ways of catering for, cosseting and beautifying our bodies. And it devotes space to discussing and suggesting ways of coping with the many problems that women may have to face at some time during their lives, from alcoholism to warts. We have not assumed that one problem is of more importance than another because, since we are all individuals, our problem will be as great or small as our reaction to it.

A little knowledge, it is often said, is a dangerous thing. We hope that THE HEALTH AND BEAUTY BOOK contains a lot of knowledge. We believe it will dispel myths, offer facts and provide new information to any woman who seeks to know more about herself. We hope it will be a guide to women wishing to be not just as healthy and beautiful as nature intended, but a little more besides.

11

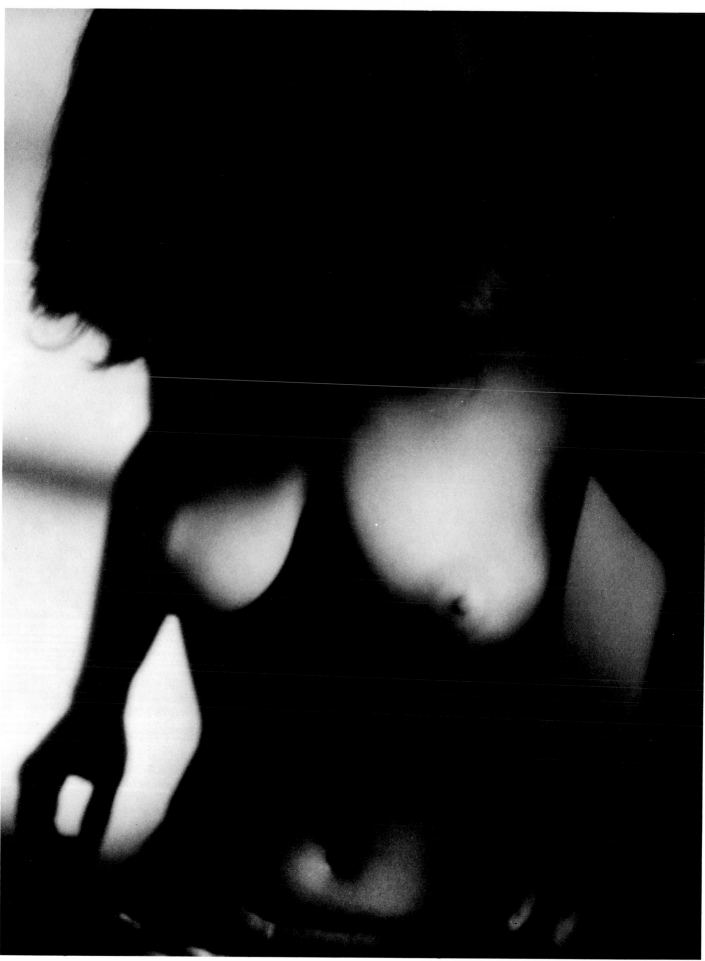

The Inner Woman

Women are narcissistic: that fact is well established. Advertising agencies have repeatedly found that you sell a product to a man by showing a naked woman – and you also sell a product to a woman by showing a naked woman. Most women are not aroused by photographs of men in the nude; but most women are interested in photographs of women in the nude. The psychologists' explanation for this is that women identify with the picture of the naked woman. All women are fascinated by their own bodies:

Narcissism in a woman can be both a good and a bad influence. It is good when it enhances her self-respect, pleases her and other people and generally adds to the gaiety of the nation. A healthy amount of self-interest brings long-term benefits not only because the individual is likely to be more fastidious and attractive than someone with none, but also in the sense that it creates a psychological resource that is helpful to the personality. Having your hair done cheers you up; buying a new dress brightens up a dank February day; losing weight, having a manicure or beauty treatment, re-fashioning yourself in some way can be genuinely renewing to the spirit. The fact that men in Western society tend to be less aware of their bodily appearance robs them of a means of relaxation and refreshment. Arranging your wardrobe for an afternoon, changing your hair colour, doing something different to your face are all forms of grooming therapy, probably akin to the grooming rituals that all the higher animals perform, and are almost certainly very good for you.

However, self-interest turns bad when it becomes a major source of distraction from other things in life, or an obsession. The academic performance of schoolgirls falls off drastically when they start concentrating on clothes and make-up, their figures and the impact that they are making, as females, on the world. Grooming in itself can never make a woman happy, and if you want the proof of that, you only need to look into the face of a great beauty who has grown old and lost everything except a fruitless preoccupation with her looks. Fulfilment, happiness, satisfaction, achievement, all the things we strive after through grooming, must begin with the inner woman and with the core of the personality. If the personality is integrated – if it is, literally, together, and functioning organically – *anything* can be achieved within the bounds of possibility. But if the personality is fragmented, under-nourished or maladjusted, then no amount of having your hair done or your face lifted is ever going to paper over the cracks. The ability to cope, to function and to blossom lies entirely with the personality, with the inner woman.

It is very easy for women today to forget this, or just not to be aware of it – bombarded as we all are with the images of the *outer* woman. Societies have always striven to create ideals in feminine beauty, and women in all societies have been exhorted to emulate these ideals: there is nothing new in that part of image-making. But never before have we had means of communication so powerful and manipulative as we have now; and never before have we had a society so relentlessly materialistic that the balancing elements of spiritual and emotional values often become outweighed. A woman in Jane Austen's time might have bemoaned the fact that she was not handsome, but she might have drawn comfort from the thought that she was considered kind and good-natured – qualities genuinely admired and constantly extolled. A woman in the last century might have feared that she was not pretty or rich enough to get a husband, but she might have been consoled by the thought that she was dutiful and useful to her family. A woman in pre-war times might have envied the great beauties who dazzled society – the Lillie Langtrys and the Isadora Duncans – yet society still respected her for being a *mother*.

The limited options open to women in the past would not seem very attractive to us because they were *so* limited, but the settled social order of other times did provide its own checks and balances. In those days a plain woman still had a harder life than a pretty one, and moreover, she could do less about it than she can today; but she had comforts and praises that she would not have today. She was told she was virtuous, she was dutiful, she was a pillar of the community – and indeed she herself would often compensate for her lack of beauty with other energies, and even find satisfaction in other achievements. Today, women are under far more pressure to be beautiful, and often feel far more anxious about their appearance because beauty, they sense, is what society values.

But then, contemporary woman has so many different conflicts to resolve; and that, perhaps, is one of the reasons why she needs, more than ever before, a balance and a perspective within her inner life. The whole driving idea behind the feminist movement which has had such an impact on the social position of women in recent years lies in the slogan adopted by the abortion lobby: *'A woman's right to choose'*. In a wider context, this is what women's liberation has been all about – the ability, before more or less reserved for men, to choose one's own path in life. To choose whether to marry or not, freely; whether to have children or not; whether to raise them oneself or to enlist help in raising them; whether to work right through one's life or to take time off for a family; and, very importantly, to choose the kind of work one does.

But what the slogan doesn't say, and what we don't always understand, is that choice always brings conflict. It always brings responsibility, dilemma and stress. And the right to choose – which is also the burden, the responsibility of choosing – has entered into almost every area of a woman's life. A few years ago, a woman in childbirth would simply have been given an analgesic as the doctor or midwife considered appropriate. But these days women are being briefed beforehand like medical students, with a lecture on the range of analgesics available, their effects, their duration, their composition, their administration. Ideally, now, the woman *chooses* what kind of birth experience she is going to have. And a very good thing this is, too, since it gives the mother more control over her own life. Yet women have been heard to mutter, coming out of such antenatal lectures, 'I wish the doctors would just decide all these things for me'; just as women who, one might imagine, should be on their bended knees thanking fate for the invention of birth control have been heard to sigh, 'I can't seem to decide whether or when to have a family – I wish it would all just happen by mistake.' Birth control is fine, but it means that women have to take the conscious decision to have a baby – and when they get to thinking about it, it's quite a burdensome decision.

When choice is expanded, life is enriched, yet it is always made more taxing, too. Making decisions takes its toll. As liberation has progressed, so have women's stresses. Alcoholism among women has trebled within a decade; while men are stopping smoking in droves, women are only quitting in dribbles. More women are taking sleeping pills than ever before; and one woman in five in Britain is taking tranquillizers. Mental breakdown is more common today than it ever used to be. All these are the indices of stress, caused by pressures with which the personality has to cope. Before we can achieve anything like the inner serenity, the 'togetherness' of ourselves, we have to be aware of the stresses which are battening upon us. We have to know ourselves – and then be able to perceive whether our inner selves are mostly in tune with the lives we lead – or battling miserably, even if subconsciously, against them.

There are some people who believe that women have a special need to be in touch with the rhythm of life, and that an environment which is highly artificial or brutally dehumanizing has a worse psychological effect on women than on men. The theory goes that because of their primary biological function in child-bearing, women have developed more tenderness than men and consequently need more tenderness themselves. The concrete jungles of new towns and high-rise blocks may indeed have a more depressing effect on women than on men, quite apart from the fact that women are imprisoned in them all day if they have children.

Then there are the ancient superstitions and taboos, based on women's menstrual cycles. Most religions acknowledge the fear and the magic associated with menstruation, for it always impressed our ancestors most awesomely that the average woman's menses are in perfect harmony with the waning and waxing of the moon – twenty-eight days. Primitive peoples assumed that this meant that women were in some mystical way in touch with

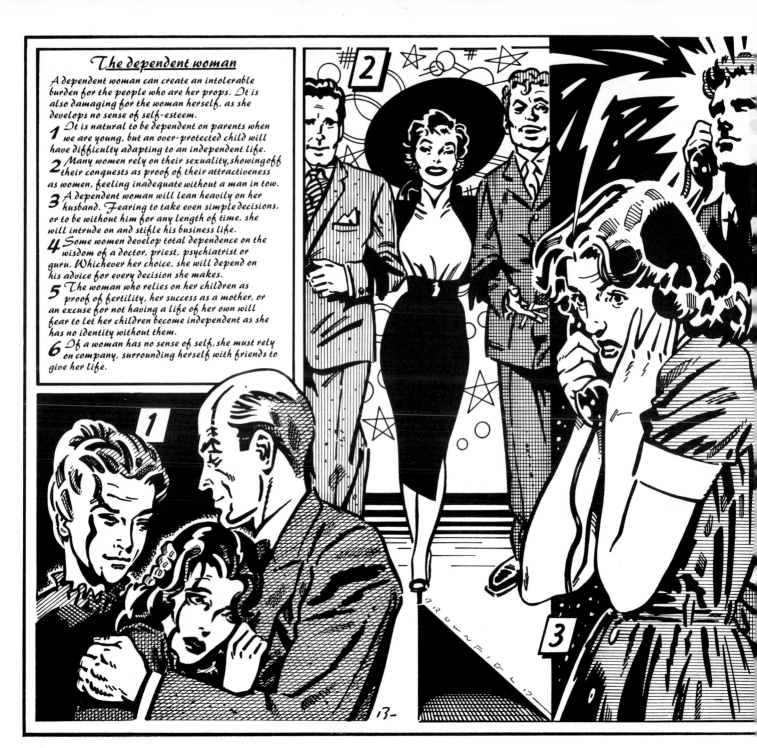

The dependent woman

A dependent woman can create an intolerable burden for the people who are her props. It is also damaging for the woman herself, as she develops no sense of self-esteem.

1. It is natural to be dependent on parents when we are young, but an over-protected child will have difficulty adapting to an independent life.

2. Many women rely on their sexuality, showing off their conquests as proof of their attractiveness as women, feeling inadequate without a man in tow.

3. A dependent woman will lean heavily on her husband. Fearing to take even simple decisions, or to be without him for any length of time, she will intrude on and stifle his business life.

4. Some women develop total dependence on the wisdom of a doctor, priest, psychiatrist or guru. Whichever her choice, she will depend on his advice for every decision she makes.

5. The woman who relies on her children as proof of fertility, her success as a mother, or an excuse for not having a life of her own will fear to let her children become independent as she has no identity without them.

6. If a woman has no sense of self, she must rely on company, surrounding herself with friends to give her life.

---

the powers of nature, and influenced by (and influencing) the great life-forces of the earth.

We smile dismissively at the simple beliefs of primitive peoples – but perhaps we ought not to write them off completely. Many an old wives' tale, because it is based on long experience and observation, has turned out to have some basis in fact – homeopathic medicine has found that out. And indeed even orthodox medicine is constantly astonished by the shrewdness of many old herbal remedies and folk cures. We should perhaps consider the question of whether women do need to be in touch with the phases of nature, and

whether it does distort, and thus add stress to, a woman's personality if she is too far removed from such rhythms.

Thus, if we suffer from something distressing like premenstrual tension, before we take drugs or other artificial medication, perhaps we should ask ourselves, 'Is my body trying to tell me something that I don't know about myself?' In mild illnesses such as the common cold, for example, the body is nearly always trying to say something; it is usually bleeping: 'Your resistance is low, you need rest, you need to lie fallow for a few days – *switch off*.' It is sometimes necessary and good to withdraw,

to be quiet and have a little tranquillity. For some people such a vital hiatus, however short, would never occur were it not for the gift of the common cold.

The more advanced we become, the more removed we become from life-rhythms. The cookery writer Delia Smith is against freezers because, she says, they make people forget that 'to every thing there is a season'. There are young housewives now who, because of the wide use of convenience foods, have almost forgotten that foods have their own proper cycles, that they are always at their best in their own season, and that the whole balance of nature is cunningly devised so

that we have this beautiful rotation of crops in our kitchens and in our cooking as well as in the fields.

In putting together our inner selves, in building the personality which will be the structural frame for our outer selves, the question of harmony is the central one. You cannot battle too much against your true nature and get away with it. You cannot, you must not, hate the person you are. You must stand up to some of the rough winds of life and be strong inside yourself. You must make decisions and live with them.

In some cases, women are made to feel guilty whatever they

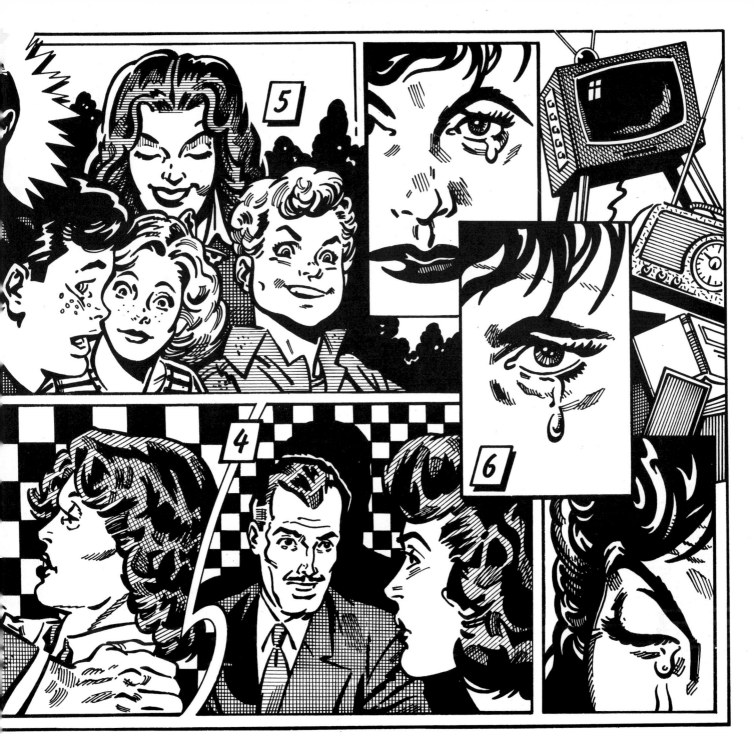

do. They feel guilty if they devote themselves to their homes and children, and equally guilty if they devote themselves to a career. It must also be said that it sometimes seems as though women are too easily manipulated by the prevailing social ethic. If one looks, for example, at fashions in bringing up children one might easily get the impression that women are slaves to the paediatricians' theology: one decade it is 'Don't give the baby any solids until he is six months old,' the next it is 'Give him solids as soon as he weighs twelve pounds.' Any contemporary mother will know, just by discussing these things with her own mother, that medical fashions in all these matters have been completely turned on their head – and women perpetually seem to follow. See how the mass switch from breast- to bottle-feeding took place as medical opinion, and commercial pressure, led it; then see how the trend is being reversed with the rediscovery that breast is best after all.

It is because of their vulnerability to guilt that women are manipulated so easily. The most persuasive advertisement for most women is still the one which says 'Bonzo washes whiter', with the underlying idea that unless you wash whitest you are *not doing your best* for your family – which always makes women feel guilty.

Guilt has its uses. We shall never be able to avoid it entirely because it, too, is part of our biological survival equipment. If someone didn't feel guilty about getting certain things done, they would never be done at all. One can also misapply the word 'guilt'. The young man who said, 'I feel guilty if I don't go and see my elderly mother sometimes,' was voicing a quite proper sense of *obligation*. And such 'guilt' for sense of obligation or responsi- bility is productive; it made him actually pay a visit to a lonely old lady. Without some guilt we might have no sense of duty.

But, in general, if you feel too much guilt you become a neurotic; if you feel none at all, you're a psychotic. The many different sorts of pressure on women today – to have successful careers, enriching marriages, nice homes, happy, healthy children – produce many more areas of guilt. There is, for many women, a continuing vague feeling of something constantly left undone. This is why one needs, perhaps more than ever, to be strong in oneself, to carry one's own convictions, to stand against too much outside manipulation of what one should or should not do. In your heart, you know what is right for you. Your first obligation is therefore to discover it.

Are women generally more vulnerable than men? The answer seems to be both yes and no; perhaps the most accurate answer would be that it depends how the woman is treated by life, it depends how she treats herself. Women nowadays tend to resent being called the weaker sex. The indications are that they are more easily hurt, physically and mentally, than men, but do not break under the strain as often. Women attempt suicide more often – but actually commit suicide less. Women use the medical services more than men, visit their doctors more often, take more days off work for sickness – yet, in the end, last longer and survive more wear and tear. It is obvious that women's physical strength, in terms of volume of weight and striking force, is less than men's, yet often their physical endurance is better, and the body of a woman can withstand more pain, extremities of heat and cold and even disease than can the male.

Yet there are very definite points of vulnerability for women. All over the 'civilized' (technically advanced) world, women suffer more from mental illness than men. In 1970 in England and Wales there were, for example, 72,000 men admitted to hospital for the treatment of mental illness, while there were a corresponding 176,000 women. Even allowing for the fact that women live longer than men, and that a fair number of mental hospital patients are elderly, there is still a marked disproportion between the sexes. Almost every study done in Europe and America indicates the same trend – virtually everywhere more women than men suffer from depression, schizophrenia, and other neuroses and psychoses.

The points in her lifetime at which a woman is vulnerable to stress and mental breakdown are known as crisis points. Among these are: leaving home, finding a new job, getting married, having a child, experiencing the menopause, and just growing old. Some societies amplify these crises more than others. For example, menopausal depression is more common in America than it is in India; it is more common in England and France than it is in Greece or Sicily. One reason why the menopause affects women more in these Western, advanced countries is, of course, that women in India may be so worried about avoiding the next famine that they simply don't have time to worry about matters like vaginal lubrication. Another reason may be that it's just not the sort of thing you go to see your doctor about – you suffer in silence. And a third reason may be that the mortality rates are so much higher in less developed countries that

there are fewer middle-aged women to go through the menopause.

Yet it is still a fact that a very important element in this phenomenon is a cultural one. Women in the West place great emphasis on their youth, on their sexuality, on what they think of as their 'femininity'; the menopause throws them into a crisis because it subconsciously means, to the woman, the loss of all these important things. Moreover, the change of life very often coincides, for a mother, with another Western distress point, 'the empty nest syndrome': the time when a woman's children grow up and leave home. Thus, for example, the women most vulnerable to menopausal depression in America have been found to be Jewish mothers, known in song and story for their particular attachment to their mothering role, which, during the change of life, they feel they are losing.

In India, however, the menopausal woman, far from losing face, is actually going up a notch in society. In traditional Indian culture, the person with least status is the young girl. She must defer to her father, her husband, her family and her in-laws. She may be pretty and attractive, but that is all she is allowed. Only when she becomes an older woman, when she becomes the matriarch in her own household, the ruling grandmother figure, does she gain authority, respect and real social position. So it is that Indian women, far from dreading the menopause as representing a loss of sexuality, welcome it as a social gain, though the person who has not experienced some regret at growing older would be hardly human.

Loss of a parent, child, spouse, partner or close friend will trigger off in the bereaved quite natural – and indeed essential and proper – depressions. Too often, such feelings of sadness are treated with drugs or therapy, as though to be sad in itself was deviant behaviour – whereas to be sad when something sad happens is both necessary and important. Loss, too, is part of the idea that 'to each thing there is a season'. One doctor's invaluable advice in these circumstances is: 'You *must* be depressed sometimes. You can't go through your whole life on a cloud of euphoria. If you weren't sometimes depressed, you couldn't, at other times, be happy. Melancholy is part of the cycle of human experience. You won't cure it by taking pills. It's good for you to go through a sober and contemplative phase, just as it is good for you to be happy. The only treatment I prescribe is: go and ring up a friend and go out and have a drink with him or her.'

Anxiety, whether real or imaginary, seems to be a necessary adjunct to survival. The impulse to worry is constructive in origin; if we didn't worry, we wouldn't achieve anything. At the most fundamental level, if parents did not worry about providing for their children they would not bother to go out in the pursuit of food.

A person devoid of anxious reflexes would be either totally nerveless or totally lethargic. Worry has its uses. Sometimes, the greater the anxiety, the greater the will to overcome. The biological root of anxiety is to galvanize us into action to survive – and it still operates in this way. For example, worrying about possible symptoms of an illness prompts us to seek treatment and thus possible cures. It is natural to worry a little about money, security, safety, survival, one's family, one's health, the passing of time and lots of other things that are symbols of survival. It is when anxiety becomes compulsive and obsessive that it becomes neurotic. Anxiety is also catching: the anxious mother transmits her feelings to the child, and makes the child timid and fearful in turn.

The trick of dealing with anxiety is to try to compartment-alize it. You must realize that some worrying is merely displacement activity. People will worry a lot about a pain in their big toe; but they would forget about that very quickly if they suddenly had a heart attack. It seems that people must worry about something, and if they can't find something big to occupy their minds, they'll worry about something small, and inflate its importance.

Very busy people who carry a lot of responsibility master the trick of compartmentalizing their worries by deferring some until the next day: 'I'll tackle this problem today, but the other two I won't worry about until Monday.' Working on a system of priorities, some worries are more important than others; if you have to get some papers to the printers this week, that's a worry to be concentrated on now. There's little point in worrying about the tax you might have to pay next year.

Never worry about something before you have to. Consider an anxiety, and ask yourself: Do I have to worry about that now? Can I take any action to remove the worry? If you're worried about a letter you haven't written, for example, the only thing to do is down tools and write the bally letter. Get what can be done, done, each day – and then try to relax. Don't put off what can be done, if you can help it; but do put off what need not be worried about yet.

Many people find help in the good old system of making lists. If you are tossing and turning at night, worrying about all the things you should do the next day, get up and make a list, and then cross them off, one by one, as you complete each task. Keep a perpetual notebook with you and add items as you remember them; this way less strain is put on your memory and the mind can concentrate on actually getting things done.

Try to separate the things which you can remedy and the things which you must accept. If the kitchen sink gets blocked up, it's maddening and inconvenient, but it's not something you should waste emotional energy worrying about. Too much precious female talent is wasted this way, and it's one of the bars to real achievement. Fragmentation and the constant feeling of things left undone if combining a job and a family, indecisiveness due to loss of confidence and self-esteem, and general fatigue from coping with toddlers all contribute to making the small worries in a woman's life seem out of all proportion. On the other hand, failing eyesight or rising blood-pressure in a difficult pregnancy are real worries which require reflection and plans, care and therapy. Worrying about them is constructive.

Anxiety which is irrational is often the most difficult to cope with. If it develops into a phobia, then it is akin to a depressive illness. But small anxieties can haunt one without actually making one ill. They can pile up and crowd in on you until you are immobilized by a general state of anxiety and find it impossible to deal with even small problems, now grown out of all proportion to their seriousness. From time to time during the day you should make a conscious effort to relax and get things back into perspective. The best way to do this is by distancing techniques. Either look at what is causing you anxiety in the context of your whole life, so that you can make a realistic assessment as to its gravity, or try literally taking off mentally, removing your mind from your body and putting greater and greater distances between them until you look at yourself from the room, from outside the house, moving back further and further until you leave behind the city, the country and finally the world itself. From out there in space you can see the dot which is you and the pinpricks of your anxieties for what they are. Having got your problems back to a size that you can cope with, tackle them – or at least some of them – immediately before they have time to grow again.

Everyone is sad sometimes; it is not necessary to reach for a pill or a psychiatrist every time you get a fit of the blues. Reactive depression – following a bereavement, an illness, childbirth, or even some great excitement such as getting married or moving abroad – is natural. Indeed, if one didn't feel sad as a reaction to loss, separation or simply great upheavals, one would be genuinely abnormal. It is human to be sad, and we deny our nature if we try to escape from that. If you are feeling low for a perfectly good reason, try to ride it out.

Use the times of natural melancholy to contemplate, to lie fallow, so that you may blossom again. Easier said than done, to be sure, but if it is the human side of our nature that makes us weep, it is the human side, too, that makes us heal.

Reactive melancholy is not, however, the only form of depression. Women are vulnerable to depression of different kinds at various stages of their lives, sometimes as a result of physical changes within their bodies. Adolescent girls, worrying about their sex-lives, and adjusting to 'womanhood', are vulnerable to the depressive illness of anorexia nervosa* – the disease of abnormal eating. Young married women with small children are vulnerable to 'housewife's depression', which is simply loneliness, isolation, too much time spent in the company of children, and a diminishing sense of self-worth.

Postnatal depression is something that almost all women who have children experience. It is definitely established that it is not a cultural phenomenon. Ugandan tribeswomen suffer from it in exactly the same way as European millionairesses. This depression is chemical and hormonal in origin – the body is undergoing dramatic and fundamental change at this time. It is as though one's nerve-ends were still exposed; the woman feels weepy and vulnerable, which she is, and the sadness of the world often weighs upon her. Added to this low emotional state is the fact that she may not be getting enough sleep, she has the responsibility of the child or children and the worries they bring, and she may still feel fat and unattractive from the effects of pregnancy. It must be said in compensation, however, that postnatal euphoria also exists, most often during the early stages of breast-feeding.

Some women also suffer from premenstrual tension – a depression which comes before a period – and of course there is the menopause, an obvious point of crisis. One woman describes it as 'a Hieronymus Bosch nightmare';

another – Sheila Kitzinger, the author of <u>The Experience of Childbirth</u> – actually claims she <u>enjoyed</u> the change of life, but most women experience some depression with the menopause, simply because it is an irreversible sign of age.

Old people of both sexes are often depressed, either from forms of senile dementia, or just from loneliness and disillusion. The old tend to be pessimistic, which underscores their depression.

Deep depression with no apparent cause which goes on for a long time is called endogenous depression and is a clinical condition. A person with endogenous depression will feel sad, miserable, weepy or suicidal constantly and without reason. Changes in behaviour may develop; the individual may avoid social contact and stay at home, and sleep rhythms, appetite, sex-drive, weight and energy may be altered. Sometimes physical symptoms occur, such as headaches, dizziness, chest-pains, palpitations or backache. Depressives may appear to reject the people around them, even those they genuinely love. They may harp obsessively on the past, or on some passage of their lives. The depression may manifest itself as a phobia, such as a totally disproportionate fear of spiders, or a fear of small places. A person may become very withdrawn or very excitable, but in some way their behaviour becomes extreme and lacks perspective. The victim may feel alienated from his or her true self.

Treatment for depression varies depending on the cause. The conventional options are anti-depressant drugs, psychotherapy, or medical treatment such as electro-chemical therapy. The usual advice given to people who feel depressed is to seek medical help. A doctor may be able to diagnose something specific such as menopausal depression and assess the possible benefits of hormone replacement therapy (see page 123) or consultation with an endocrinologist (specialist in glandular problems). But, unfortunately, medical treatment for depression is still limited. A doctor may prescribe anti-depressant drugs, but many depressed people seem just as wretched on barbiturates as they are without them.

Perhaps the most positive development for the depressed is the fact that depression is now accepted as an illness. The growth of group therapies has also helped since a great deal of depression is caused by loneliness, and many depressives benefit from talking out their problems with other like-minded people.

Talk to another human being.'

Mental illness is broadly divided between the neurotic and the psychotic. People who are psychotic are genuinely ill – as ill as anyone with TB, cancer or multiple sclerosis. The victims form a relatively small and constant percentage in any given population and they need treatment in just the way a person with a physical illness needs it. Neurotics are more ambiguously ill. The best definition of a neurotic is someone who sees things out of perspective; it is a behavioural inability to take a rationally objective view. Any of us may at one time or another be slightly, or emphatically, neurotic. After all, who takes 'a rationally objective view' of everything, all the time? The cleverest people can be fools with no judgement at all when it comes to something near to their passions.

We can control neurosis to some extent since there are social and environmental factors attached to its development. But the question is *how* to control it. We know, for example, that the depression which preys so much on young women is the depression commonly called 'housewife's disease'; it is the depression of isolation. People need people to talk to. Yet the whole tendency of modern life is to isolate, even perhaps alienate. When you take a bus, you stand in a queue with other people, jostle along with them, and are part of a group experience; when you take your car, you shut yourself up in your own little box. When you go to a local shop, you chat with the people behind the counter and meet neighbours on the way in and out; when you go to a super-market, you can shop for an hour without exchanging a word with anyone. When you go to your amateur dramatic group, your choral society or local political party, it may not be very sophisticated as entertainment, but you are making contact with other people; when you watch your magnificent colour television, you watch it alone. Thus the more technically advanced we are, the more we are cut off from the human group, because the aim of technology is to use machinery rather than people. We strive towards a materially improved standard of living, not realizing all the while that we are very possibly eroding deeply-rooted patterns of human contact.

When women are behaving neurotically, it is often because they have shut away, or not acknowledged or realized, a subconscious demand which may be very simple and fundamental – like the need for companionship. Or the need for challenges. Or the need to give love. Sometimes we

fail to recognize a very obvious crisis point in our lives. Reactions of depression and stress can affect a person months after the high point of the crisis seems to have passed, so that the symptoms are not understood for what they are.

The important point is that, instead of reacting neurotically, or simply negatively, to a crisis point in our lives, we should be able to use it for growth. Strange as it may seem, anxiety, unhappiness, stress and conflict can also be means of intellectual and emotional growth. If we never lived through, and survived, distress and difficulties, we would be hopelessly childish and undeveloped people; and if we accept crises too passively, taking it for granted that we are simply 'depressed' and there is nothing to be done except take pills, we also close off the potentiality for growth from the experience.

Freud observed that women were more rigid in their attitudes than men, and noticed that they often lost their capacity for intellectual and emotional growth much earlier. A man of thirty, he noted, was just at the beginning of his 'flowering' as a personality, while a woman of the same age often seemed incapable of further intellectual development, and was already a 'closed' personality. This was very probably an accurate observation in nineteenth-century Vienna; Freud, however, considered his observations immutable to all time and all cultures. He saw women's limitations not in terms of the social curbs that were put on their development, but as inherent in women, and linked to their sexuality: 'It is as though', he wrote, 'the whole process has been gone through and remains inaccessible to influence for the future; as though the difficult development which leads to femininity has exhausted all the possibilities of the individual.'

We know that this isn't true; we have empirical evidence that women frequently develop *most* in their thirties and forties, and that this is often a fascinating growth period for them. Yet there is often an uncomfortable, niggling shaft of truth in Freud's observations, and women have to guard against letting their inner selves atrophy. If, as Freud claims, such intellectual and emotional stagnation takes place because the woman has pinned her identity on her sexuality, then the road to growth must be not to concentrate one's whole identity on one's sexuality, but to build up reserves of other sources: an intellectual interest, family, friends, a job, a hobby, a peer group, a community.

Sex is a double-edged gift for women. We have learned, more than previous generations, that it

17

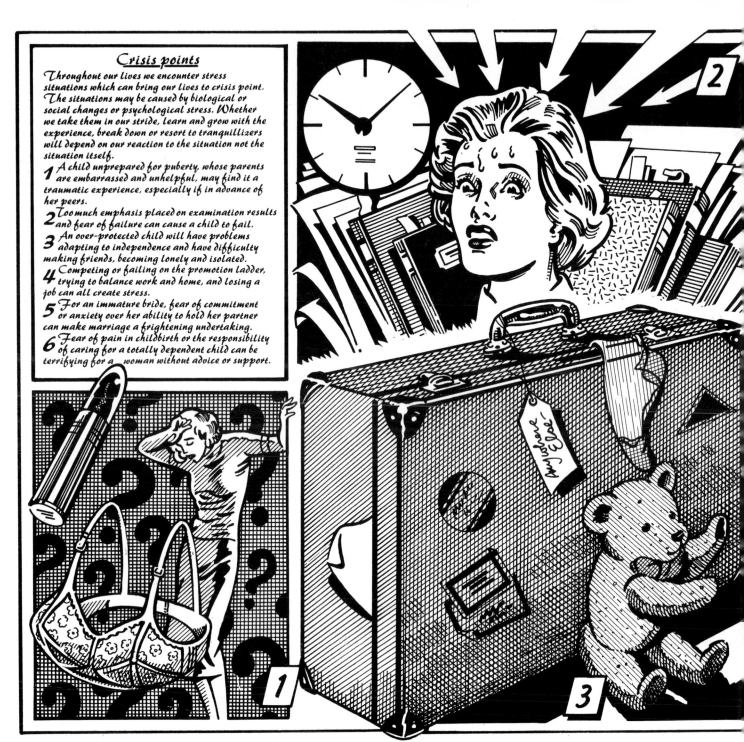

Crisis points

Throughout our lives we encounter stress situations which can bring our lives to crisis point. The situations may be caused by biological or social changes or psychological stress. Whether we take them in our stride, learn and grow with the experience, break down or resort to tranquillizers will depend on our reaction to the situation not the situation itself.

1 A child unprepared for puberty, whose parents are embarrassed and unhelpful, may find it a traumatic experience, especially if in advance of her peers.

2 Too much emphasis placed on examination results and fear of failure can cause a child to fail.

3 An over-protected child will have problems adapting to independence and have difficulty making friends, becoming lonely and isolated.

4 Competing or failing on the promotion ladder, trying to balance work and home, and losing a job can all create stress.

5 For an immature bride, fear of commitment or anxiety over her ability to hold her partner can make marriage a frightening undertaking.

6 Fear of pain in childbirth or the responsibility of caring for a totally dependent child can be terrifying for a woman without advice or support.

is an instrument of pleasure – a pleasure, indeed, to which one has a right. Formerly, women were more inclined to be acquainted with its problems and pains. We have now learned the desirability of being sexually free and open, demanding if necessary, unhypocritical. Yet, as the problem page of any magazine testifies, sexual freedom is not without its risks. It is all very well for us to be proud of our sexual equality, but 'equality' is always a theoretical, abstract concept: who, exactly, is equal to whom in this world? All men and women cannot be sexually equal, by the law of human variability, and in some cases – perhaps in most – women

are still more vulnerable than men. They are physically vulnerable to the dangers of pregnancy: even birth control isn't risk-free, and abortion is often traumatic in some way. Emotionally, women have to protect themselves against being used too much: 'too much' because in human relationships there is nearly always some manipulation. But it is deeply hurtful to women to feel they have been used and cast aside, and if that hurt is inflicted too often it builds up until it becomes a neurosis and a source of terrible unhappiness. Many a woman who seems to manifest some kind of sexual dysfunction – frigidity or promiscuity or sexual inversion of

some kind – is simply deeply hurt by the way she has been treated, by rejection or insensitivity from someone else.

At the core of all personal development lies self-esteem. Again, Freud believed that men were born with more of it – with a 'superego' – and that in women it was merely something derived from the outside. It is certain that it is all-important to all human beings, however they get it. Perhaps the best, the most perfect way of having self-esteem is simply to be greatly loved and encouraged as a child and given a high sense of one's own worth; certainly many people believe that their lack of self-esteem is the direct result of

a childhood rejection.

But again, that law is not immutable, since some people who were adored as children are nevertheless totally lacking in confidence as adults; while others who have had lonely childhoods with apparently little love have developed the necessary personal belief in themselves. Self-esteem may be something which can be built up, yet which can be lost again, temporarily or permanently; self-confidence – the partner of self-esteem – is certainly a matter of practice and even of relating to society and the other people around one. Think of that phrase which should be banned from everyone's vocabulary: 'I'm only a

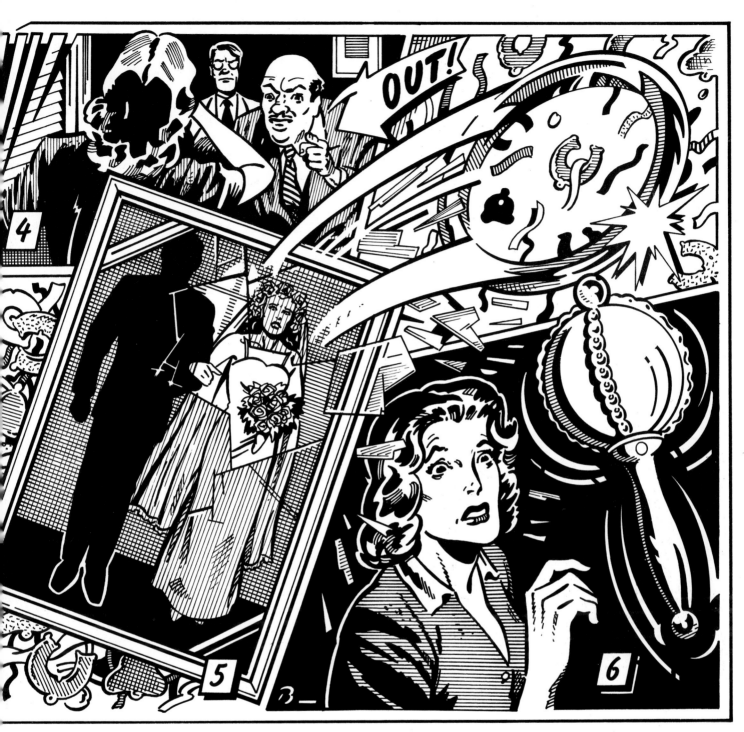

housewife.' Consider how that reflects the speaker's subconscious lack of esteem for the role that she is playing at the moment. Yet a couple of years earlier, that 'only-a-housewife' might have been a high-powered saleswoman in a successful business; a few years later that 'only-a-housewife' might again be doing something in which she takes pride and will then no longer be belittling herself or her role. No woman should ever say she is 'only' anything. Putting yourself down is bad for you: like cigarette smoking, it can damage your health.

However, the 'only-a-housewife' is also reflecting how she thinks society views her. In

Mrs Beeton's famous book of household management, the confident, authoritative tones of that Victorian Superwoman make it quite clear that she considered the job of running a home extremely serious, a full-time job, and a genuine case for professionalism. But housework in itself has been so denigrated, not least by the feminist movement, in more recent years that women are scarcely to be blamed if they conclude that it is only fit for the mentally deficient. Why is it so denigrated? It can be boring, it is repetitive and frustratingly fragmentary but, like everything else, it has its positive side, too. It can be comforting, it can make

you feel brisk and organized, and it can give you pleasure to see that you have created a pleasant atmosphere in which your family may live happily.

Perhaps, however, the root of its poor status is that it is usually not paid for, since in our world everything is judged by its commodity value. In India, street-sweeping and garbage-collection are done by Untouchables who are virtually unpaid, and the work is regarded with contempt. In Britain and America, garbage-collectors have used the strike weapon to great effect; they are now highly paid and most people respect them and are extremely grateful for their services. The more money

that is paid for a service, the more people tend to respect it.

Similarly, the housewife's job is a *job*. But because we don't pay for it, we tend not to regard it well. This derogatory image feeds back to the 'housewife' herself, and in spite of the fact that she has something valuable to do, her self-esteem is drained away by society's attitudes. It is hard to battle against this, and so comes the paradox that in order to be a successful housewife today you actually have to be a very confident, intelligent person, with well-developed inner resources. The idea that a happy housewife is a mere cabbage is the opposite of the truth; the happy housewife is

19

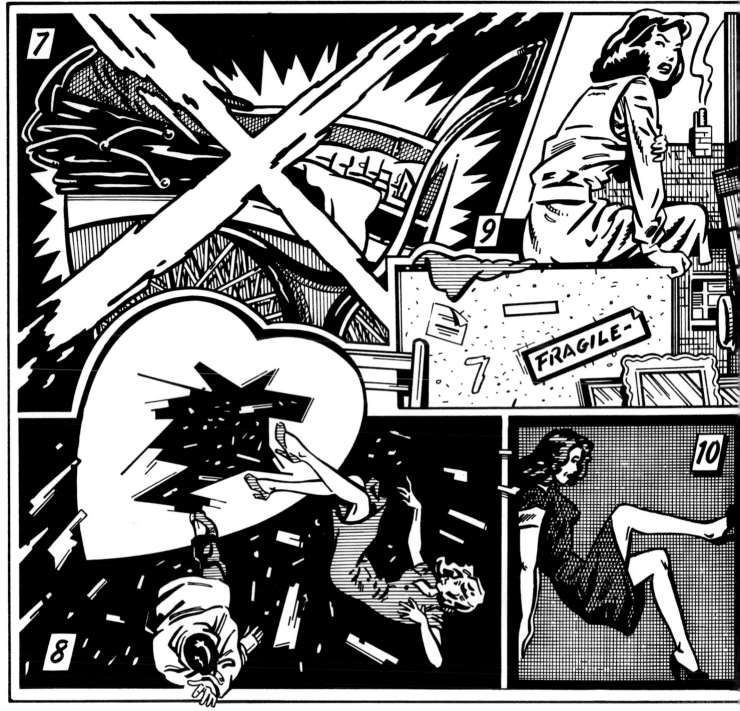

almost always a very reflective person with an admirable sense of self, of what is right for her.

Self-esteem should not depend on a 'role', though too often it does for both sexes. Impotence, for example, is a common problem among men who have lost their jobs. Fundamental self-esteem comes from the proper evaluation of oneself as a *person*, independent of job or social role. The enemy of woman's self-esteem is in part her altruistic nature: her urge to 'give' herself to her husband and her family, to erase her own identity for their sake. Women are notoriously bad at keeping up with their friends after marriage. If a man doesn't like his

wife's best friend, the wife will, in most cases, drop the friend. Men, on the other hand, rarely change their friends or intimates on marriage. The mutual friends of a couple will tend to be the friends of the man.

Compulsive togetherness brings over-dependency; over-dependency robs one of one's own identity; lack of one's own identity makes self-esteem impossible. And yet, here is another paradox. The ultimate bringer of self-esteem is – old-fashioned, sentimental *love*. The winning of someone's love, someone you love in return, bolsters the personality as nothing else. Unfortunately, it is the

person with low self-esteem who most needs love, yet that is the very person who finds it most difficult to get, on account of the low value she puts upon herself. People who think little of themselves are often spiky and rejecting, because they are always seeking out people who will reject them. This is the Groucho Marx syndrome: 'I'd never want to join any club that would be common enough to accept the likes of me.' The person with little self-confidence believes that anyone who could love her couldn't possibly have any judgement.

Weight-watching is an interesting example of the same kind of paradox. To care for one's

body, to see that it is trim and healthy and not distorted by fat, is a sign of self-esteem; but to be obsessive about dieting is an act of self-rejection. To punish one's body too much in the pursuit of a cultural idea of beauty and size is to show that one has not accepted some fundamental things about oneself. 'There are a lot of things that can be done to change a woman,' Eileen Ford of the famous Ford Model Agency in America once said. 'You can bob your nose, change your hair colour, make yourself lose weight and give yourself a first-class *maquillage*. But you can't change your basic structure. You will never change an endomorph shape

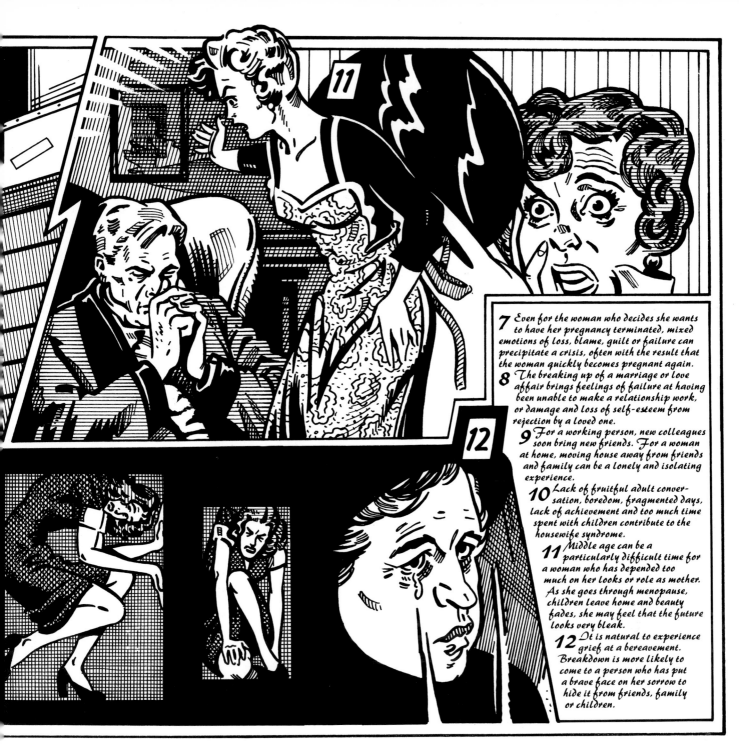

7 Even for the woman who decides she wants to have her pregnancy terminated, mixed emotions of loss, blame, guilt or failure can precipitate a crisis, often with the result that the woman quickly becomes pregnant again.

8 The breaking up of a marriage or love affair brings feelings of failure at having been unable to make a relationship work, or damage and loss of self-esteem from rejection by a loved one.

9 For a working person, new colleagues soon bring new friends. For a woman at home, moving house away from friends and family can be a lonely and isolating experience.

10 Lack of fruitful adult conversation, boredom, fragmented days, lack of achievement and too much time spent with children contribute to the housewife syndrome.

11 Middle age can be a particularly difficult time for a woman who has depended too much on her looks or role as mother. As she goes through menopause, children leave home and beauty fades, she may feel that the future looks very bleak.

12 It is natural to experience grief at a bereavement. Breakdown is more likely to come to a person who has put a brave face on her sorrow to hide it from friends, family or children.

[round-body structure] into an ectomorph [angular body structure].' In other words, you can make the best of yourself, to be sure, and that helps self-confidence, but you cannot become a different person, and to want to be a different person is to have not a weight problem, but a personality problem. If you are dieting too much or too obsessively, perhaps the questions you should ask are: Am I rejecting myself? Is the problem more with self-esteem than with actual body shape? Is it something I should be tackling in another way?

Susie Orbach, who runs a women's therapy centre in London and has written a book about weight problems, battled for years with her own weight, starving herself then eating obsessively. One day she stopped, deciding instead to be herself, and her weight simply 'settled', quite spontaneously, at an acceptable average, while her appetite automatically regulated itself. Very often problems to do with our living habits are connected with deeper, subconscious things. In order to stop smoking or drinking, for example, it is often necessary to ask oneself *why* one smokes or drinks, to carry out an examination of conscience before one can find a way of stopping. Excessive, self-destructive smoking or drinking may be more than an unhealthy habit: it is a sign of unhappiness at some deeper level.

And that is the nub of it all: to know, to value and to grow towards a true realization of yourself. That is how the inner woman is built. Yet one of the many contradictions of life is that in finding yourself you do not just seek within yourself. The old laws of scriptures may be right when they direct man towards self-realization by doing the *opposite* of what might be obvious: 'It is in giving that we receive, it is in dying that we live.' Thus it is very often the people who have most occupied themselves with others who discover the greatest depths of self-realization.

Intense narcissism doesn't, curiously, tell you very much about yourself. You learn about yourself through stretching your intellectual and emotional muscles, by sustaining relationships, living in a community, nourishing a group of people around you, challenging yourself to learn various disciplines and working and filling your life with useful things, while leaving time for contemplation. Work, play, reflect; try to balance contrasting activities in your life. Never cut yourself off from people, for people are the channel to yourself. Try to be true to what you believe is your real nature.

THE DEPENDENT WOMAN

Historically, with one or two notable exceptions such as the legendary Amazons or the inhabitants of the island of Lesbos, women have always taken second place to men in society. We have taken second place because it has always been assumed that we are not as strong, as clever, as aggressive or as brave, and so we have had to look to man to support us. We have been, in a word, dependent.

Latterly things have changed. Western woman wanted the right to be equal to and not necessarily dependent on man, to vote and to enjoy equality at work and play. To a large extent we have won much of what we wanted. But we are new to the notion of equality. Centuries of dependence leave their mark and many of us still look to men and to the children they give us for our identity. Though marriage may no longer be an end in itself, we still seem to rely on 'catching' our man in the first place if we do want marriage or children. We still depend on our looks, on being sexy and desirable and staying that way, for in a society where divorce has become a relatively easy process we cannot rely on the fact that our men will remain our husbands, especially as we grow older. Small wonder that the cosmetics and fashion industries continue to thrive, and that women still depend heavily on creating a desirable and youthful image. We continue to depend on our children, too, sometimes simply as a reason for living. We may live vicariously, through their achievements and failures, or do all we can to give them a good start in life. Either way, the break when it comes and they leave the nest can hit us very hard, especially if in becoming over-dependent on them we have failed to develop other interests.

Few women, one suspects, would wish to return to a situation where they were owned body and soul by a man. The majority, if statistics relating to marriage and cohabitation are relevant, want a situation where they have the right to be an individual, plus a partner who supports them in this and at least shares in their emotional, physical and material needs. Achieving this happy compromise is not easy, as divorce, separation, nervous or physical breakdown, and our increasing dependence on drugs such as alcohol or nicotine demonstrates. One extremist view is that, unable to cope with the liberation which technically at least we can achieve, we revert to the ingrained habit of dependence; since we can no longer 'depend' on men, we find substitutes.

A more tolerant view is that women today have to cope with stress situations in a way they never had to before - being working mothers, single parents, striving to maintain their identity in a marriage or to hold on to a husband for whom divorce is a relatively simple procedure. To cope with stress you need to be strong and sure of yourself, to have a healthy ego and a profound sense of self-preservation. For many women, that is a tall order.

The steady and alarming increase in alcoholism among women is often cited as an example of the fact that women find life today difficult to cope with. Many of the taboos which once prevented women from being at risk of becoming alcoholics have now been lifted. Women can and do drink openly, in bars, restaurants or at home, and they can do so unaccompanied by men. A woman working in a high-powered job alongside men may not only want to join them in a drink, but may feel she has to prove her equality. At the other extreme is the woman who sits alone at home and feels unused, unfulfilled. Perhaps her children have grown up and gone away, or her husband is never around, or she simply feels at a loss for ways of passing the days and nights. A solitary drink at lunchtime to cheer oneself up can lead to two, three, and eventually a bottle. Alcoholism has insidious beginnings and, like so many diseases, it is often only recognized as such when the disease has progressed to a chronic stage. Similarly, an addiction to nicotine starts in an apparently harmless way. The odd cigarette after a meal or with a drink does no damage, but all too often smoking cigarettes becomes a regular habit and finally a compulsion.

There are still other types of dependence or addiction which have as yet not acquired the stigma of alcoholism, for example, but which are nevertheless an indication of the fact that many women simply cannot cope with their lives. The use and abuse of tranquillizers* have escalated incredibly among women in the last decade. The widescale intake of such drugs is unquestionably a barometer of stress, whether real or imagined, and the medical profession is aware of and worried by this fact. The use of sleeping pills as an automatic accompaniment to going to bed is also steadily increasing among women, yet this is another area where no stigma is attached to the practice and so the dependence is less easily recognizable.

Of course, there are women who do not resort to any of the drugs mentioned; maybe they spend a lot of time drinking cups of tea and coffee, both addictive but ultimately less harmful, over-eating or starving themselves, or perpetually spring-cleaning their houses. And maybe many of them avoid these 'dependent' forms of behaviour altogether and lead full, satisfying, healthy lives. But one has only to look around, possibly no farther than one's own home, to realize that many of us do depend on some kind of drug at some time in our lives, be it a 'real' drug such as alcohol or a 'placebo' such as food. The important questions we have to ask ourselves are why we have the dependence and what we can do to be rid of it.

If we drink or smoke or dust, polish and clean to excess, it could simply be that we have time on our hands and have not yet woken up to the fact that there are hundreds of alternative and more fruitful ways of using time. It is a terrible cliché, but true, that habit is habit-forming and we may need to make some radical changes in our lives to break those habits and dependencies that are non-productive or wasteful. Never before have there been so many opportunities for women to go out and get what they want, though the effort needed to do so might be great. We can read for extra-mural degrees, be re-trained for new careers, develop entirely new aspects of our personalities. There is literally no need for us to be bored and, if it is boredom that is causing us to depend on drugs we can alter the situation.

However, the reasons why we turn to drugs for help may be far more complicated. We may be suffering from stress and yet be unaware of the fact. Or we may be caught in a dilemma which we know about but which appears insoluble, such as a marriage that is cracking up, difficulties with our children, fear and sadness at the prospect of getting old, loss of job or status. All these can send us to our particular poison in the hope, vain though it is, that we will somehow feel better or be more able to cope. Drugs *are* useful for specific and short-term problems. A stiff drink can give you the courage you need temporarily to face a situation; a sleeping pill can promote eight hours' desperately-needed rest after an exhausting week; a cup of coffee can help get you on your feet when you need to be. But once we start using drugs on a habitual basis, and thereby become dependent on them, we are in an extremely dangerous situation.

It is with good reason that doctors, psychiatrists, marriage-guidance counsellors, or any of the multitude of groups who aim to discover and promote self-awareness attempt to cure a problem by getting to the root cause or causes. The process may be painful and a palliative drug may seem preferable to trying to unveil a situation which may be even more so. But drugs and the dependence they create are no real alternative to facing up to facts and learning to deal with them. Learning to love oneself – which means respecting the fact that one is a person to be cared for and respected, warts and all – is the key.

Learning to be honest with oneself – if, to begin with, nobody else – is the first step towards independence. Changing what can be changed and accepting what cannot is the second step. If in all honesty we can accept that we are addicted to or over-dependent on something we are halfway to taking the next step, which is getting rid of the addiction. There are numerous individuals and groups whose sole aim is to help people who find themselves dependent on a habit which they wish to break.

DRUG DEPENDENCE

When we talk of drugs in connection with dependence we tend to refer to those that belong to two main categories: depressants – which include the barbiturates and opiates – and stimulants – the amphetamines, caffeine and cocaine. But a drug is literally any substance, either organic or inorganic, used alone or in combination with others, as a medicine. Alcohol is a drug, as is caffeine (found in tea, coffee, cocoa and cola drinks) and nicotine (found in tobacco).

Alcohol

Alcohol is considered to be the most serious drug problem in modern societies, with up to 5 per cent of the population affected - a growing number of whom are women. Alcohol taken in excess is literally a poison. Liver, kidneys, heart, veins, arteries and bones can all suffer, and the brain may be irreparably damaged. The chronic alcoholic differs from the heavy drinker in one vital respect, namely that he or she is totally dependent on drink.

The onset of alcoholism may only be recognizable to a skilled observer and rarely is to the person involved. The first stage of alcoholism, which may last for anything from a few months to five or even ten years, is one where drinking gradually becomes a regular part of the daily routine. Usually it is 'social' drinking, with others at fixed times, say in the pub, over lunch or after work, but sometimes it may include drinking alone. Then, almost imperceptibly, the drink becomes a need. It is turned to to relieve stress or tension and consumption inevitably increases. Alternatively, the social drinking pattern gets heavier: instead of two gins and tonic, six or seven become the rule.

The second stage comes into effect when, instead of simply wanting or even needing a drink, it becomes an urgent compulsion. Very often the day cannot begin properly until several drinks have been consumed. Times when a drink is 'allowed' become more fluid. The vicious circle of hangovers and therefore a 'heart-starter' the following morning is set up. Whilst the social drinker may continue to do so openly, he or she will also be drinking surreptitiously, as will the person who drinks at home. She will probably lie about the fact and the amount that she has been drinking, and although often privately worried or guilty will continue to do so.

The third stage has arrived when, in spite of fear of losing face or guilt, drinking becomes a continuous activity and the drinker cannot stop until totally intoxicated, with the concomitant loss of consciousness or nausea, slurring of speech, and incoherent or uncontrolled behaviour. Memory lapses, where the drinker has no recall of the events surrounding the drinking, are frequent. During this stage she may try again and again to 'moderate' the drinking, or stop altogether, without success. Lying continues and false promises are made, while she tends to let her self, family, work and play all go – putting drink before all other requirements. She will probably have little or no appetite, and her appearance will reflect the actual poisoning of her body which is taking place.

The fourth stage, when the drinker is a chronic alcoholic, is typified by total self-neglect and a need to drink which will often stop at nothing – begging, stealing, conniving – to gratify itself. The alcoholic's tolerance level, which will probably have decreased in the third stage, will now be very low and one drink may be all it takes to make her drunk. Finally, there will be physical and moral collapse, fantasies, paranoia and delirium tremens.

The reasons why one person remains a heavy drinker and another becomes an alcoholic are various and complicated. Certainly personality, background and possibly the metabolism itself are involved. Some people will be chronic alcoholics within five years of taking their first drink; others will be in the third stage after drinking for twenty years.

The prognosis for cure is best when alcoholism has been diagnosed, recognized and accepted by the sufferer, and there is a fundamental desire to be cured. It you suspect, or secretly know, that you are an alcoholic, even if only in the early stages, you must take action immediately.

Try to cut down. If you can't, try to stop altogether for a while. If you are unable to do either, you must seek professional help.

Support systems are vital: help and sympathy from friends, family and doctor. Many alcoholics find that joining Alcoholics Anonymous helps; there are branches in most large towns. Actual treatment may involve the withdrawal of alcohol from the system, usually medically supervised, vitamin supplements, and tranquillizers and other drugs to counteract the inevitable unpleasant withdrawal symptoms. Antabuse techniques, where the patient takes drugs that produce violent nausea if alcohol is then consumed, hypno-therapeutic techniques and back-up psycho-therapy can all help to rehabilitate the alcoholic. But with this disease, as with all others, prevention or at least recognition of the early-warning signs offer more hope than last-ditch attempts at recovery.

Nicotine

There can no longer be any doubt that excessive cigarette smoking is dangerous. The risks to health are not only in the increased chances of developing something as serious as lung or throat cancer, a greater propensity to bronchitis, hardening of the arteries and therefore an increased risk of heart disease, accelerated heartbeat, and a number of other less serious aesthetic problems such as dull skin and discoloured teeth. The dangers to the foetus of a pregnant woman who smokes are also greater: at birth, the child of a smoking mother will weigh up to several pounds less than it would have done otherwise. If a person becomes dependent on nicotine, it may be very difficult to lose that dependence. The greater the number of cigarettes smoked and the more years that smoking has been a habit, the more difficult it will be to lose. All medical opinion is agreed on one point, that the *desire* to give up smoking is the critical factor. Once that has been established, a number of techniques may help to put the desire into effect. These include gradual withdrawal, antabuse materials which induce a feeling of sickness or actual vomiting on smoking, hypnosis, group support therapy, and reward or substitute systems. Nevertheless, many of those who have been successful in giving up generally agree that smoking one cigarette could mean that they acquire the habit again. Like all drugs which cause dependence, nicotine should be approached with caution and pre-ferably not taken in the first place.

Aids to giving up or cutting down smoking

☛ Read all the literature you can, look at pictures, watch films which demonstrate just how damaging smoking can be to your health.

☛ Tell yourself how much better you will feel and function (YOU WILL) if you stop.

☛ Put aside the money you would have spent on smoking and treat yourself or your family on the proceeds.

☛ Try hypnotism or aversion therapy.

☛ Take up some form of *enjoyable* exercise - swimming, tennis or dancing - and set yourself success targets in these. If you can stick to them, you will find you have to cut down or give up altogether if you are to compete at all.

☛ Buy half your normal daily ration of cigarettes and refuse to buy any more when you've smoked them (don't cheat and smoke other people's). You can repeat this process and halve the amount again after a period of time.

☛ Give yourself fixed times of the day when you can smoke and stick to them.

☛ Take only a few puffs of a cigarette and then *grind* it out (otherwise you may re-light it).

☛ Leave your cigarettes at home when going on short journeys, and then make it a rule never to smoke while travelling or when away from home.

Barbiturates

Barbiturates work as depressants by reducing impulses to the brain. They may relieve anxiety and tension and induce sleep or anaesthesia. Abuse of barbiturates can lead to addiction, a problem that has become increasingly common among the middle-aged, particularly women. Consequently, members of the medical profession now prescribe barbiturates with more caution than they once did. Overdoses of barbiturates are common causes of suicide, though death may be accidental if they are unwittingly taken in excess with alcohol. Withdrawal from barbiturate addiction produces symptoms at least as bad as with-drawal from alcohol or heroin.

Opiates

The opiates include opium itself, heroin, morphine and codeine (derivatives of opium). Like barbiturates, the opiates depress the nervous system, but act particularly on the sensory centres, promote sleep and alleviate pain. In large doses they act on the hypothalamus* and give rise to feelings of euphoria, happiness and safety. Opiates create tolerance and subsequently dependence. Withdrawal symptoms include stomach cramps, diarrhoea, nausea, vomiting and sweating with streaming nose and eyes. Panic, trembling and insomnia* are also usually present, accompanied by acute depression. Codeine is the least effective of the opiates and therefore the least dangerous in terms of creating dependence. It is followed by opium and then morphine, which is of great benefit in the control of pain but has to be administered with great care to avoid overdose or possible later addiction. Heroin, which is three times as strong as morphine, is extremely dangerous. Although the initial effect of sniffing or injecting with heroin is one of acute pleasure, withdrawal symptoms are commensurately bad. It takes only one grain (60 mg) of heroin over a period of two weeks or less to create a dependence on the drug.

Cannabis

Cannabis or Indian hemp is a drug with opiate properties which is illegal in Great Britain and the United States, although pressure groups are trying to legalize its sale and use. It is found either as cannabis resin or as 'grass', the dried flowering tops of the female plant, and is smoked in cigarette or pipe form or eaten. Like all the opiates, cannabis affects the sensory centres, often promoting relaxation, heightened perception, sexual desire or sleep. It can also bring on hallucinations. Cannabis has not been proved to be an addictive drug, nor are the side-effects generally held to be harmful, but it remains illegal to possess, use or sell the drug.

Amphetamines

Unlike the barbiturates, amphetamines stimulate the nervous system, inducing increased adrenalin (epinephrine) production so that the heart beats faster, blood sugar levels are raised and muscles tensed. The effects are a greatly increased sense of well-being, accompanied by hyper-activity and physical symptoms of trembling, sweating, reduced appetite and possible dizziness. Withdrawal from the drug produces feelings of fatigue and depression, with the result that the user desires more to put her back on a 'high'. Because of their strongly addictive nature, the prescription of amphetamines is now rarer than ten years ago. Chronic dependence not only weakens the body because of the excessive stimulation, and therefore activity, but may also induce psychotic behaviour such as schizophrenia. Overdosage can result in death.

Cocaine

Cocaine produces symptoms similar to those described above and dependence can lead to the same results. Its anaesthetic properties, if correctly administered, are medically useful however. Overdose can result in paranoia, hallucinations and physical illness largely due to malnutrition, convulsions and, in extreme cases, death.

How well do you know yourself?

In the last ten to fifteen years, women have learned to see themselves in a way quite different from their ancestors. We are gradually growing used to the idea that what we make of ourselves and of our lives is not in the hands of the men around us but, in so far as it is in the hands of anyone, it is in our own. We can decide who we are, what we do, where we live and with whom, in a way formerly open only to men. We are being offered the chance to be as totally responsible for ourselves as any human being can be. What are we going to make of it? That is one side of a woman's position today. The other has always been with us, and we can't escape it: the biological aspect of being a woman. We do, however, want to make it as successful, as enjoyable, as much part of our lives as possible. The fact that we are asking for equal rights and equal opportunities with men doesn't mean that we abrogate the right to be ourselves biologically and sexually. We are looking for an extension of our horizons, not for an exchange of one landscape for another.

The aim of this book is to offer a review of the various aspects of feminine humanity. What we suggest is that, at this point, you should ask yourself some questions. These are not the sort of questions you will meet in a magazine quiz, designed to give you a score at the end from which you discover whether you are extrovert or introvert, generous or mean, a career girl or a home-maker; they are questions to which there are far more than one or two neat, tidy answers. But they are questions which we should all ask ourselves from time to time, in order to discover where we are in our lives and where we are going next.

HOW ADULT ARE YOU?

Do you like to have your own way, but do you also blame other people when things go wrong?

How far are you prepared to take responsibility for yourself?

Do you let your emotions rule your decisions with too little regard for practical realities?

Do you fall in love with people, things or schemes, and demand instant gratification, but later find that you have acquired a totally unsuitable man, object or undertaking?

Do you know your own vulnerable points?

It would be ridiculous to ask 'Do you ever make mistakes?' because we all do – making mistakes is part of the experience of living. Much more important is 'Do you learn from them?'

While we are still children, we assume that anyone with a 'grown-up' body also has a grown-up mind. As we ourselves approach and reach physical maturity, we discover that this is anything but the truth. We all retain some childish charac-teristics, which may or may not be obviously part of our make-up. We don't exhibit them all the time, but they are nevertheless there. They may be charming – enthusiasm, energy, flexibility – or they may be maddening – unreliability, total dependence, irrationality. How they affect our behaviour as adults will depend on our ability to suppress reactions at times when they are inappropriate. It may be perfectly all right to exhibit childish enthusiasm over a game, a new project, a holiday or a new friend, but it is less than charming if losing the game or disappoint-ment over the project, holiday or friend is always expressed in the childish terms of 'It's everyone else's fault, not mine!'

WHAT DO YOU FEEL ABOUT HEALTH?

Do you understand how your body functions? Does it work to your satisfaction? Do you suffer from it, ignore it or enjoy it?

Do you have indigestion, constipation, odd aches and pains? Are you permanently snuffly, breathless or coughing? Do you always feel tired and listless, under the weather?

How much do you worry about your physical functions? More important, what do you do about the problems you have?

Do you have regular medical and dental check-ups?

Are you sorry for yourself? When you catch a cold, bruise or wound yourself, do you find that no one is sufficiently sympathetic? Are you the only person who seems to care?

Are you over-stoical? Do you refuse to give up till you can't hold out any longer? Do you despise all possible medical help, refuse to take painkillers, even, perhaps, enjoy being a martyr?

Do you ever use ill-health as a form of controlling other people? Do you plead a headache to avoid sex, or ill-health to avoid doing something disagreeable or that you feel you can't cope with?

Do you use your health as blackmail: 'You know that going to visit your mother always gives me migraine'?

Do you see yourself as basically healthy, an invalid, or someone who has to be careful? Is this a true assessment of your present health? Are you as well as you used to be, or alternatively, are you delicate?

Some illnesses or physical disabilities are not immediately susceptible to treatment, others are. The important thing is to discover whether or not you can be helped, and if you want to be. It is stupid to harbour chronic indigestion if diet or medicine can relieve it, or to allow yourself to be crippled by a headache which is due to faulty glasses. On the other hand, if your trouble is, for one reason or another, incurable, then you have to learn how to live with it and to allow it to disrupt the sort of life you want to lead as little as possible. We all know 'professional invalids', people who make ill-health their main occupation, their excuse not to face life, so it is useful to ask yourself what attitude you take towards your health, or its absence, and whether you are in touch with the way you are now.

And what about the care of your body? Fortunately, most of the body's functions are self-regulating and don't leave us much choice as to whether we keep them running or not. For example if our energy supplies run low, hunger makes us eat. But there is a choice in the way in which we treat or maltreat the various physical systems. We can eat too much, drink too much, stay up too late, endanger our breathing apparatus with nicotine. We can allow our muscles to become flabby through want of use, our teeth to decay, our feet to suffer from lack of attention or badly-fitting shoes. From time to time we should do a mental and, if possible, physical check-out, just as we should for any house-hold or industrial machine, to find out whether the parts are in good working order or whether any need expert attention. If we learn to function as efficiently as possible on this level, we are likely to find that our mental and emotional functioning is good, too.

HOW DO YOU LOOK?

Are you comfortable with your appearance? If not, why not?

Do you feel that what other people see when they look at you is the true expression of what you are really like? For instance, do you perhaps look more or less feminine than you feel? More clever or less clever? More or less helpless, demanding, sexy?

Do you feel that your success or failure depends on one feature you possess? Do you consciously make the most of this if it is good, or try to hide it if it is not up to standard? Do you tend to cover a big mouth with your hand, or try not to present the profile of a beaky nose or receding chin?

Have you a standard of looks to which you compare yourself? Do you model your hairstyle, make-up and dress on a world-acclaimed beauty, to whose type you think you approximate?

Do you follow beauty advice in women's journals to correct or change your features, so that your face conforms as nearly as possible to current standards of fashion?

If you have stopped wearing make-up, did you do so because you feel happier completely natural? As a feminist gesture? Because you gave up trying to look pretty and decided people should accept you warts and all? Because you don't feel it necessary now you are married or have reached a certain age?

Do you wear a particular colour or do your hair in a special way to please your husband or boyfriend, or because someone once said it suited you?

How often do you take a look at yourself as a whole, in a good light, before a full-length mirror, assessing not a detail or two, but asking yourself what the total impression is?

There are very few women who are totally satisfied with their looks. Since each of us is the person most intimately concerned, we have had more opportunity to study advantages and faults in our bodies than any outside observer. We are also likely to be more critical. We know that the nose is just that little bit too long, that the two halves of the face don't balance perfectly, that we have fat thighs, thick ankles, ugly knees, the wrong sort of hair, too much/not enough bosom. But asking ourselves what is wrong is not enough. We should also ask: What do I do about it? Is it practical to try to remedy the fault? The answer will depend on the degree of its gravity and on the time and money necessary to correct it. For instance, if it is adolescent acne, which can persist into the twenties, we should try following medical advice, since this won't involve any great expenditure. If it is an ugly nose we may consider plastic surgery. If it is bad posture we might go in for remedial exercises. But let us suppose that the offending feature can't be changed. Then how do you cope with it?

We all know the woman who, when complimented on what she's wearing, says, 'Oh this old thing? I've had it for ages!' – a rejection of both the compliment and the speaker's taste. Women who are uncomfortable with some aspect of their appearance often do much the same thing; they eagerly point out to others the offending feature, as if this were the most noticeable thing about them. If you find yourself doing this, you are probably in reality asking for a denial, or some comforting remark such as 'No, it hardly shows.' But do you really need this reassurance? Does your ability to make friends depend on whether or not they can accept this unfortunate feature? The answer, of course, is that if you yourself can accept it, consider it a built-in part of the whole of you, no one else is going to bother about it. Try to remember what you notice about other people when you first meet them. If it has been a favourable impression, it probably wasn't the symmetry of both the noses or mouths or the length of their eyelashes that you remarked, but the whole person: appearance, yes, but also posture, movements, tone of voice, and a lot of other things you would never notice if you were busy matching them up with some conventionally correct model.

HOW DO YOU FEEL ABOUT YOUR AGE?

Do you tell your true age, if you are asked? Do you try to disguise signs of age by tinting your hair, or wearing dark glasses to hide wrinkles and bags under the eyes? Do you try out 'youth-preserving' skin creams?

Do you regard the deterioration of your looks as inevitable and use the process of physical ageing as an excuse for giving up the attempt to look and feel as good as possible?

Do you keep an eye on your weight? Do you exercise regularly? Do you take note of and correct your posture?

Do you from time to time survey your clothes, your hair-style, your make-up, and consider whether they go with your face and figure today, rather than your appearance of a year or two ago?

The point of asking yourself these questions is to try to discover what you really feel about your own age. Sometimes time seems to stand still for years, sometimes there's a nasty jolt when you notice the first white hair, catch sight of the beginnings of a second chin, realize that your muscles aren't quite as resilient as they were a year or two ago and that you are more easily tired. At the present time there is so much emphasis on youth that any indication that we are not going to stay twenty-five for ever seems particularly unwelcome and frightening. There is an implicit message in the media that youth is good, growing older is bad, but we need to resist and question this.

If we could retain the elasticity and physical strength of youth and at the same time have the benefit of our experience, then we should have an ideal condition. But, if we are honest, most of us will probably admit that life in our early twenties was not unadulterated bliss, and if we are wise we will accept that there are compensations as well as disadvantages in ageing.

This doesn't mean that we should give up, resign ourselves to being dependent or out of touch with the younger members of society; we have to strike the balance between presenting ourselves as eternally young – which means mutton dressed as lamb, both in our physical appearance and our emotional attitudes – and the other extreme of allowing our minds and muscles to degenerate for want of use. Again, this entails being honest with ourselves. We shouldn't pretend to go along with currently fashionable beliefs and opinions if they are not really ours, just as we shouldn't compete physically with people twenty years younger than we are. It is more comfortable both for ourselves and others if we can accept how we are *now*. And it's reassuring to note that in spite of the present cult of youth – or perhaps because of it – middle age now seems not to start till the end of the forties or even later, and old age is now pushed back to the over seventy-fives or eighties.

Mentally and physically, our bodies inexorably age with the years, so from time to time we should look into the mirror, not to make sure that our hair, make-up and dress are right for the occasion, but rather to look and ask: Is this right for *me*? It is terribly easy to continue to wear the clothes and keep the hairstyle which suited us at a younger age. The question is: Is my appearance appropriate to my age? Of course, you don't have to dress according to your years if you happen to look twenty years younger in face and figure; the important thing is that face, figure and dress should harmonize. This assessment should be done in full daylight and in a full-length mirror; cheat the world on this score if you like, and if you can, but don't cheat yourself.

HOW DO YOU FEEL ABOUT YOURSELF AS A WOMAN?

Has the revolution in the last fifteen years, during which women have fought for equal opportunities and sexual freedom, changed your view of yourself as a woman? If so, in what ways?

If circumstances forced you to choose between a career and a family, which would you choose? Do you resent the fact that men rarely if ever have to make this choice?

Do you believe that a childless woman must be either unfulfilled or lacking in femininity?

Do you believe that for women sex must be an expression of a one-to-one, deep and lasting commitment between two people? Do you think that sex is, or should be, this for men?

Does the sexual aspect of your body make you feel pleased, guilty, ashamed, proud?

How much do you think you need to know about how your body functions in order to have a successful and enjoyable sex life?

Whether safe contraception has been the chicken or the egg in the history of women's emancipation doesn't really matter. What is important is that women today find themselves in a position of unprecedented freedom: freedom to choose their careers; freedom to choose whether or not to marry; freedom to choose whether to have children and if so, how many; freedom to become financially and socially independent; freedom to discover what they are like as individuals.

But freedom brings the responsibility of choice and the necessity of making decisions, and decisions about what lifestyle will be appropriate for any one of us involves self-knowledge. In former days, very few women asked themselves if they wanted to become mothers or if they were suited for the job; they knew that whatever their wishes or fitness, they were likely to find themselves bearing and rearing (and burying) children. They weren't consulted or instructed about their sexuality; sex when and how a husband demanded was the price of the financial support not otherwise generally available. The choice of a career was similarly limited, and even as recently as the Thirties the 'career girl' was looked upon as something extraordinary and likely to be unattractive to men.

It was limiting, but it was simple. Today we can't afford to take such a passive attitude towards life. We have fought not to be victims, now we have to order our own directions. We have to inquire into what we, ourselves, really want. It is no longer good enough to gripe against the husband and children we opted for, because their presence makes it more difficult to pursue a career. We must discover, too, what we feel about our own sexuality. Are the old stereotypes of male and female attitudes right for us? Or have we feelings which don't fit? Now that sex is not a taboo subject or a forbidden activity, can we be honest – and not pushed in any direction by current fashion – about the part sex plays in our relationships with others? And are we in danger of over-exposure to the subject, so that we trust what the experts write about it, rather than our own feelings?

Finally, in this age of equality, shouldn't we women borrow one of the more attractive characteristics of men? Men don't assume that their personalities are to be judged by their conformity to a standard of male good looks. They don't link their sex-appeal to their flawless complexions, their sylphlike figures, their lustrous eyes or hair. Imagine Humphrey Bogart or Edward G. Robinson protesting that they weren't pretty enough to be movie stars! Suppose Arthur Rubinstein had felt that as a small, fat, elderly man he wasn't attractive enough to make platform appearances! Women tend to use the male demand for female beauty to excuse their own attitude towards their appearance, and to equate good looks with personality. But this really is not fair. If men have exploited women in this particular way, they have been helped towards doing so by women's acceptance of their attitude. Maybe it is time we stopped adopting the innocent victim pose and, instead of abusing men for forcing us into the submissive position, learned to present ourselves to the world not as slaves or rebels, but as people who just happen to be women.

For your complete body check see pages 26–31.

FOREHEAD

Frown lines? What causes them: tension, headaches or eyestrain? Page 142. Should you try camouflage with a fringe? Page 173. Or massage? Page 141.

EYES

Sparkling or dull and tired? Eyestrain? When did you last have them tested? Dark rings or bags before your time? Reassess your living habits: fatigue or constipation will take their toll. Massage gently and use cooling eye pads. Page 141. If you wear glasses, try new frames or contact lenses. Page 199. How good is your eye make-up? Fashion changes quickly. Page 164. Pale lashes? Why not dye them? Page 169. Clogged lashes? Try a new mascara or buy an eyelash brush. Page 162.

EYEBROWS

Sleek and arched or bushy and untidy? Work on the shape. Page 130.

NOSE

Too long, too retroussé, too bumpy or just too big? Shading can help. Page 147. Plastic surgery is drastic, but would it make you happier? Page 207. Do you breathe properly? Page 57. See your doctor about persistent colds, sinus trouble or hay fever.

MOUTH

Smiling or turned down and sulky? Page 155. Elegantly outlined in pencil and coloured, or smudged and indecisive? Would a coloured gloss make a change from lipstick? Page 166. Do you always protect lips from the elements? Do you smile enough?
Moustache. Does it need a depilatory cream, bleaching or electrolysis? Page 130.

CHEEKS

Cheek-bones lost in a chubby curve? Accentuate with highlighter and shader. Would blusher bring a glow to pallid cheeks? Page 147. Broken veins, flaky skin or open pores? How good is your skin-care routine? Page 139. What about a facial or make-up lessons?

EARS

Have to hide them with hair? Do they really stick out? Thought about plastic surgery? Page 207. Are they rather beautiful? What about a swept-up hairstyle? Page 184. Ear-piercing? Page 212. A little rouge on the lobes?

TEETH

How long ago was your last check-up? Are teeth stained by smoking? What about a change of toothpaste? How old is your toothbrush? Are you brushing gums, too? Page 201. Fight to get dodgy teeth crowned rather than extracted. Page 203. Sour breath? Could be caused by tooth decay or gum disease. Page 201. Or it might be a health problem. Page 127. Deal with it!
Jaw line. Single or double chin? Slack jaw line from crash dieting? Exercise every day to tighten it up. Page 63.

HAIR

Condition. Healthy, shiny and silky? Too dry? Oily? Lank and lifeless? Plagued by dandruff? Frizzed by perms? Roughened by chemicals? Page 174.
Style. In need of a trim? Looked the same for over a year? Still suit your face and personality? Spoiled by changes in the weather? Page 179.

Colour. Is natural colour dull colour? Are you a secret redhead? What about more warmth, some highlights? Check for root retouching. Page 178.

How well do you know your body?

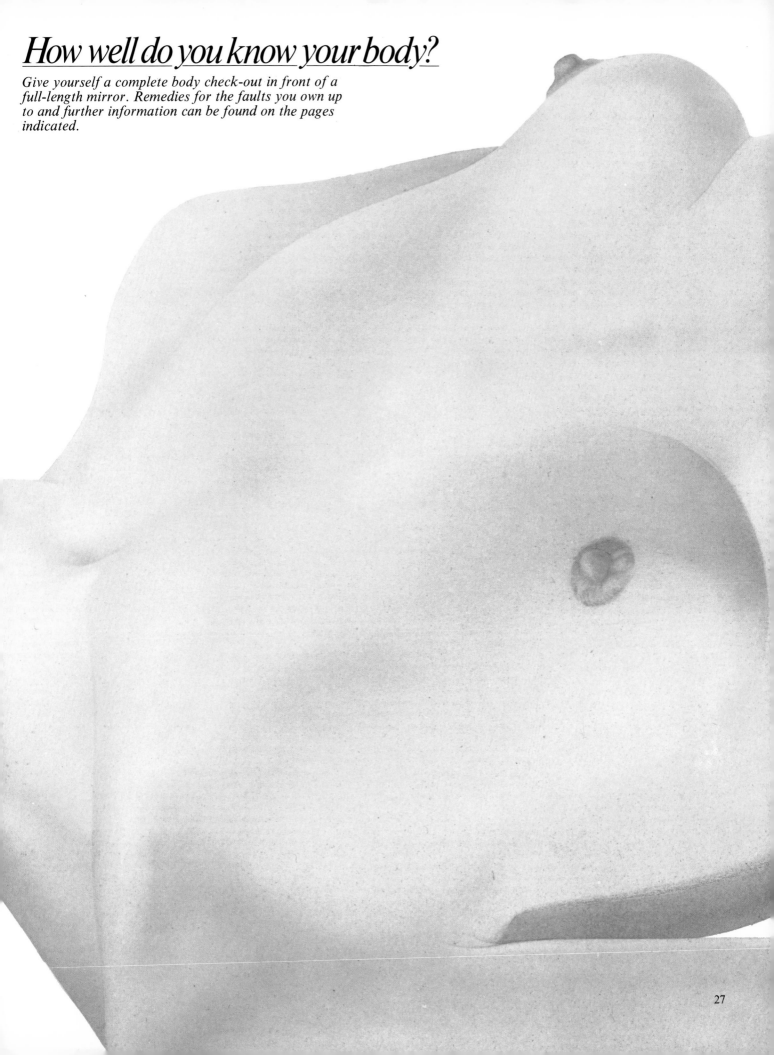

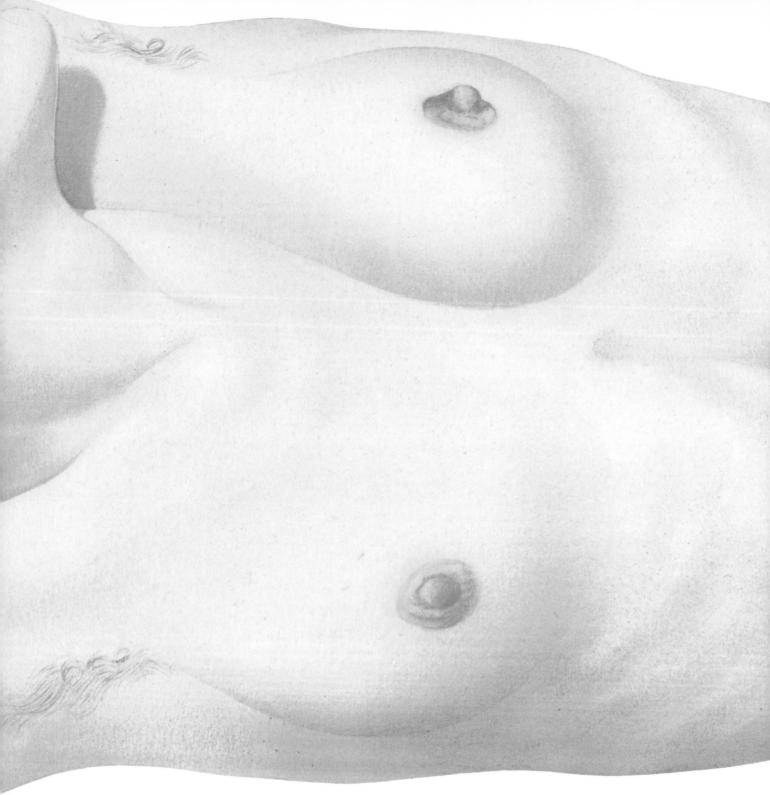

UNDER-ARMS
Have you decided whether to go hairless or not? Well do, in-between just looks scruffy. If you choose a naked armpit then make it just that - no stragglers. Page 130. If you opt for hair, keep it clean and silky. Fresh and odourless? If your deodorant isn't doing the job, it's time to switch. Page 126.

NECK
Worth showing off or a bit dingy? More thorough cleansing needed? Surely your face mask doesn't stop at the chin? What about a rich night cream to protect against wrinkles? Page 138. Do you hold your head up? Exercise is a vital treatment for headaches resulting from muscle tension. Page 75.

BREASTS
Firm and pretty or not what they used to be? Exercise won't change the shape but it will help to lift them a little. Page 63. Would a shop-fitted bra help? Hairs round nipple? Lots of people have them, but if they really worry you they can be removed by electrolysis. Page 133. Had your yearly check-up? Every woman should know how to do a basic breast examination herself. Page 222.

BACK
Out of sight out of mind? Take a mirror and look at your back view. If the skin looks spotty and sluggish, use the loofah and a tough back brush to get the circulation going properly. Page 126. Posture erect, or slouched with bottom sticking out? Stand up straight; you'll feel better and be less likely to get backache. Page 55.

WAIST
Measured it lately? Was it larger or smaller? Odds on it was larger, but why? How much weight have you put on? You should know, but if not hop on the scales now. Choose a diet that's right for you and start shedding. Page 53. If slackness is due to idleness, start exercising. Page 60. It's easy to tighten up a waist. Get out your old hoola-hoop.

INTERNAL
Do you know how your body functions? Page 87. Are you bearing menstrual pain unnecessarily? Page 92. Are you happy with your contraceptive or experiencing side-effects? Page 101. Do you have a regular check-up with your gynaecologist? Are you confident of your knowledge of pregnancy and childbirth or do you feel you are being kept in the dark? Page 109. Do you suspect you might be entering menopause? Page 123.

PUBIC HAIR
Straggling up the tummy or down on to the legs? Waxing or bleaching will help. Electrolysis will remove stray hairs permanently. Page 130. Is your pubic hair rough and unkempt? Why not brush and trim it?

STOMACH
Checked sideways for stand-up sag? Is it a postnatal problem that's gone on a bit too long, or is it just slack muscles and overweight? Choose your diet and exercise programme and swing into action. Page 52ff. Meanwhile, would a one-piece be better than a bikini this summer? Is skin dry instead of glossy and supple? Oil in your bath water will help. Page 125. Use cream on your body as well as hands and face.

29

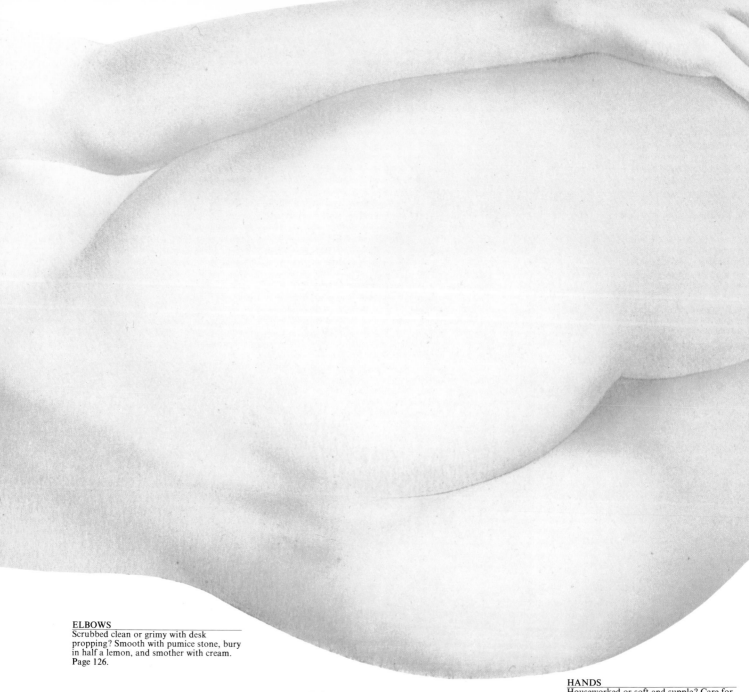

ELBOWS
Scrubbed clean or grimy with desk
propping? Smooth with pumice stone, bury
in half a lemon, and smother with cream.
Page 126.

ARMS
Slender and graceful? Or getting a bit
flabby? Start exercising daily. Page 62.
Choose dresses with a small sleeve. Too
hairy? What about bleaching? Page 130.
Wear a Cleopatra bracelet on a pretty
upper arm.

HIPS
Taut and trim or starting to spread? Is it
over-weight pudge? Try the pinch test. If
you can grab more than a generous inch
(2.5 cm), you're too fat. What are you
waiting for? Shed some weight and start
exercising! Page 60. Dingy or spotty skin?
Don't just sit on it in the bath, stand up
and scrub.

HANDS
Houseworked or soft and supple? Care for
them with night creams and barrier creams
and protect them with rubber gloves.
Page 191. Disgusting nicotine stains?
Eliminate immediately; pumice and lemon
juice will help to bleach them away. Try
exercise to loosen up the finger joints.
Page 65.

THIGHS
Slim as a young boy's and free of flab?
Lucky! You can get away with short
shorts. If thighs are bulging and spoiling
your shape, try a special salon massage;
at home give them a good pinch and scrub
in the bath. Exercise? Page 66. And what
about taking up jogging or a regular
walking programme?

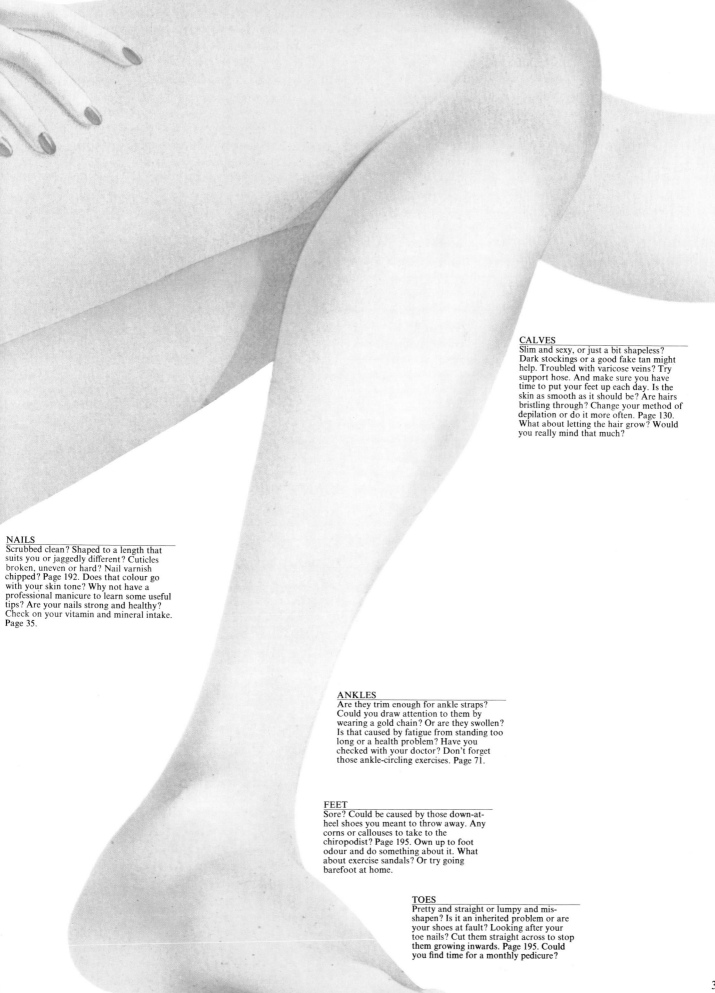

CALVES
Slim and sexy, or just a bit shapeless?
Dark stockings or a good fake tan might
help. Troubled with varicose veins? Try
support hose. And make sure you have
time to put your feet up each day. Is the
skin as smooth as it should be? Are hairs
bristling through? Change your method of
depilation or do it more often. Page 130.
What about letting the hair grow? Would
you really mind that much?

NAILS
Scrubbed clean? Shaped to a length that
suits you or jaggedly different? Cuticles
broken, uneven or hard? Nail varnish
chipped? Page 192. Does that colour go
with your skin tone? Why not have a
professional manicure to learn some useful
tips? Are your nails strong and healthy?
Check on your vitamin and mineral intake.
Page 35.

ANKLES
Are they trim enough for ankle straps?
Could you draw attention to them by
wearing a gold chain? Or are they swollen?
Is that caused by fatigue from standing too
long or a health problem? Have you
checked with your doctor? Don't forget
those ankle-circling exercises. Page 71.

FEET
Sore? Could be caused by those down-at-
heel shoes you meant to throw away. Any
corns or callouses to take to the
chiropodist? Page 195. Own up to foot
odour and do something about it. What
about exercise sandals? Or try going
barefoot at home.

TOES
Pretty and straight or lumpy and mis-
shapen? Is it an inherited problem or are
your shoes at fault? Looking after your
toe nails? Cut them straight across to stop
them growing inwards. Page 195. Could
you find time for a monthly pedicure?

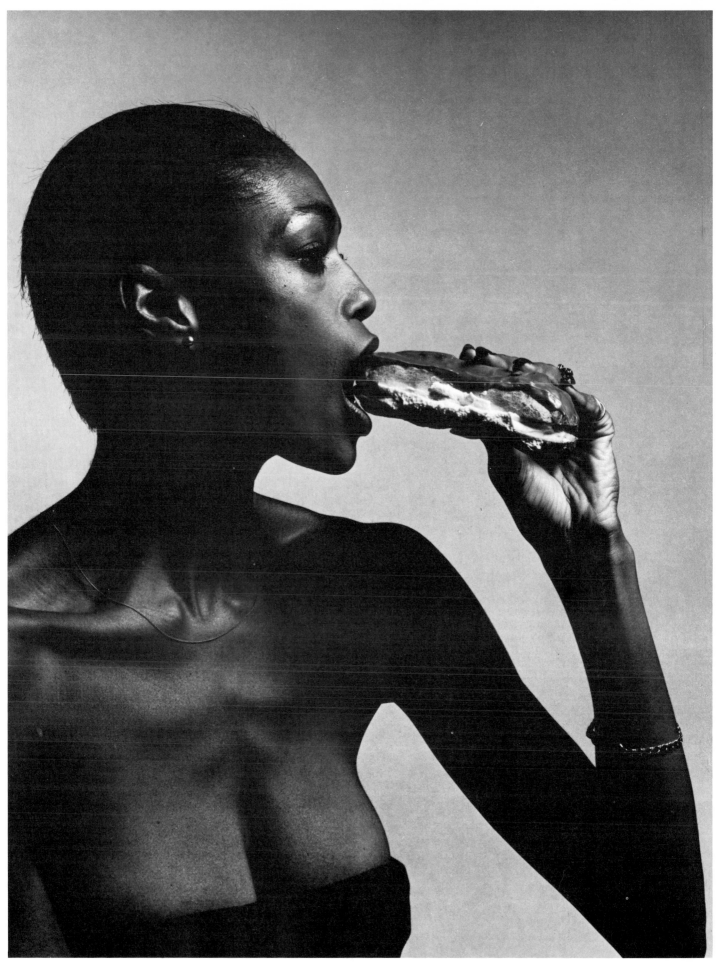

A Healthy Body

If a friend asked you right now whether or not you were fit, you might – unless you were a health fanatic, chronic hypochondriac or knew yourself to be genuinely unwell – find the question difficult to answer. Being fit is something most of us take for granted: if we weren't, we argue, how could we cope with the business of living – getting up in the morning, putting in a hard day's work for ourselves or our employers, or coping with the demanding task of bringing up a young family? In as much as we are able to perform the numerous and often onerous tasks demanded of us during the course of each day, we are by definition if not fit, then functioning. The two are not synonymous. The fact that our bodies manage to get us through the business of the day does not mean that they are strong and healthy, as fatigue,

backache and indigestion bear witness. Our bodies are like machines, and as such need to be kept in good running order if they are to function at maximum efficiency. Like cars, they need sound parts and thorough servicing. They also need the right kind of fuel and regular runs at the speed for which they were designed. Ideally the bodywork should be in gleaming order, but the engine that it houses needs most attention. So, in considering whether we are fit or not, we must ask ourselves whether we are fuelling and exercising our body machine correctly. If we are, not only will it function better but we will also feel better and, very important to most women, look better. No amount of careful dressing or make-up can disguise a body that is slack or skin that has become tired and dingy.

Perhaps at this point we should give ourselves a thorough check over to see what sort of shape we are in and then we can set about the job of getting back to the health and vitality we took for granted in our teens.

1 Take a good look at yourself in daylight, without clothes, in a full-length mirror. How does your body look, <u>honestly</u>?

If you do not look as good as you think you could, then now is the time to take action.

2 Weigh yourself. Do you weigh considerably more than you did when you were twenty, or when you remember being able to take a more or less constant weight for granted? Compare your weight with the chart on page 50. Is your weight within the 'accepted' norm? What weight would you like to be?

Are you significantly over- or under-weight? To be over-weight is far more common. If you weigh more than 7 lb (3.2 kg) over the average for your height and age (see page 50) or more than the weight at which you were most comfortable, you should think about dieting. It is a fact that women and men who are over-weight are more prone to a variety of illnesses than people who are not. You may be able to work out quite simply the cause of your excess weight (you know you eat too much, have a sweet tooth which you indulge, eat when you are fed up or unhappy, finish off the children's left-overs). You become over-weight when you consume more calories than you need, though hormonal imbalance may sometimes be responsible. One warning note, however. Being slim as opposed to fat is healthy. But being, or trying to be, leaner than you were meant to be can be as dangerous as over-eating.

3 How supple are you? Can you bend down and touch your toes keeping your knees straight? Sitting down with legs straight out in front, feet together, can you

touch your toes and put your head down on your knees? Do you get breathless? Can you walk up a steep hill or sprint for a bus without panting? Can you hop on one leg, skip with a rope for more than a minute, or dance to pop records without flagging?

If you cannot do any one of the various 'test' activities with ease, then you are not as fit as you should be. Getting fit when you are out of condition requires effort and will-power. It has been proved that ten minutes' brisk walking or jogging daily, or a regular exercise routine, is far more beneficial than an occasional burst of physical activity. You will also find that the more consistently you exercise the more you will be able to undertake. It is partly a matter of habit and partly that the fitter you get the fitter you can become. But don't rush it. Start to exercise now, even if you can only manage ten minutes a day. Keep it up and you will be amazed at your increased suppleness and stamina a month from now.

If you smoke, even moderately, physical exertion will prove more difficult for you. And if you are both over-weight and a smoker your ability to perform what should be fairly easy tasks, such as climbing stairs, will be even more impaired.

4 Do you feel tired or worn out nearly always, often, occasionally? At what time of the day do you tend to feel most fatigued?

We all feel tired sometimes for no apparent reason, or because we have quite literally over-exerted ourselves. A healthy person, however, who eats sensibly, takes a reasonable amount of exercise and sleeps soundly, should not suffer from regular tiredness. Unless you can immediately pinpoint the cause of persistent fatigue (a young baby who needs night-time feeds, cramming for an exam, looking after a sick and

demanding relative), you should visit your doctor to see if there is any medical or psychological reason for your tiredness; boredom and a lack of stimulation can often be the cause. People get tired when the sugar level in their bloodstream drops. This is to some extent a normal occurrence, as for example when you have gone too long without anything to eat or drink. A deficiency of iron or vitamins, perhaps due to a poor or unbalanced diet, can also be responsible for lassitude.

However, it is also a fact that different people function better at different times of the day. The owls come alive late in the evening and are able to work happily whilst their fellows are snoring soundly. The larks can wake at dawn and get half a day's work done before most people have finished their breakfast. Habit and the demand of certain occupations (night nurses and milkmen, for example) may have a lot to do with the hours when we function best, but we should also be aware of our natural rhythm and try to work with it and not against it.

In many women tiredness and fatigue are related to their menstrual cycles (see page 89). Whatever the cause, if tiredness is a permanent companion you must seek medical advice. There may be a simple answer – or it may be more complicated. It is a fact, for instance, that people suffering from depression, particularly if it is undiagnosed, complain of being permanently tired.

5 Do you find it easy to go to sleep naturally, without the aid of pills or some form of night-cap? Do you wake easily and refreshed, or are you still tired?

If you find it hard to sleep it could be that you are not taking enough exercise or are eating too late (see Insomnia, page 215). Our sleeping hours are crucial if our bodies and brains are to rest and

recharge. Our dreams* are vital, too, in ways that have still not been definitely analysed, but we know that deprived of our dreams for any length of time we can become mentally ill. If you feel tired when you wake after a reasonable number of hours asleep, which will vary from person to person, then again you must trace the root cause.

6 Do you take the Pill as a form of contraceptive?

Much research has been done into the effects of the contraceptive pill. For the majority of women who use it, the Pill represents a safe, trouble-free form of contraception (see page 101). But some women are unsuited to it. If you have been taking the Pill for more than five years, if you smoke heavily, or if you have any history of heart disease or thrombosis, then you should immediately visit your doctor or gynaecologist and discuss whether you should use some other contraceptive. There is also evidence suggesting that some forms of contraceptive pill can cause depression and even suppress sexual drive. Whatever the reason, if you are at all worried and think the Pill may be affecting your health, visit your doctor.

7 How often have you been ill this year with flu, colds or a general feeling of being 'run down'?

If you have had only the odd cold, or fallen victim to a flu epidemic, then you are probably typical of millions. If, on the other hand, you have been constantly under the weather, it could be that you are not looking after your body properly. Insufficient or unsuitable food providing less than the necessary amounts of nutrients, vitamins and minerals, combined with lack of exercise, can cause your body machine to become run down and prone to infection.

8 Do you take stimulants or tranquillizers.* regularly or

occasionally or for emergencies?

Most women are prescribed stimulants or tranquillizers at some time during their lives; many feel that they are handed out too freely. If, however, the doctor does prescribe them and you find you are becoming dependent on the drug, either to calm or to stimulate you, you should go back to your doctor immediately, Some drugs are habit forming and, like any substance which alters the body's natural functioning, they should be treated with respect and taken with care.

9 How much alcohol do you consume each day? Are there regular times when you feel you like, want or need a drink? Or does this depend on social circumstances?

Some of the healthiest, best-looking women in the world never drink alcohol; others, equally beautiful, do. A few, but unfortunately a growing number, drink far too heavily. Alcohol, contrary to popular belief, is a depressant and, whilst a few drinks may induce a sense of well-being or elation, taken in excess alcohol depresses. It can also damage not only your looks but your body and brain as well. Kidneys, liver and heart are vital organs which alcohol can attack and damage, sometimes irreversibly. Alcohol also destroys much of the nutritional value of the food you eat and if you drink daily you may well need supplements of Vitamin B complex and Vitamin C. Drink by all means in moderation, which of course does not preclude the odd party or celebration (when you may take too much), but if you find that alcohol is damaging your looks and life then take heed and cut down. If you find you cannot cut down seek help, you have a drinking problem (see page 22).

10 Do you smoke? If so, how many cigarettes a day? Are you a habitual smoker or do you smoke only on certain occasions?

There is absolutely no doubt that smoking is harmful to your health. The odd cigarette will probably not harm you but regular heavy smoking, which can mean anything over ten cigarettes a day, *is* harmful. If you smoke heavily, try to cut down, or better still stop altogether. Heavy smoking is an addiction and as such is hard to break. See page 23 for tips to help you stop.

11 If you don't look as good as you know you should, do you assume this is because you are getting older or have had babies?

If you have been completely honest in your stocktaking and have found yourself wanting, then you should by now have some clues as to how you can improve the situation. Work on it. There is all the difference in the world between living in a healthy body and one which is running even slightly below par.

EATING FOR HEALTH

We live in a society where the outpourings of newspapers, magazines, radio and television keep us, whether we like it or not, constantly and almost obsessively informed about food. Advertisements vie with each other to sell particular products; consumer programmes talk of 'best buys'; nutritionists lecture us on the contents of foodstuffs and how our bodies use them; documentary programmes ask questions about the political and humanitarian ethics of our eating habits; magazines tell us to be slim and beautiful and suggest innumerable diets and ways of becoming so; psychiatrists discuss food as sexual sublimation, solace or revenge; family-orientated articles tell us how to be good mothers and feed our families to the best of our budget; food columnists recommend this restaurant and disparage that one. There is cuisine minceur, cordon bleu, economique, familiale. If we didn't constantly remind ourselves, apart from the fact that food can be enjoyable and mealtimes important family occasions, we might just forget that if we didn't eat and drink we would eventually die. We are approaching the stage where we can feel worried or guilty about eating anything in case it harms us in some way, although fish and chips eaten happily will probably do you much more good than yoghurt and lentils eaten in a spirit of self-sacrifice.

Quite simply, like all animals, we need food and the nutrients it contains to build, restore, repair and process our bodies. Like any machine, the body can only function if it receives the substances it needs to keep it in working order. We *can* actually survive for a certain length of time without it, and we can function, albeit inefficiently, on a less than adequate diet, as millions of under-nourished people in the world bear witness. However, because in the Western world there is enough food to eat, and because most people have sufficient money to purchase food, we are lucky enough to have a choice in our diet. But that choice is dictated to a large extent by forces beyond any one person's control. Food production is now an industry, whether it is the manufacture of loaves, the trawling for fish or the rearing of livestock. In addition, we are all influenced by a mixture of habit, circumstance and current food theory. We eat bread, butter and certain meats, fish, fruits and vegetables because our parents did or because they are readily available. During the Second World War, mothers of small children were perpetually worried not only about the amount of food they could give their families, especially babies and young children, but about the quality of that food. With meat, proteins and fat-based foods in short supply, they were concerned that their offspring's growth and development would be impaired, being unused to the idea that the basic wartime diet of strong bread, eggs, cheese and vegetables could be very nourishing. In the post-war years, once the rationing of food ceased, there was a boom in the purchase of high protein foods, as though people were trying to make up for lost growth. Today, while no nutritionist would undervalue the importance of proteins in a well-balanced diet, many would claim that we eat, and erroneously believe that we need, too much protein. Also, in recent years, the evidence that saturated fats, such as butter and lard, may be harmful to our bodies or that too much cholesterol, also found in saturated fats, eggs and cream, can be similarly damaging has led to changes in many people's eating habits. We now need to remind ourselves of what food is, how it helps us to function, and how to eat to keep healthy without becoming food faddists.

THE FOOD WE EAT

Food is basically anything with a chemical composition that can provide the body with material from which to produce energy and heat; material for use in the growth and repair of bone and tissue; and substances to regulate the process of energy production, growth, reproduction and repair. The human body needs proteins, carbohydrates, fats, vitamins, minerals and water. For energy, the body uses carbohydrates, fats and proteins; for growth and repair, it uses proteins, minerals and water; for the control of its functions, it uses proteins, vitamins, minerals and water. Eating and drinking are therefore vital activities and, in our attitudes to the foods and liquids we consume and the ways in which we do so, this fact should not be forgotten.

Carbohydrates

Carbohydrates – sugar and starch – provide the body with energy, which if not required may be converted into body fat. Starches provide a major form of food for a large part of the world's population. Many nutritionists believe, however, that in the West we consume too much carbohydrate and definitely too much sugar. One hundred years ago, the average consumption of sucrose in Europe was estimated at $4\frac{1}{2}$ lb (2 kg) per person per year. Today, in Europe and the United States, the average consumption is nearer $112\frac{1}{2}$ lb (50 kg) per person per year, twenty-five times as much as our great-grandparents ate. And, although sugar can provide us with energy, nutritionally it has no other benefits; it contains what are called 'empty calories'. On the other hand, foods containing starch, such as bread, rice and potatoes, do have nutrients. In addition to its starch content, bread provides us with proteins, B vitamins and calcium, and potatoes are a source of Vitamin B, Vitamin C, Vitamin K and potassium.

Over-consumption of either starch or sugar, eating or drinking more than we need, leads to obesity which is, of course, unhealthy. In the West we probably eat less starch than we did perhaps fifty years ago, and it is the increase in sugar consumption that now causes concern. Not only does too much sugar make us fat, but it can also contribute to heart disease and tooth decay. Ideally, our diet should include a reasonable amount of starch, minimal amounts of sugar – we can obtain all we need from fresh fruit and vegetables – and fibre or roughage, which is present in cereal husks and the fibrous tissue of fruit and vegetables.

Fats

Fats may be saturated (animal fats, such as lard and butter) or polyunsaturated (vegetable fats, such as maize and sunflower oil); they provide energy and may be converted into body fat. Nutritionists divide them into 'visible' fats, such as butter, margarine, cooking oils and the fat on meat, and 'invisible' fats, contained in milk, lean meat, nuts or cheese. Weight for weight, fats provide us with a more concentrated form of energy than either proteins or carbohydrates, and make up most of our energy reserves. They not only improve the texture and palatability of food but also, because they are digested comparatively slowly, give us a feeling of being well fed. Furthermore, fats usually contain certain other nutrients: animal fats have Vitamin A, Vitamin D and cholesterol, while vegetable fats can contain carotene, which the body can convert into Vitamin A, and Vitamin E.

It is very unlikely that anybody will suffer today from a deficiency of the essential fatty acids that the body is unable to manufacture by itself. An adult needs about 1 oz (28 g) a week and these acids are present in so many foods that our needs will almost inevitably be met. It is far more likely that we will eat too much fat, and especially too much saturated fat. The trend away from eating quantities of butter, lard and cream towards vegetable margarine or oil is based on scientific evidence that too much cholesterol, an essential constituent of the body in small amounts, can ultimately cause heart disease and heart attacks. Scientists now believe that the less cholesterol we consume, the more probable it is that our blood cholesterol will stay at a safe level.

Proteins

Proteins provide us with amino acids, which the body needs for growth and repair. There are two types of amino acid: those known as essential amino acids, which cannot be made in sufficient quantity in the body itself and must therefore be supplied by food, and non-essential amino acids, which can be made in the body from any excess of certain other amino acids. There are only about twenty amino acids, but in different quantities and permutations these build many thousands of proteins. To ensure a healthy supply and sufficient variety of all the amino acids, it is important to include a wide range of protein foods in your diet.

Proteins can also be converted into carbohydrates and used to provide energy. Most food contains protein in varying quantities. At the bottom end of the scale, for example, a lettuce has between 1 and 2 per cent protein, while at the top end of the scale a hen's egg or a piece of cheese contains between 20 and 30 per cent. Egg is the only protein which has all the essential amino acids at the required levels. All other proteins are limited in quality by one or more of the essential amino acids. Most animal proteins are more complete than vegetable proteins; they also contain vitamins B12 and D which are absent in a strict vegetarian diet. In a balanced meal, proteins will come from different sources and the essential amino acid which is lacking in one protein will be supplemented by a surfeit of that amino acid in another. Thus the classic combination of bread and cheese provides more complete protein than either bread or cheese eaten alone. The average adult human needs about 10 oz (280 g) of protein a week. Babies and growing children need rather more, as does a pregnant woman, and some diseases demand a high protein intake. However, in the Western world, most of us consume far more protein than we actually need.

Minerals

Fifteen minerals known to be essential to the human body are derived from food. Most important are iron, calcium, phosphorus, magnesium, sodium, chlorine and potassium. Small amounts of fluorine, iodine, chromium,

HAIR
Vitamin A
Vitamin B2
Vitamin C
Copper
Iodine
Iron
Zinc

EYES
Vitamin A
Vitamin B2

TEETH
Vitamin A
Vitamin C
Vitamin D
Calcium
Fluorine
Phosphorus

TONGUE AND GUMS
Vitamin B3
Vitamin C

THYROID GLAND
Iodine

HEART
Vitamin B1
Potassium

NAILS
Vitamin B2
Vitamin D
Calcium
Gelatine
Iodine
Iron
Potassium

ADRENAL GLANDS
Vitamin B5

LIVER
Vitamin A
Vitamin B Complex
Vitamin C
Copper
Iron
Phosphorus
Zinc

NERVES
Vitamin B1
Vitamin B2
Vitamin B5
Vitamin B6
Vitamin B12
Choline (B Complex)
Calcium
Iodine
Magnesium
Phosphorus
Potassium

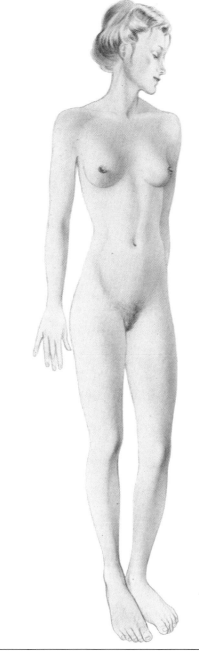

SKIN
Vitamin A
Vitamin B3
Vitamin C

BONES
Vitamin C
Vitamin D
Calcium
Fluorine
Magnesium
Phosphorus

MUSCLES
Calcium
Iodine
Magnesium
Potassium
Sodium

BLOOD
Vitamin B6
Vitamin B12
Folic acid (B Complex)
PABA (B Complex)
Vitamin C
Vitamin E
Vitamin K
Calcium
Chlorine
Chromium
Cobalt
Copper
Iodine
Iron
Potassium
Sodium

ANTIBODIES
Vitamin A
Vitamin B6
Vitamin C

ENZYMES
Vitamin E
Copper
Magnesium
Manganese
Phosphorus
Zinc

ENERGY
Vitamin B1
Vitamin B2
Biotin (B Complex)
Iodine
Iron
Phosphorus

CELLS
Vitamin B1
Vitamin B12
Choline (B Complex)
Magnesium
Potassium
Phosphorus
Sodium
Sulphur

---

cobalt, copper, manganese, sulphur and zinc also play an important role in maintaining the body. The minerals have three main functions. First, they provide the constituents of bones and teeth; the minerals responsible for this include calcium, phosphorus and magnesium. Second, they control the composition of the body cells and body fluids; sodium and chlorine are necessary for the fluids, such as blood, and potassium, magnesium and phosphorus for the cells themselves. Third, they are essential for activating enzymes and proteins, to enable energy to be released and used; magnesium acts as an agent in the utilization of Vitamin C and calcium, and iron is the most important mineral in the

formation of haemoglobin. If a well-balanced diet is followed, there should be no problem in ensuring that our bodies receive the minerals they need. However, where the diet is lacking, or the body has to contend with a particular disease, deficiencies in certain minerals can occur. The minerals most commonly subject to deficiency are iron, calcium and iodine. A diet lacking in iron may eventually lead to anaemia;* insufficient calcium may cause poor teeth and brittle bones, and increased premenstrual tension; and a deficiency in iodine may lead to goitre, a swelling of the thyroid gland.* Deficiencies in sodium and chlorine, which are found in salt and are lost from the body in excessive perspiration, can

result in muscular cramps, which is why if you take part in athletics or live in a very hot climate salt tablets may be required.

Vitamins

Vitamins are organic chemical compounds which are essential in the diet in relatively small, but critical, quantities to maintain health. If the body is seriously deficient in one or more vitamins, there will be a breakdown of normal bodily activity and certain illnesses will occur, or symptoms such as fatigue, nervous irritability or lack of growth in children may be experienced. There are basically two types of vitamin: those that are soluble in fat, A, D, E and K, and those that are soluble in water, the B vitamins and Vitamin C. If a well-balanced diet is followed, there should be no need to take extra vitamins in tablet or any other form. It is far better to adhere to a healthy diet than to take the lazy way out with a poor diet supplemented by pills; a poor diet, low in vitamins, will almost certainly be low in vital minerals as well. If, however, you know that your consumption of fresh fruit or vegetables has been lacking, a course of Vitamin C can do no harm. Some doctors recommend regular C supplements, particularly before the winter months, to help ward off colds and flu. Although there is no positive scientific proof that it is beneficial, it will certainly do no harm.

FOOD FADS

Today we have more choice about the food we eat than we have ever had before. As well as food which we have traditionally used as the basis of our diet, our supermarkets are stacked with an enormous range of products – many from other countries – a variety that our great-grandparents could not have imagined. In the past few years we have also seen the establishment and expansion of what we loosely term 'natural' or 'health' foods, many of which would have been familiar in content if not in packaging to a housewife shopping sixty years or so ago. In a technological age that can scarcely keep pace with itself, it was perhaps inevitable that we should pause, and look back, in order to compare what we have gained with what we have lost. After all, 'simple' foods and remedies sustained our forebears, who milled their own flour and baked their own bread, grew vegetables and fattened cattle without the aid of sophisticated techniques and, many people now believe, may have been the healthier for it. There is nothing simple about bread production these days, nor about the rearing of poultry and livestock for that matter. But the basic question we have to ask ourselves is: Does the fact that the food we eat today is largely grown or reared in a highly organized, intensive manner, with all the knowledge that scientific progress has brought, really matter? Are we in fact as healthy as we would have been at the turn of the century?

Much mileage has been made out of the phrase 'you are what you eat', yet strictly speaking the statement is true. For instance, those who believe for either moral or religious reasons that it is wrong to consume the flesh of other animals can logically say of those of us who do that our bodies are 'made' from other animals. But, moral reasons apart, meat eaters can say of *them* that their bodies, in the final analysis,

contain the same elements as ours, whatever the source. For instance, they may get the proteins they need from vegetables, nuts or flour; a regular consumer of meat will get much of hers from animal produce. Then there are the housewives who insist on whole-wheat flour to make bread and pastries, use only brown sugar or honey as sweeteners, and never eat anything from a tin or a deep freeze, while others rely largely on 'convenience' foods to feed their families. Is one household any healthier than the other? In recent years we have been so bombarded with differing and often contradictory theories about nutrition that, at this point, it might be helpful to look at some of the current theories about certain kinds of foods and see what, as far as scientific research has established, is fact and what fiction or fashion, bearing in mind that it is an excess of anything which is dangerous.

Organically versus chemically grown foods

Methods of growing food – grain, fruit and vegetables – have changed radically in this century. Today most crops are grown with the aid of chemicals, fertilizers and pesticides, geared to the production of the greatest number of the highest quality foods. Increasingly, there has been concern not only about the fact that such foods as these 'contaminate' our bodies in some way, but also that in the long term by using them in our soil and in the atmosphere we may be altering the proper balance of nature. A certain pesticide, for instance, will kill certain insects that are harmful to certain vegetables; but in removing those insects we may also be removing a source of food for other insects, animals or birds, thereby reducing their numbers, and they too have a role to play in the overall food cycle. We worry also because the animals we eat have consumed chemically grown crops as well, so we may be taking in even more of these chemicals. Research is continuous into their effects not only on the soil, but also in relation to the human body. So far, there has been no conclusive evidence that controlled amounts of chemical added to the soil or atmosphere are damaging to us, but only time will tell.

Organic methods of growing food, used for centuries, rely on enriching the soil with natural manure: animal droppings or composted vegetables. Few farmers would argue that, if the demand for food production had not become so great, these methods would not be adequate or for that matter ideal. However, from the plant's point of view, the nutrients it requires are absorbed

from the soil in the form of inorganic salts, and whether organic or inorganic in origin, the fertilizers or manure have to be broken down into these salts before the plant can benefit from them. And there is still no evidence at all that plants grown with the aid of organic fertilizers are in any way nutritionally better than those grown by inorganic methods.

If you still feel that you prefer to eat organically grown fruit and vegetables, make sure that they really are what they claim to be. A potato covered in earth is not necessarily an organically grown potato, any more than an egg with a few feathers adhering to it comes from a free-range as opposed to a battery hen. You will find genuine produce in specialist healthfood shops and market gardens, or you can grow your own, but a great deal of profit has been made by cashing in on the trend towards natural foods.

Vegetarian versus meat or fish-based diet

The human body falls about midway between a herbivore and a carnivore. It has incisors and canine teeth for meat eating and molars for vegetables. It is equipped with an intermediate length intestine and lacks the enzymes that would be needed if totally vegetarian, to break down the cellulose in grass. The emotional arguments in favour of vegetarianism are many and convincing: the fact that a great deal of land is needed to grow vegetables to feed livestock which only a minority of the world's population can eat; the appalling conditions for factory-farmed animals for ever-greedy people; and even the fact that meat is dead tissue full of fat and chemicals that the animal has eaten. Yet, in spite of these arguments, most of us still find vegetarianism somewhat 'faddish'.

There are basically two kinds of vegetarian: those who will eat anything apart from the flesh of animals or fish, and a more radical group, vegans, who will not eat any animal produce at all, including milk, eggs or honey, nor use wool for their clothes or leather for their shoes. A vegetarian diet can be nutritionally as sound as any other, provided certain facts are taken into consideration.

Proteins are an essential part of our diet, vital for body building and repairing. You don't have to eat meat to include proteins in your diet. In the West we eat too much protein anyway, but meat is the best of all food sources of iron as well. Meat, fish, eggs, cheese and milk are all excellent sources of protein. Pulses and nuts provide an

excellent source of vegetable protein and also contain minerals and vitamins. Whether vegetarian or not, we should all try to include these sources of protein regularly in our diet. A vegetarian will tend to have a lower overall calorie intake than a meat eater and may need to supplement meals with some high calorie food such as nuts. Vegetarians will also take in more water than non-vegetarians, since vegetable foods tend to have a higher water content, and will probably consume less fat; this may be ultimately beneficial to the vegetarian, since water is the purest and most essential liquid our bodies need and fat, particularly animal fat, if taken in too large a quantity can prove positively harmful. Another advantage of a vegetarian diet, if large amounts of *raw* whole food are eaten, is that the consumer will get plenty of roughage which may be lacking in a largely meat-based diet.

The strict vegan diet, however, does have several inherent disadvantages. It does not contain Vitamin B12, essential for the blood, since this is made by bacteria in the animal intestine, and stored in the liver, and cannot be made by plants. A vegan, therefore, should take regular amounts of this vitamin, even though there may well be a sufficiently high level of Vitamin B12 already stored in the liver to last the body for several years. The lack of Vitamin B12 over a prolonged period can cause anaemia and nervous disorders.

Vitamin D is also absent from a vegan diet. Although adults do not need this vitamin, it is important for the development and growth of strong bones in children. However, the vitamin is synthesized by sunlight under the human skin and, if children get sufficient sunlight, they will be able to manufacture it; otherwise, they should be given Vitamin D in tablet form.

Bran: beneficial or not?

Bran is the outer husk of wheat, removed from all but 100 per cent wholemeal bread and flour. Although it has no nutritional value as such, being literally indigestible, the roughage it provides is increasingly believed to be beneficial to our bodies. It expands in the intestines and helps to push all foodstuffs through, assisting their expulsion as faeces. It is undoubtedly helpful if you suffer from constipation and should be taken by anyone on a diet which consists mainly of refined, rich or fatty foods, which by themselves leave the intestinal system only with some difficulty. Many doctors now believe that roughage, which is also obtained

36

from raw, fresh fruit and vegetables, prevents major diseases of the colon and rectum, and may help to flush excess cholesterol from the bloodstream, thereby reducing the likelihood of heart disease. A tablespoon of bran sprinkled on breakfast cereal or fruit every morning can do no harm and will probably do you a lot of good. However, if you are eating a well-balanced diet it should not really be necessary.

Saturated versus polyunsaturated fats

Cholesterol and the three fatty acids – stearic, palmitic and oleic – comprise the fats stored in our blood. They are all released by the pancreas during times of high activity, stress, love and anger, when the body demands more adrenalin. If they are not burned up by the body, the fats are stored in the body tissue and are recognizable as the familiar bulges we so often wish to lose. The word cholesterol is Greek in origin and means literally 'solid bile', or the more commonly used 'gall stone'. Each of us generally has about 6 oz (168 g) of cholesterol within the body, which helps to build brain tissue and sex hormones. There is increasing evidence, however, that there is a close relationship between cholesterol and heart disease. Too much cholesterol in our systems results in a build-up of fats and blockages in the arteries which, in an artery supplying blood directly to the heart, can cause a heart attack. Since cholesterol is stored in animal fats, as well as our own, whenever we consume these fats we are adding to the cholesterol level in our blood, hence the trend away from saturated (animal) fats towards polyunsaturated (vegetable) fats. The cholesterol level of eggs is also very high. Although the exact relationship between cholesterol and heart disease has not as yet been clearly established, it would seem advisable to eat as few animal fats as possible, since prevention is always better than cure.

Brown versus white

Just because a loaf is brown, it does not necessarily mean that it is more nutritious than if it were white; it may simply contain colouring. Only wholemeal flour – 100 per cent whole wheat, maize, rye or whatever grain it is, husks and all – can be classed as totally and naturally 'brown'. Other 'brown' flours may be a combination of refined white flour and a percentage of whole flour. Refined white flour has become increasingly popular in the West over the past century, but in recent years more people have taken to using coarser varieties. However, the soft, sticky, sliced, white processed loaf remains top of the shopping list. Some vitamins and minerals are automatically lost in the refining and processing of white flour, but bakers in the UK are now required by law to replace these, so a white loaf is virtually as nutritious as an unrefined brown one. Processing does, however, remove the roughage, the grain husks themselves, which most nutritionists now believe is an important part of our diet.

Brown rice, brown spaghetti, brown macaroni and brown flour for pastry and cakes are also now widely available. They are an acquired taste but make a nice, and nutritious, change from the white varieties.

The sugar controversy

White sugar is almost 100 per cent sucrose and contains no vitamins. Brown sugar is less highly refined sucrose, which contains traces of other sugars, minerals and sometimes colouring. Honey is also a concentrated form of sugar and, although it has been used for centuries either alone or in conjunction with other liquids as a soothant, if not a remedy, for such ailments as sore throats and colds, nutritionally speaking it is no more valuable than either white or brown sugar. The most that can be said for sugar is that it provides the body with a quickly-absorbed, concentrated source of energy. As such, it does occasionally have its uses – if the sugar level in the blood has dropped below its normal level, for instance, after too much alcohol has been consumed. The fact remains, however, that in the West we eat and drink far too much sugar. It is literally an acquired taste, an addiction, and one that tends to increase in proportion to the amounts we eat and drink. All the heavily sugar-sweetened foods and drinks we consume – squashes and colas, ice-creams, sweets, tinned fruit, cakes and buns – could disappear from our diets tomorrow with only good results. Sugar can cause our teeth to decay and our bodies to become fat, and there is some evidence that it increases the risk of heart attack. We can acquire all the sugar we need from fruit and certain vegetables.

Uncooked versus cooked food

We cook certain foods not simply to make them more palatable, but also because in an uncooked state they would be indigestible. A diet of raw fish, meat and potatoes, for example, would be highly indigestible, although other foods – most fruits, many vegetables and nuts – can be eaten easily without subjecting them to the cooking process. But often, if we cook food, we make it more appetizing – it will look more attractive, and may smell and taste better. The many ways in which we cook food can make what is a basic necessity an enjoyable pastime and an integral part of family life. In addition, cooking some foods actually kills micro-organisms which would otherwise be harmful to our systems. Nevertheless, in the West we often over-cook unnecessarily, and in so doing destroy many nutrients that are present in raw food.

We are most culpable in the cooking of vegetables, a major source of Vitamin C, which is destroyed by prolonged cooking. We boil vegetables for too long, in too much water, and often compound this by soaking them in water beforehand. We are also guilty of robbing vegetables such as potatoes of the valuable proteins which lie beneath their skins when we peel them. Salting water before we cook vegetables, or meat before cooking it, also releases valuable juices which contain vitamins. And boiling food for any length of time results in minerals, soluble in water, being lost.

Below you will find a few basic rules to bear in mind when cooking. These should lead to happier digestive tracts, healthier eating and therefore healthier bodies.

1 Only cook what you have to; eat plenty of raw foods, with peel as this provides roughage.
2 If cooking vegetables, use the minimum amount of water possible, salt the water just before you finish cooking rather than earlier, cover pans with a tightly-fitting lid, and steam in preference to boiling to retain more vitamins and minerals.
3 Add a drop or two of acetic acid – lemon juice or vinegar, whichever is appropriate – when cooking peeled fruit or vegetables. This helps to prevent discoloration and slows the Vitamin C breakdown process.
4 Retain the water in which you have cooked any fruit or vegetable and drink or use as basis of stock, sauce or soup. The liquid contains some of the vitamins and minerals which 'escaped' from the fruit or vegetable.
5 Although too much animal fat can be harmful, leave enough on meat when cooking to ensure it retains its natural juices. You can remove the fat when cooking is completed.
6 'Seizing', i.e. subjecting to fierce heat for a few moments to form a 'skin', helps to retain the juices and vitamins in the food, particularly meat and fish.

Food additives

All food is, as we know, chemical. The mixture of proteins, fats, carbohydrates, minerals and vitamins needed in our diet is basically a mixture of chemicals. Some of these chemicals can be found in natural foodstuffs and others can be artificially prepared. With the trend, essentially a good one, towards a greater consumption of 'natural' foods has come an increasing awareness of what we eat and a greater concern with what we should not eat. This has generated a mood of near hysteria over the dangers of chemical additives to food. People worry about the often almost incomprehensible list of ingredients in convenience foods, such as prepared soups and sauces, preserved meats and ready-mix cakes, as though the food industry were deliberately trying to poison us all, and forget or are unaware of the fact that there are government agencies which operate strict controls and constantly monitor such foods to ensure that only permitted additives, safe for human consumption, are included. Chemical additives are under continuous scrutiny for possible toxic side-effects and suspect substances are immediately withdrawn from the permitted list.

PRESERVING FOOD

Very few countries are agri-culturally self-supporting today, and population growth throughout the world has meant that all countries import and export some food. Whether it is vegetable or animal, if not consumed within a certain time food will decay and become inedible, toxic and dangerous to the human body. So certain foods have to be preserved. Many methods of preserving, such as smoking and drying, are centuries old, but if the process is done in a factory it is not necessarily any the worse – and may be positively better.

Drying

Drying is one of the oldest methods of preserving foods and *must* be done at the right heat. Occasionally in the past it caused considerable damage to foods, such as meat and fish, which were dried slowly in the sun when both temperature and humidity were high. However, on the whole drying took place, and still does, in the right season and in countries where the climate was suitable. Today, the foods which are most commonly dried include fruit – currants, sultanas, raisins and apricots – and certain vegetables – such as peas, lentils and beans.

A relatively new process, known as freeze drying, is often used to preserve such foods as eggs, prawns and coffee granules. Freeze drying involves two processes, freezing the product and then evaporating the ice away, so it is a comparatively expensive method. However, it has the advantage of retaining not only all the flavour of the product, but also most of the nutrients.

Freezing

Freezing is also an expensive

method of preserving foods, although for anyone able to buy in bulk and use a home freezer costs can be reduced. All frozen vegetables are blanched and pre-cooked for a few minutes, which renders the enzymes inactive. Subsequent cooking time will be less than for fresh vegetables and, although the blanching process removes some of the B and C vitamins and minerals, frozen vegetables are nutritionally as good as boiled fresh vegetables, which also lose some nutrients in the cooking. Meat, fish and fruit, unlike vegetables, do not have to be blanched before they are frozen. All foods should be frozen quickly, to avoid damage and nutrient loss, and although freezing may be an expensive process it is very effective in preserving the quality of food.

Canning
The principle of heating food in a sealed container, can or bottle, as a method of preservation was discovered at the beginning of the nineteenth century. The process was developed further throughout the century and still more refinements have been made in recent years, such as subjecting the container to shorter heat treatments, which results in higher quality products, and inventing tops which are easier to open. In the canning process, foods are first cleaned, and fruit is peeled and blanched, and then heating is continued for long enough to cook them. The can is then sealed and made airtight, so that oxidization and contamination by bacteria in the air cannot occur. The temperatures at which canning is done vary: foods with a high acid content, such as tomatoes, can be sterilized at boiling point, 212°F (100°C), while foods lower in acid content, such as meat and fish, need heating under pressure to 250°F (121°C). Food which is canned properly can be kept for years and this is one of its major advantages. Although some vitamins are lost in the process, canned food is nutritionally only slightly less valuable than fresh food, and is positively better than over-cooked fresh food.

Bottle preserving
This method is generally used for fruit, some vegetables and jams. It is similar to the canning process, in that the food is contained in airtight conditions and frequently subjected to heat. However, certain foods, mainly vegetables such as cabbage or onions and occasionally animal foods such as herrings, can be preserved without cooking, through the addition of sufficient quantities of vinegar and usually salt.

Pasteurization
Pasteurization is the process of heating milk to a temperature of 162°F (72°C) for fifteen seconds,

followed by rapid cooling, to kill the organisms which can cause disease, including the bacteria responsible for tuberculosis. The process takes its name from Louis Pasteur, who pioneered the study of micro-organisms and 'discovered' inoculation. A newer method of treating milk, so that it will keep for longer periods, is to heat it to 270°F (132°C) for one second and then pack it in foil and polythene-lined cartons. This milk will keep for several months. Homogenized milk is also popular. After pasteurization, this is forced through jets which break down the fat globules so they do not rise to the surface. Most of the dairy produce that we consume – milk, cream, butter, cheese and yoghurt – is pasteurized; after 1980, with the exception of goats' milk, all dairy products in Great Britain will have to be pasteurized by law.

Smoking
Today, in the West, smoking is used more often for the flavour that it produces than for the preserving effect. There are two kinds of smoking: cold and hot. In cold smoking, the food is hung or placed in ordinary smoke for varying lengths of time; in hot smoking, it is placed in the smoke from a fierce source of heat and literally cooked at the same time. Traditionally, wood smoke is used in the process from a fire burning oak or beech; conifers are not suitable because the high level of resin in the wood produces a very acrid smoke and therefore taste. Many foods that are smoked are cured beforehand, i.e. soaked in brine, a saline solution. These will keep for much longer than if they have been smoked only.

PLANNING A GOOD BASIC DIET

A good basic diet is one that provides us with the materials we need to build (especially important for children), repair, and supply our bodies with the energy to carry out the various tasks demanded by our lifestyle. If we consume more food than we need to carry out these various functions, we become fat; if we take in too little, we lose weight. Ideally, our consumption of food should be such that we have enough of the right kind to ensure that our bodies 'tick over' at maximum efficiency, and no more.

If we consume more calories – units of heat – than we can use, we lay down stores of surplus fuel, rather as we fill a petrol tank in a car, the difference being that in humans the store is laid down in fatty deposits.

We all burn fuel, i.e. food in human terms, at different rates, which depend not only on the amount of fuel needed for a particular activity, but also to some extent on our individual

make-up. However, as long as we are alive, even if we are only asleep in a warm atmosphere, we have to burn fuel, or to put it more commonly, use up calories. The rate at which we consume these calories for the essential purpose of keeping alive is known as the basal metabolic rate (BMR) and it accounts on average for two-thirds of our daily energy. Other forms of activity such as exercise, whether necessary or pleasurable, account for the remaining third. If all over-weight people had a low BMR it might account for their condition: their 'tick over' would be very efficient, and so their energy requirements would be low and easily exceeded. However, not all those who are over-weight do have a low BMR; there are some who appear to consume less than their measured BMR and still put on weight. Such people probably depress their energy expenditure during the night in the same way as hibernating animals, but it is not yet known why or how.

A good basic diet is therefore one which provides us with our necessary energy requirements, however we use them. It also implies the right proportion of the various kinds of fuel needed to sustain our bodies in the most efficient and enduring way possible. Too much of certain kinds of fuel may have harmful effects, such as regular overdoses of sugar or animal fat, just as too little of others, such as protein, may be equally damaging. Most adults, for instance, generally need about 10 per cent of their daily calories in the form of protein, and children need rather more. Fatty acids should make up 1 to 2 per cent of our total calorie intake and vitamins, minerals and adequate amounts of water are also important.

For 'basic' read 'simple'
A basic diet is essentially a simple one: it contains water in un-restricted quantity, proteins, fats, carbohydrates, vitamins and minerals. The biblical phrase 'man cannot live by bread alone' may have been philosophical in intention, but it is also true. And although it would be narrow-minded and stupid to recommend that we stick to simple, un-adulterated diets all the time, it is useful to remember that our needs are different from our pleasures; that food is necessary to keep us alive apart from being a delight; that most of us over-eat a lot of the time, because we can afford to and because custom and social circumstances sometimes make it awkward to refuse food.

If, to pursue the analogy we used earlier in the chapter, you think of your body as a machine, it will help you to buy and eat the right kinds of food. The fuel you

need should be adequate in quantity, high grade in quality. Follow the rules below for healthy eating.

1 Eat raw, fresh fruit and vegetables as often as possible, washed but unpeeled whenever sensible.

2 Drink plenty of water; it is a vital body fluid and also helps to flush out waste matter, for example through the kidneys.

3 When cooking foods, remember that vegetables should be cooked for as short a time as possible with a lid on the saucepan, in as little water as possible to prevent vitamin loss, and that frying in vegetable oil is preferable to using animal fat.

4 Eat or drink as little sugar as possible. Several pieces of fruit a day should be quite sufficient to supply all the sugar you need.

5 Try to include wholemeal or wholegrain products in your diet: bread, pasta and pastry. They will provide you with roughage and, although nutritionally not proven to be much better than refined white flours and pasta, they are infinitely more satisfying.

6 Listen to your body. If only we ate when we were hungry and stopped when we were full, few of us would be over-weight. It is possible to re-educate an appetite that has come to expect three large meals a day, with several snacks in between. Many dieticians believe that little and often is the best way to eat. This does not mean that you can nibble away all day, but that four or five *small* meals can be eaten in the course of a day. A small meal could, for example, be a piece of cheese and an apple, a glass of milk and a slice of wholemeal bread, a lamb chop and a green salad, or a raw carrot and a dip.

7 Think through your daily routine and work out which parts of the day demand the most exertion (see page 56 for calorific expenditure for different activities). If, for example, most of your work is done in the morning, you should eat a good breakfast, which does not necessarily mean that it should be heavy or rich. If, on the other hand, your day is relatively undemanding but you have to work at night, an early evening meal should be designed to provide you with the energy you will need. Try to get out of the rut of cooking and eating at traditional times if these have no relevance to your lifestyle. Russian athletes, for example, probably amongst the fittest men and women in the world, eat large, high protein breakfasts, have a light lunch and a snack before bedtime. Eating in this way gives them all the energy they need at the right time of day and does not overload their stomachs in the evening. Their digestive tracts are

not grappling with a large food intake whilst they are asleep, a sin that many of us in the West are guilty of when we eat our biggest meal at the end of the day.

8 Keep a sense of proportion about food and drink. Don't become a food fanatic or bore, refusing to allow yourself the occasional splurge on a chocolate gateau or ice-cream, embarrassing your hostess by rejecting her canard à l'orange followed by zabaglione because you think it's too rich. As long as you bear in mind that in the long term simple food is often the best, your body will be well looked after. But remember also that we all need variety, and now and then even excess, in our eating and drinking habits as much as in other areas of our lives.

9 If you over-eat or drink too much one day, and you *know* when you have, simply cut down on your consumption the following day. Listen to what your body is telling you: noisy stomach, feelings of being bloated or sluggish, slight headache. Your digestive system is asking for a rest. Give it one.

The healthy balanced diet set out here should give you all the nourishment you need and, if you are a normally active person, will not put on weight. If you follow this plan you will certainly look and feel better and will be on the way to a healthier pattern of eating. Allowing yourself the inevitable exceptions, such as when you go out to dinner, entertain at home or indulge in celebrations, try to keep to the plan for all normal mealtimes.

SENSIBLE SHOPPING

The ad hoc way in which we shop and eat is, as much as anything else, responsible for unbalanced diets. If we have to dash round the supermarket after work on Friday, or buy food only when we run out, we are less likely to choose wisely and therefore eat less well. Planning ahead may seem like a time-consuming activity, but it will in fact save time in the long run and provide a much healthier and better balanced diet. A few rules of thumb can help to ensure that we get the best value for money as well as the best nourishment for our bodies.

1 Try to set aside thirty minutes each week in which to plan what you will need for either yourself or you and your family. It helps to have a calendar or cook book which tells you, weather and other circumstances being equal, the best seasonal buys, particularly with regard to fruit and vegetables, though meat and fish are also at their freshest at certain times of the year. Food is always best for taste, nourishment and cost when it is in season. Buying seasonal

Breakfast

1 slice wholemeal bread or small portion cereal such as muesli (preferably home-made)
1 tablespoon bran
½ oz (14 g) margarine or butter
1 egg or grilled sardine or rasher of lean grilled bacon
4 fl oz (120 ml) fresh fruit juice (minimum) or an orange or grapefruit
3 fl oz (90 ml) milk with cereal or less in cup of tea or coffee (optional)
From this breakfast you will receive proteins, a small quantity of fats, carbohydrates, sucrose, vitamins and minerals.

Mid-morning

1 raw vegetable, e.g. carrot or stick of celery, or 1 piece fresh fruit
or wholemeal biscuit
or small portion natural yoghurt
1 cup tea or coffee with a little milk (optional)

Lunch

Raw vegetable salad, not more than 6 oz (168 g), e.g. cabbage, celery, peppers, chicory, onions, tomatoes, and possibly a small quantity of cooked potato and/or leeks
1 or 2 eggs or not more than 4 oz (112 g) lean ham, chicken, grilled or steamed fish, liver, oily fish such as sardine, herring or mackerel, or cheese (preferably low-fat)
1 slice wholemeal bread and small scraping butter or margarine (optional)
4 fl oz (120 ml) fresh fruit juice
Again, you will be taking in proteins, fats, carbohydrates, vitamins and minerals.

Afternoon

1 piece fresh fruit or vegetable
1 wholemeal biscuit or 2 oz (56 g) wholemeal cake (optional)
1 cup tea with lemon or a little milk

Dinner

4 oz (112 g) lean meat, beef, lamb, poultry or ham, liver or fish
Once a week at least prepare a vegetarian dish, e.g. lentils, red beans, rice, currants and beans, vegetables and brown rice, pasta, omelette, cheese soufflé
Green leaf vegetables, steamed, boiled for only a few minutes, or quick fried in vegetable oil
1 potato, preferably baked in its jacket, or small portion pulses or other root vegetable or rice
2 oz (56 g) cheese of your choice (maximum) plus small piece fresh fruit or small portion yoghurt
Small slice wholemeal bread, roll or biscuit (optional)
1 glass fresh fruit juice or 2 glasses dry red or white wine (maximum)
Proteins, fats, carbohydrates, vitamins and minerals are all contained in this meal as well.

foods also ensures a good variety and rotation of foods to eat.

2 Buy fresh foods wherever possible, *if they really are fresh*. A wilting lettuce, over-ripe tomato or dull-looking herring will do no more, and probably less, for you than the frozen equivalent.

3 If you have a deep freeze, you can buy foods when they are at their best and freeze them yourself. Always follow instructions on the proper way of freezing different kinds of food, whether cooked or uncooked, to avoid losing nutritional value.

4 Make sure that your larder or cupboards are always stocked with basic ingredients, such as salt, flour, rice, pasta, eggs, milk, cheese, vegetable oil, pulses, dried and fresh fruit, and vegetables.

5 Store food appropriately, in hygienic conditions, and at the right temperature and humidity to ensure maximum life span.

MEALTIMES

Mealtimes for many families today are not what they were. All too often we rush them or, if we are under pressure, miss them altogether. Hectic days when there just doesn't seem to be enough hours to get everything done, convenience foods, and the intrusion of television into our daily lives have all contributed to ways of eating that our great grandparents would have found unthinkable. Obviously, there are times when the family cannot all sit down together to enjoy a meal, but we often do not make the most of the opportunities we do have. For example, many young mothers at home with children fall into the habit of feeding the children separately as though they were kittens or puppies on a special diet, instead of sitting down and sharing a meal with them. You should, after all, be following a similar diet if you are to be healthy. Sitting at a table with your family or a friend and eating a proper meal, even if it is a light one, is beneficial in more ways than one. Not only do we tend to eat more slowly, which means better absorption, involves less risk of indigestion and contributes to a feeling of fullness, but we also have an opportunity to talk, share ideas, discuss the day, or even argue, in a situation which is by definition amicable. Centuries-old traditions such as breaking bread together and sharing salt stemmed not only from necessity but from a desire to share, and we should try to maintain this tradition. If you live alone, make a point of asking a friend round and cooking a meal for both of you, or try to meet friends in a restaurant. Sharing a meal is as important for your personality as for your stomach.

When referring to the list below to plan a well-balanced,
healthy diet, bear in mind that the nutritional value of a food depends
both on its composition and on the amount eaten.

Vitamins

A

liver
kidneys
cod liver oil
asparagus
carrots
beans (French,
  runner, broad)
broccoli
Brussels sprouts
cabbage
parsley
peas
green peppers
spinach
spring greens
tomatoes
turnip tops
watercress
avocado pears
apricots
prunes
bananas
cherries
peaches
sweet potatoes
cheese
cream
eggs
butter
margarine
milk

B1. THIAMIN

liver
beef
lamb
pork
bacon
asparagus
haricot beans
peas
potatoes
brown rice
wheatgerm
bran
wholemeal bread
Brazil nuts
peanuts
brewer's yeast
milk
eggs

B2. RIBOFLAVIN

liver
kidneys
beef
lamb
pork
rabbit
meat and yeast
  extracts
avocado pears
beans
mushrooms
peas
spinach
wheatgerm
wholemeal bread
yoghurt
cottage cheese
milk

B3. NICOTINIC ACID

liver
kidneys
beef
lamb
pork
chicken
turkey
tuna fish
sardines
salmon
halibut
mackerel
dried peas
vegetable and
  yeast extracts
wholemeal bread
wheatgerm
peanuts

B5. PANTOTHENIC ACID

liver
kidneys
mushrooms
bran
brewer's yeast
peanuts

B6. PYRIDOXINE

liver
chicken
mackerel
bananas
bran
wheatgerm
wholemeal bread
Brazil nuts
walnuts
eggs

B12. CYANO-COBALAMIN

liver
kidneys
rabbit
beef
cod
haddock
tuna fish
sardines
herrings
oysters
soya beans
milk
cheese
eggs

BIOTIN

liver
kidneys
cauliflower
leeks
blackcurrants
rolled oats
dried milk
egg yolks

CHOLINE

heart
fish
beans
lentils
wheatgerm

FOLIC ACID

liver
oysters
cod
peas
beetroot
cauliflower
chicory
cucumber
lettuce
potatoes
spinach
sweet corn
avocado pears
oranges
lemon juice
bran
wheat
almonds
hazelnuts
peanuts
walnuts

INOSITOL

sesame seeds
oats
bran
wheatgerm
nuts

PABA

liver
kidneys
broccoli
cabbage
kale
brown rice

C

liver
asparagus
broad beans
broccoli
Brussels sprouts
cabbage
cauliflower
leeks
lettuce
parsnips
potatoes
radishes
spinach
spring greens
plantain
tomatoes
turnips
avocado pears
watercress
onions
parsley
peppers
blackcurrants
lemon juice
melon
pineapple
strawberries
raspberries
oranges
tangerines
grapefruit
bananas

D

sardines

herrings
mackerel
canned salmon
cod liver oil
milk
butter
eggs
sunshine

E

tuna fish
cod's roe
cod liver oil
asparagus
parsley
sweet potatoes
carrots
cabbage
celery
leeks
tomatoes
apples
blackberries
sunflower seeds
sunflower seed oil
olive oil
rolled oats
muesli
wheatgerm
wholemeal bread
eggs

K

broccoli
Brussels sprouts
cabbage
cauliflower
potatoes
strawberries
wheatgerm
oats
eggs

Minerals

CALCIUM

pilchards
sardines
clams
sprats
mussels
shrimps
parsley
spinach
broccoli
haricot beans
watercress
dried figs
sesame seeds
black treacle
bran
almonds
Brazil nuts
yoghurt
milk
hard cheese

CHLORINE

fish
meat
carrots
celery
lettuce
spinach

tomatoes
watercress
salt
milk

CHROMIUM

shellfish
chicken
green vegetables
fruit
wholegrain cereals
bran
honey
nuts
brewer's yeast

COBALT

meat
green vegetables
fruit
wholegrain cereals

COPPER

liver
shellfish
bran
wheatgerm
wholegrain cereals
Brazil nuts

FLUORINE

seafood
fluorinated water

IODINE

seafood
shellfish
spinach
lettuce
watercress
seaweed
sea salt

IRON

liver
kidneys
meat
sardines
sprats
shellfish
mussels
parsley
spinach
peas
watercress
haricot beans
dried apricots
dried figs
sunflower seeds
black treacle
cocoa
curry powder
bran
wheatgerm
Brazil nuts
peanuts
walnuts
eggs
red wine

MAGNESIUM

seafood
meat

avocado pears
haricot beans
muesli
wholewheat cereals
bran
wheatgerm
Brazil nuts
almonds
peanuts

MANGANESE

kidneys
lentils
parsley
watercress
apricots
bran
wheatgerm
almonds
walnuts

PHOSPHORUS

liver
fish
meat
wheatgerm
brewer's yeast
cheese
eggs

POTASSIUM

dried butter beans
dried haricot beans
dried lentils
potatoes
spinach
soya beans
dried apricots
dried figs
bran
wheatgerm
almonds
Brazil nuts

SODIUM

meat
seafood
carrots
celery
lentils
peas
spinach
dried pulses
bran
salt
water

SULPHUR

chicken
fish
haricot beans
soya beans
nuts
cheese
eggs
milk

ZINC

liver
shellfish
sunflower seeds
bran
wholewheat flour
eggs

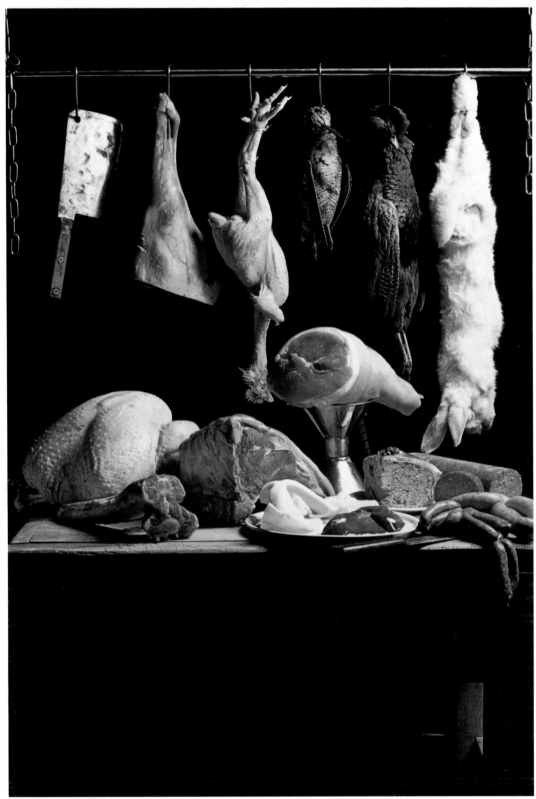

Meat is a vital part of our diet, as it is one of the best sources of protein, but most people eat more than they need and neglect other important protein foods such as fish, eggs, cheese, pulses, grain and nuts. However, meat is also high in the B vitamins and iron. Try to choose meat which is relatively low in fat, as there is now evidence that too much animal (saturated) fat increases the level of cholesterol in the body, giving a predisposition to heart problems. Cook meat in its own fat, then drain, skim off or remove excess fat before eating. Do not add fat when cooking unless absolutely necessary; then use a minimum of vegetable oil. Vary your choice of meat to include poultry and offal at least once a week.

Beef. This is an important source of protein, the B vitamins, iron and phosphorus. Select lean cuts.

Lamb. Although as good a source of protein as beef, lamb is almost as high in fat as pork.

Pork. Although an excellent source of B vitamins and protein, pork is particularly high in fat.

Veal. This is low in fat and a good source of protein.

Rabbit, venison, hare, grouse, pheasant and partridge. All are high in protein and low in fat. Goose and duck are higher in fat.

Turkey and chicken. These are an excellent source of protein, low in fat if you remove pads of fat inside.

They are also high in B vitamins, iron and phosphorus.

Offal. Very high in protein and low in fat, liver and kidneys contain Vitamin A, plenty of B vitamins, iron and other minerals; liver is also a source of Vitamin C, Vitamin D and Vitamin E. Tripe is lower in protein than many other cuts of meat, while oxtail is high in protein but also usually high in fat.

Pâtés, sausages and salami. Generally higher in fat than protein.

41

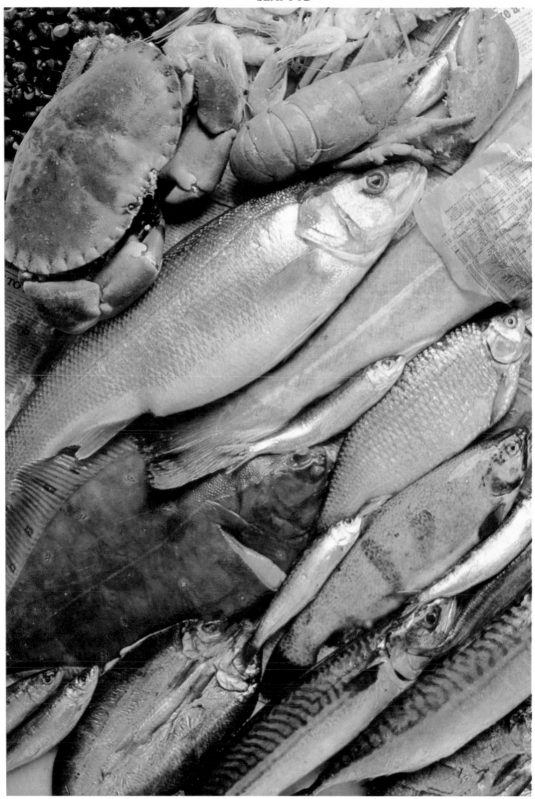

Fish is an excellent and much neglected food which should be included in a meal at least once a week. It is an important source of protein and contains a wide range of the minerals that we need, if only in minute quantities. By varying your choice of fish you can add plenty of calcium and iron to your diet, as well as fluorine, magnesium, potassium, sodium, phosphorus, sulphur and iodine. Fish also supplies Vitamin A, the

B vitamins, Vitamin D, Vitamin E and Vitamin K, and fish roes are a source of Vitamin C. It is best to grill, steam or boil fish. Cooking in lemon or vinegar releases valuable additional calcium from the bones of the fish.
White fish: cod, plaice, sole and whiting. A good source of protein and low in fat, these are not so good for vitamins, iron and calcium.
Oily fish: herring and mackerel. These have a high nutritional

value and provide protein, Vitamin A, the B vitamins, Vitamin D, Vitamin E, Vitamin K and minerals; but they are high in fat content.
Salmon. This is high in protein and a good source of B vitamins. Sardines. High in protein, but also very high in fat, sardines provide vitamins A, D, E and K.
Crustaceans: crabs, prawns, shrimps and lobster. All are excellent sources of protein,

vitamins and minerals and are low in fat.
Shellfish: cockles, winkles, whelks and mussels. All are high in protein, low in fat and valuable sources of minerals, especially iron and calcium.
Oysters. These provide protein and supply plenty of B vitamins.
Roes: cod's roe and herring's roe. Roe is particularly high in cholesterol, but provides protein and Vitamin C.

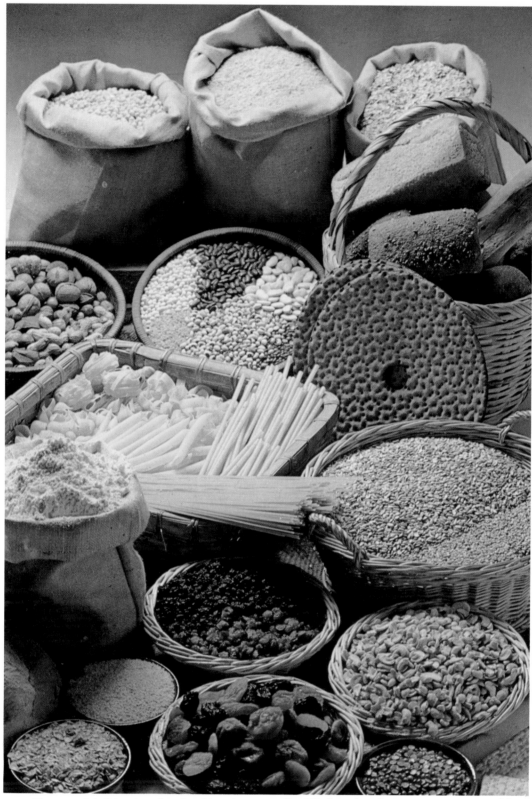

Grain, nuts and pulses provide us with carbohydrates which give us energy, but an excess is stored in the body as fatty tissue. It is important, therefore, to limit your intake to what you need and to select those carbohydrate foods which also provide vitamins, minerals, proteins and vegetable fats, so that they can be a valuable addition to the diet.

Grain. Although some vitamins are usually added to refined products,
it is fair to say that the whiter the bread, flour, rice or pasta the lower the nutritional value. Wholemeal versions of these foods are an acquired taste, but are generally more satisfying to the appetite and provide valuable roughage which helps the digestive system. By eating wholemeal foods, brown rice, muesli or rolled oats instead of sweet, manufactured breakfast cereals, there should be no need for the fashionable addition of bran to
our diet. Wholemeal products, wheatgerm and brewer's yeast provide the whole range of B vitamins in quantity, which because they are water soluble must be replenished every day. They are also valuable sources of vitamins E and K and contain a wide range of minerals, as well as proteins, which in conjunction with other vegetable proteins from nuts and pulses provide the necessary range of amino acids for those who do not
eat meat or dairy products.
Pulses: lentils, dried peas, soya beans, chick peas and haricot beans. A good source of vegetable protein, these also provide iron and other minerals and the B vitamins.
Nuts: Brazil nuts, almonds and peanuts. Valuable as a source of vegetable protein, these also supply B vitamins, iron and other minerals and are high in vegetable fats. All nuts provide protein, but those mentioned are especially nutritious.

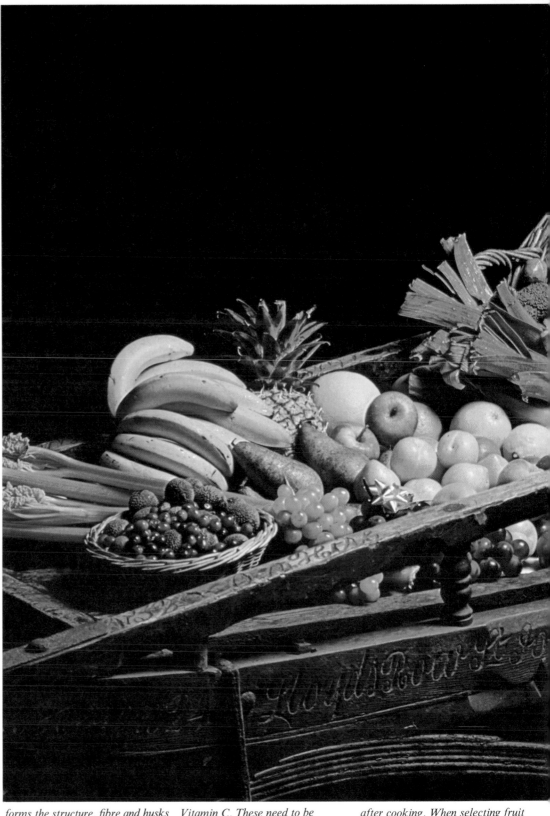

Fruit and vegetables should represent the largest group of foods in our diet, providing all three of the carbohydrates which we use. The sugars in fruit are an immediate source of energy; the starch in root and tuber vegetables is converted by the body into glucose to provide more energy (any excess of either of these, however, will be stored as fat); and cellulose, which

forms the structure, fibre and husks of the plant, provides valuable fibre or roughage which helps the body to excrete waste material, preventing constipation and other disorders of the lower digestive system. Fruit and vegetables also contain many of the essential vitamins and minerals required for health. The most important are the water-soluble B vitamins and

Vitamin C. These need to be replenished on a daily basis, since the body does not store them as it does the fat-soluble vitamins – A, D, E and K – but excretes any excess in urine or perspiration. The water-soluble vitamins can be reduced or lost altogether by over-washing or too much soaking, by boiling for too long or in too much water, or by leaving to keep warm

after cooking. When selecting fruit and vegetables vary your choice as much as possible, taking the seasons into account to ensure that the foods are at their best and freshest and have not been stored or forced. Eat fruit and vegetables raw and in their skins whenever practicable. If cooking, do so for the minimum amount of time and eat immediately. Particularly valuable are the green

44

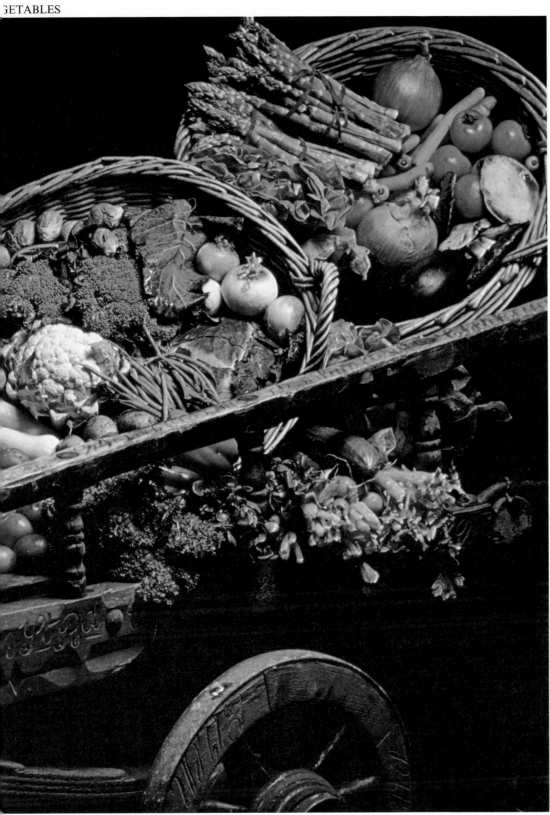

leafy vegetables – broccoli, cabbage, sprouts, kale, lettuce, parsley, tops of vegetables such as turnips, spinach and watercress. Include plenty of these in your diet, varying your choice, and they will provide much of the body's need for Vitamin A, the B vitamins, Vitamin C, Vitamin E and Vitamin K, as well as iron, iodine and other valuable minerals. Radishes,

parsnips, turnips and onions all provide Vitamin C, radishes being a particularly good source. Cauliflower, leeks, avocadoes, peas, mushrooms, potatoes, French beans and runner beans provide many of the B vitamins; peas also contain iron and Vitamin A; cauliflower, leeks and avocadoes have Vitamin C; beans contain Vitamin A; and potatoes supply Vitamin C and

Vitamin K, as well as good quantities of potassium. The colourful vegetables – carrots, tomatoes and red and green peppers – all provide Vitamin A; carrots also contain Vitamin E; and peppers and tomatoes have Vitamin C. Among the fruits, all the currants – with blackcurrants highest on the list – provide Vitamin C, as do the citrus fruits,

such as grapefruit, oranges, lemons and tangerines, the berries, such as raspberries and strawberries, and pineapple. Apples are a moderate source of Vitamin C, while bananas contain Vitamin A, the B vitamins, Vitamin C and several minerals. Peaches and apricots are also well stocked with Vitamin C and minerals. Dried fruits retain their sugar but lose Vitamin C.

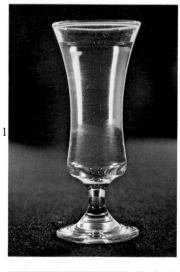

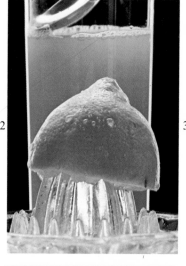

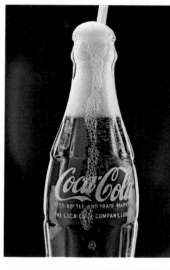

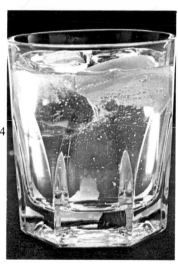

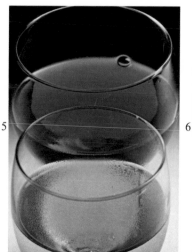

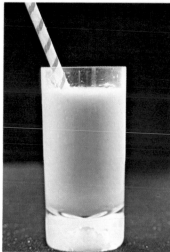

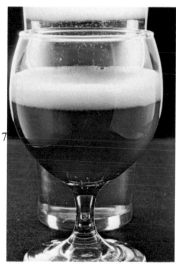

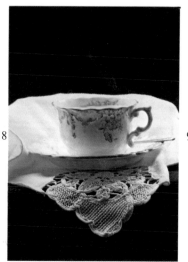

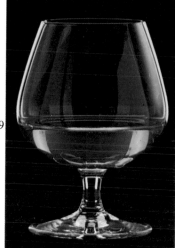

Water is vital to a healthy human body, second only in importance to the air we breathe. We can survive without food for many days, even weeks, but without water we would soon become dehydrated and die. Under normal circumstances, we need to drink about $1\frac{2}{3}$ pt (1 litre) of water a day, but the amount is almost always more, since we also take in water with our food: fruit and vegetables, for example, are 90 per cent water. Provided our kidneys are functioning properly,

no matter how much fluid we drink the level of water in our bodies will stay constant, although some women find that they retain more liquid just before menstruation. The most healthy way of taking in the fluid we need is by drinking plain water. All other drinks contain extra calories, usually in the form of sweet carbohydrate which is surplus to our needs. A few drinks may contain some minerals or vitamins, but these do not contribute to our dietary needs in

any significant way. Alcohol is swiftly absorbed and converted into energy; but taken in excess, food intake is reduced causing vitamin deficiencies.
1   Sherry is high in carbohydrate and of insignificant nutritional value.
2   Fresh lemon or orange juice is high in Vitamin C, can be diluted with water if desired but without sugar if possible.
3   Colas and canned drinks are high in sweet carbohydrate, mostly

coloured and flavoured with chemicals. They are of no nutritional value and are harmful to teeth.
4   Gin and vodka contain only a trace of carbohydrate and no additional nutrients. There are probably more calories in the mixers than the spirits.
5   Wine contains small quantities of B vitamins and minerals; dry red wine provides iron. The sweeter the wine, the higher the carbohydrate content.

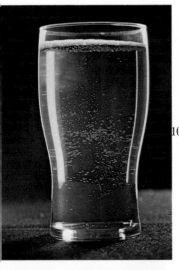 10

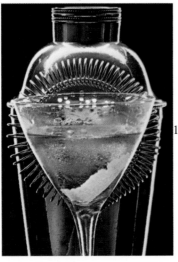 11

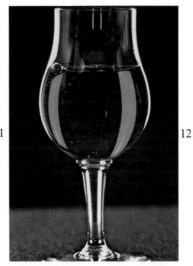 12

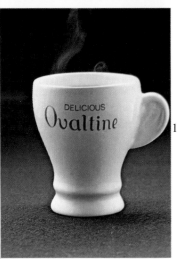 13

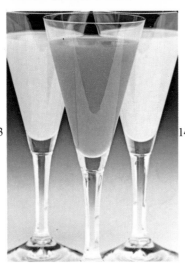 14

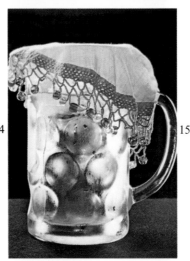 15

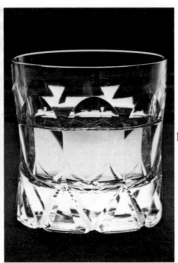 16

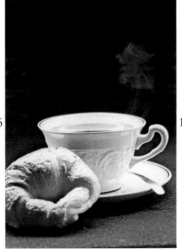 17

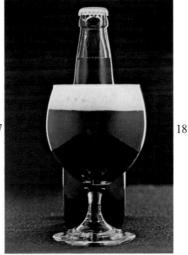 18

6   More of a food than a drink, milk contains animal fats, proteins, carbohydrates, vitamins and minerals. It is a useful source of calcium for children and pregnant women. Skimmed milk contains the same nutrients but less fat.

7   Lagers and barley wine have some B vitamins, but a high carbohydrate value.

8   Tea contains the drug bromine, is a diuretic and stimulant, can induce nervousness and insomnia if drunk in excess and is mildly addictive. Take with lemon if dieting.

9   Brandy is highly alcoholic and a stimulant, with no nutritional value.

10 Beer provides B vitamins, but is high in carbohydrate.

11 Vermouth is of little value for vitamins or minerals. The sweeter it is, the higher the carbohydrate content.

12 Port is high in carbohydrate, but contains some iron.

13 Chocolate milk drinks contain many calories. Can be used to persuade a child to drink milk.

14 Bottled or canned fruit juices contain Vitamin C and often sweeteners and chemical preservatives. Squashes usually contain chemical colourants and flavourings, and sometimes vitamins are added.

15 Tap water, particularly in hard-water areas, contains trace minerals, especially calcium. Fluoride is sometimes added to help prevent tooth decay. Mineral waters are usually no more beneficial than tap water, as the minerals are generally provided in a balanced diet.

16 Whisky is a dry spirit with no additional nutrients.

17 Coffee contains caffeine, a mildly addictive stimulant drug, has the effect of reducing appetite and is a diuretic. If drunk strong and in quantity, coffee can cause insomnia, nervousness and irritability.

18 Stout contains some B vitamins, but is high in carbohydrate.

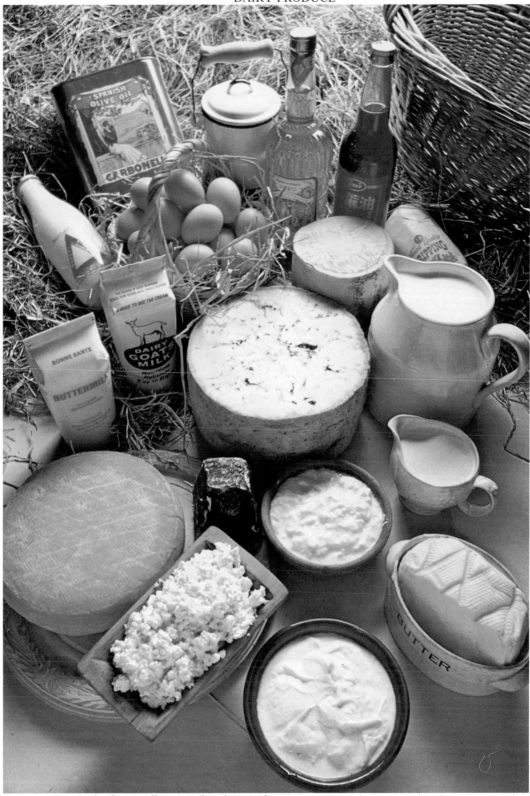

Fats provide the most concentrated source of energy in our diet, reducing the amount of carbohydrate we would otherwise need to consume. They also constitute a good source of the fat-soluble vitamins, A, D, E and K. Like carbohydrates, fats are composed of carbon, oxygen and hydrogen. In fats these form three fatty acids and glycerine. Animal (saturated) fats are usually solid at room temperature, vegetable (polyunsaturated) fats usually remain liquid. Animal fats contain cholesterol in varying quantities, vegetable fats do not. Because of the cholesterol in animal fats, and the link between increased cholesterol levels and heart problems, it is wise to limit the amount of animal fats we consume in dairy products and where possible to avoid using butter or dripping for cooking, replacing them with the polyunsaturated vegetable oils.

We can also reduce our intake of animal fats by choosing less creamy milk or by substituting cottage cheese for cream cheese. However, dairy products contain high levels of calcium, vital for growth, several other minerals, Vitamin A, the B group of vitamins and Vitamin D. Milk, yoghurt and cheese, particularly hard cheeses such as cheddar and parmesan, are high in protein and wholemeal pasta with parmesan cheese or cauliflower cheese with a sauce made from grated cheddar and reconstituted dried milk would make a nutritious meal. Eggs, together with human milk, are top-value proteins. Although eggs have suffered greatly in the cholesterol controversy, they are an excellent food taken in moderation, providing proteins, vitamins and minerals in good quantities. A boiled egg and wholemeal toast make an excellent start to the day.

WEIGHTS AND MEASURES

Your body shape and weight are to a large extent dictated by genetic inheritance. If, for example, your parents are both tall and slim, there is a good chance that you will be also. If, on the other hand, neither parent is above 5 ft 6 in (1.68 m), it is unlikely that you will grow to Amazonian proportions. Nevertheless, our genetic inheritance is complicated and it is not simply our parents, but their forebears also, who are responsible for our shape and size. It is not uncommon to hear someone referred to as a 'throw-back', meaning that they are unlike their parents or siblings but resemble an aunt or grandparent. Also, in the West, we are growing slightly taller and heavier with each decade: nutritionists believe this is largely due to the fact that we are eating more of the essential body-building foods than ever before. Our body shape will depend too, on whether we are naturally endomorphs, ectomorphs, mesomorphs, or a combination of these body types. Endomorphs are basically rounded, heavily built with quite a lot of fat; ectomorphs are thin and angular, with less muscle; and mesomorphs are muscular and rather athletic. Your general attitude to food and eating and your BMR (basal metabolic rate), the rate at which you burn the calories which you consume (see page 38), will also have an important influence on your size.

YOUR NATURAL WEIGHT

Living in an almost obsessively weight-conscious society, with photographs of slender model girls smiling out of every magazine and down from every hoarding, it is easy to lose sight of your natural weight and to imagine you are over-weight simply because you do not look like them.

If you look at the chart on page 50, you will see the range of weights according to height and bone structure that insurance companies, for whom lists were originally prepared, accept as 'normal', that is to say healthy. These figures, however, are only guidelines. You may see that a weight of 140 lb (63.5 kg) is considered acceptable for a woman of medium frame who is 5 ft 6 in (1.68 m) tall and yet if *you* are that weight and height you may know that you are slightly *over-weight*, that for you 133 lb (60.33 kg) is better. There is no rule of thumb by which to gauge your individual natural weight, except perhaps to say that it is one at which you are the most comfortable, at which you feel

healthy and look good, and which keeps more or less constant on a normal healthy diet. A slightly rounded tummy and chubby legs do not necessarily mean that you are not at your natural weight, but rolls of fat bulging over your waistline *do*.

Women put on weight for many reasons, and although occasionally the reason may be beyond our control – for example, a glandular malfunction, a side-effect of taking certain drugs, such as steroids, or the Pill – we usually become heavier quite simply because we are eating more food than we need. Gaining weight can be a slow process, at first almost imperceptible. A woman of thirty who weighs 126 lb (57.15 kg), who is happy, fairly active and eats reasonably, may not give her weight a thought. Five years later, when she cannot understand why she can no longer wear the same size dress, she gets on the scales and sees that she now weighs 135 lb (61.24 kg) and wonders how it happened. It could be quite simply that her food intake in calorific terms has remained constant but the amount of exercise she takes has diminished; or that she is on the Pill where she previously wasn't; or that she has given up smoking and to rid herself of one habit has adopted another, eating sweets or even apples as a substitute. Another factor to be taken into account is that as we get older we need less food and a small surplus each day over several years can result in a slight though continuing weight-gain. There are also certain times in a woman's life when her weight is likely to fluctuate and when, if she is not careful, a temporary weight-gain may become a permanent one.

Baby

Although the effects of over-feeding can be corrected later, a fat baby is likely to become a fat adult, so *don't* over-feed. In tests carried out with infants old enough to feed themselves, in which one group was fed a regular, well-balanced diet and the other was allowed to choose from a wide range of foods, ranging from beetroot to milk, the results showed that the babies who fed themselves were just as healthy as those whose diet was prescribed. Amongst other things, this has been interpreted to mean that even at an early age, given a choice of foods, we know not only what we want but also what is good for us; that we can 'listen' to our bodies even before we can talk. As the baby becomes a toddler, resist emphatically the temptation to offer her ice-cream or chocolate bars as a cure for grazed knees or as treats, rewards or just to keep quiet. Our attitudes to food are learned from babyhood and eating

for solace can develop into a compulsive eating habit later.

Young girl

Try as we might, it is difficult to stop our daughters eating at least a certain amount of sweets, cakes and ice-creams. Even if they do not have them at home, grand-parents or parents of other children inevitably offer them. The danger in over-consumption of sweet things is not only the damage which we inflict on our teeth, and in later life perhaps the risk of heart diseases or diabetes, but also the harm we do to the taste buds and appetite which come to demand and depend on larger intakes of sugar. Try to counter advertisements for sweets, colas and chocolate bars with your own campaign: without nagging, tell your daughter that all these increase her chances of bad teeth, and lots of fillings; show her pictures of really fat girls and then of slim ones, and ask which she would prefer to be. To use a cliché, a lesson well-learned when she is young will be better remembered when she grows up. Quietly keep an eye on her weight and, without making a fuss, adjust your family diet if you think she is getting too fat. Make sure that the healthy food you offer her at home is at least as exciting as the ice-cream and chocolate cake that she is offered elsewhere. A carefully-planned packed lunch of whole-meal bread, salad, cheese or a cooked chicken leg, fruit and yoghurt is often better than stodgy school meals if she is allowed the alternative.

Teenage girl

At the onset of and during puberty, a girl's body undergoes many changes. As she grows from child to woman her body will reflect the process: lean hips will become broader, breasts will develop, and she will put on weight in other places, too – arms, legs, tummy and face. Some lucky girls make the transition easily, no spots or puppy fat, while others experience both. This is a time when a mother should be at her most understanding. If your daughter suffers from puppy fat and is worried about it, help her by planning a diet which will assist in keeping her weight under control – and if necessary follow it with her. If she refuses to eat a meal with you because she thinks it is fattening, don't laugh at her or insist. Set aside a tray with fresh orange juice, a salad and some wholemeal bread and stick a piece of paper on the tray showing the calories contained in her meal and those in yours (with any luck, there shouldn't be *too* great a discrepancy!). Give her books to read which explain why she is plump at this stage, so that she can both accept and cope with the fact. If she shows signs of

anorexia nervosa* you *must* seek professional help from your doctor immediately. On the other hand, if she is feeling a bit miserable and self-conscious with spots or puppy fat, or because of the changes that she is experiencing, she may well take to sitting around and eating chocolates, cream cakes or crisps for solace. If this is the case, do your utmost to make her feel prettier: a new hairstyle, something nice to wear, or help with her skin may be the answer. Make sure also that she is busy doing something interesting, and see that the 'nibbles' available in the house are of the healthy variety and not those which will exacerbate weight and skin problems.

Single working girl or student

Not all single girls move away from home once they start a job or embark upon a further education course, but many do. The single girl who continues to live with her family will probably eat proper meals because her mother will continue to prepare them for her along with the rest of the family, so even if breakfast is skipped and lunch inadequate there will be a 'square meal' for her in the evening. If her family eats healthy foods, she is unlikely to put on weight at this time, but danger lies in the situation where her mother insists on her having a cooked breakfast, she eats a stodgy canteen lunch, and then has to face three courses with the family at night. Many mothers are over-zealous in insisting on plying the working members of a family with substantial meals, 'to keep their strength up'.

The girl living away from home, either alone or sharing a flat with friends, has different problems. She has to rely largely on herself for shopping, preparing and cooking her own meals. Having flat-mates is probably an advantage, in that there will often be someone else around with whom to share the work and the meals. If she is quite alone she is less likely to eat well, since few people really enjoy cooking or preparing a meal which only they will consume, and the temptation is to rely on convenience foods or take-away meals which are often high in calories and low in nutritional value. A busy social life will more or less guarantee that she eats sometimes, but if she spends much of her spare time alone, it is all too easy either not to bother to eat or, if she is lonely, to eat far too much of the wrong things for comfort.

The single working girl may neither lose nor gain weight, but if any one of the circumstances above applies, and her weight has changed for the worse, she should look for ways to resolve the problem: tell her mother kindly but firmly that though she loves her cooking she is getting fat because she is eating too much of it; collaborate with flat-mates in planning nutritious, healthy menus for the week; if alone, perhaps put in a cooking session once a week to prepare her own supply of ready-to-eat nutritious meals.

Young married woman

Living with and cooking for another person can be exciting, exasperating and time-consuming, particularly if you have married a man who loves nothing better than mother's steak-and-kidney pudding or apple turnovers. If you are really strong-minded, and are prepared for marital battle, you can try to re-educate him in his eating habits, but it takes a tough newly-wed to do this. It is more likely that you will try to give him the food he likes, and if it happens to be of the rich, high-protein, fat and carbohydrate variety, you certainly risk putting on weight. The danger of this happening will be even greater if you have given up work and are more sedentary than you used to be. If you then have a child, and have the extra task of feeding him or her as well, you may feel that a large part of your day is taken up with preparing food. In this situation it is easy to eat too much. You may not think that finishing the baby's rusks or stewed prunes will matter, or that in eating similar quantities of the beef stew and blackberry pie as your husband you are doing anything more than enjoying the fruits of your well-earned labours, but those extra calories will gradually contribute to a spreading waistline.

Pregnant woman

There was a time, not so long ago, when the whims of pregnancy – wanting strawberries and cream or chocolate gateau in the middle of the night – and an increased appetite were put down to the fact that you were 'eating for two'. The theory seemed logical enough – after all, there *were* two of you to feed. But now it is accepted that over-eating in pregnancy is not a good idea. Provided that the expectant mother eats well and wisely, a diet high in protein and vitamins and low in carbohydrate is considered desirable, both she and the baby will be healthy. Gaining too much weight in pregnancy can put the health of both mother and baby at risk. Ideally, the extra weight that a pregnant woman is carrying at term, when the baby is fully matured and ready to be born, should amount to the actual weight of the unborn child, the weight of the placenta from which it feeds, the weight of the amniotic fluid* in the uterus,* plus the weight of the increased volume of breasts and blood (see page 115). A few extra pounds may not prove serious, but a gain of more than

IDEAL WEIGHT CHART
for women over the age of twenty-five

HEIGHT in bare feet		SMALL FRAME		MEDIUM FRAME		LARGE FRAME	
ft in	m	lb	kg	lb	kg	lb	kg
4' 8"	1.42	92–98	41.73–44.45	96–107	43.55–48.53	104–119	47.17–53.98
4' 9"	1.45	94–101	42.64–45.81	98–110	44.45–49.90	106–122	48.08–55.34
4' 10"	1.47	96–104	43.55–47.17	101–113	45.81–51.26	109–125	49.44–56.70
4' 11"	1.50	99–107	44.91–48.53	104–116	47.17–52.62	112–128	50.80–58.06
5' 0"	1.52	102–110	46.27–49.90	107–119	48.53–53.98	115–131	52.16–59.42
5' 1"	1.55	105–113	47.63–51.26	110–122	49.90–55.34	118–134	53.52–60.78
5' 2"	1.58	108–116	48.99–52.62	113–126	51.26–57.15	121–138	54.89–62.60
5' 3"	1.60	111–119	50.35–53.98	116–130	52.62–58.97	125–142	56.70–64.41
5' 4"	1.63	114–123	51.71–55.79	120–135	54.43–61.24	129–146	58.51–66.22
5' 5"	1.65	118–127	53.52–57.61	124–139	56.25–63.05	133–150	60.33–68.04
5' 6"	1.68	122–131	55.34–59.42	128–143	58.06–64.86	137–154	62.14–69.85
5' 7"	1.70	126–135	57.15–61.24	132–147	59.87–66.68	141–158	63.96–71.67
5' 8"	1.73	130–140	58.97–63.50	136–151	61.69–68.49	145–163	65.77–73.94
5' 9"	1.75	134–144	60.78–65.32	140–155	63.50–70.31	149–168	67.59–76.20
5' 10"	1.78	138–148	62.60–67.13	144–159	65.32–72.12	153–173	69.40–78.47

Average weight ranges are based on statistical data commonly used by insurance companies. It is difficult to gauge an ideal weight because different factors are involved, such as energy consumption or metabolic rate, quality and quantity of diet, age and mobility. However, the ranges given are based on the size of your bones, limbs, hands and feet (e.g. small, medium or large frame), and they correlate to weight, height, body size and health standards. If you are uncertain about the size of your body frame, measure your wrists: 5½ in (13.75 cm) signifies a small frame, 6 in (15 cm) a medium frame, and 6½ in (16.25 cm) a large frame. If you are within your range there is a minimum health risk. If you are obviously over-weight or under-weight, you do face a health risk and should seek advice. In middle and old age there should be little or no change. Women between the ages of eighteen and twenty-five should deduct 1 lb (0.45 kg) for each year under twenty-five. Weights are inclusive of indoor clothing and shoes; deduct 6 lb (2.72 kg) if you weigh naked.

28 lb (12.6 kg) implies that the pregnant woman has put on more than she should have. It is also a fact that, if you do gain weight during pregnancy, it will be harder and take longer than usual to lose.

Middle-aged woman

We need less food as we grow older. The lifestyle of a young mother with several children and a husband becomes less strenuous as her children grow up and become largely self-sufficient, though for a working woman coping with the demands of a home and a job life may not change very much. Middle age is a difficult term to define: it means literally half way through your life span, but it is also associated with patterns of behaviour, the menopause and other factors. Biologically speaking, during and after the menopause the female reproductive system undergoes changes as drastic as those experienced at puberty, except in reverse. If she has come to terms with her own personality, and environment, a woman will find the inevitable changes in her body and in her way of life easier to cope with. There is no reason to suppose that because you are forty or fifty years old you have to adopt the attitudes of a 'middle-aged' woman. But do remember that, in nutritional terms at least, your calorific requirements will be less; there will be a tendency to over-weight if you do not bear this fact in mind when planning meals.

DIETING

Some women are habitual dieters. They may diet several times a year, often before a holiday, lose some weight for the occasion, and then promptly put it back on until the next time. Others are always on a diet but never seem to lose any weight, although they talk all the time of tomorrow when they will. To lose weight, you have to have the will to succeed and many women, whilst bemoaning their extra pounds, do not have this will. Some finally prefer the pleasures of food to the pleasure of being slim, others con themselves into thinking that the scales are wrong or the dress has shrunk, and for a number of women there are emotional or psychological reasons far stronger than their apparent desire to slim which prevent any real progress being made in dieting. Among this group are those who use dieting and the constant challenge it presents as a substitute for other challenges, such as finding a job, letting their children 'go', or facing up to a difficult marriage, because they are unable to battle with the real problems they face. Others pretend – even to themselves – that they are on a diet, stoically refusing to eat anything but a lettuce leaf and stick of celery in public, but privately gnawing their way through cakes and other goodies. Very often such women are basically distressed and unhappy and are punishing themselves for some private failure, real or imaginary, or punishing others for letting them down. Like many addicts, they are genuinely incapable of owning up to or recognizing their addiction and the reasons for it: 'Feel sorry for me, I don't eat and I'm still fat,' or 'I know you can't love me because I'm fat (but try).'

The fear of failure, particularly if the fear is reinforced by experience, is also a great deterrent to successful dieting. If you've tried several times to lose weight without success, it is all too easy to say: 'It didn't work last time, so it won't now.' And actual failure, when the scales refuse to register the expected weight-loss, can turn a determined dieter into an angry over-eater.

Diets fail for social as well as personal reasons. For instance, it is customary to woo, though perhaps seduce would be the better verb, friends and family with food and drink. At home a mother may play on a family's guilt by insisting that they eat what she has offered, not to do so means they don't love her, and she also has to eat to make sense of the blackmail. Husbands who arrive home late from work or the pub are presented with vast plates of food and daughters who have left home are told they need feeding up because they no longer receive mother's four square meals a day. In this case, a mother who has become over-weight herself but whose daughter is still slim may subconsciously envy the girl and try to make parity by 'helping' her to put on weight.

Social occasions also contribute to the difficulties of dieting. Going out to see friends or inviting them into one's home is usually the signal to offer or be offered hospitality – anything from tea and cake, alcoholic drinks and appetizers, to a full-scale meal. When you are out at a dinner party, it is awkward to refuse whatever the host or hostess has prepared for fear of appearing rude or unappreciative. Equally, if *you* are the hostess you will try to please, impress, and encourage your guests to eat as much as possible; not to do so might be interpreted as meanness. Even at work colleagues with a sweet tooth can invite your collaboration in laying down extra pounds by offering to share their biscuits, sweets or nuts and, if they are touchy, implying that you are stand-offish if you refuse. It takes determination and politeness to resist all the temptations that social intercourse constantly puts in your way when you are trying to lose weight, without becoming a social outcast or a diet bore, and many would-be dieters founder in the attempt.

One of the saddest aspects of breaking a diet, apart from the nasty taste of failure, is that people tend to fall back into their old eating habits. One reason for this is that they were setting themselves an impossible target in the first place. They were aiming at too great a weight-loss in too short a time, hoping for miracles by using dietary gimmicks such as special 'diet' foods, often cellulose-based products which give the impression of fullness but have little or no nutritional value and do nothing to re-educate the stomach to expect smaller quantities of food, or following a crash diet based perhaps on bananas and milk, boiled eggs, grapefruit, avocado, or whatever. The boredom factor alone has to be taken into account when considering how often diets such as these fail.

HOW TO SUCCEED ON A DIET

Knowing that you are over-weight is not difficult; deciding that you want to get rid of the extra pounds requires little effort; actually *losing* weight demands common sense, will power and very often a great deal of determination. A few women will be able to get on the scales, see that they are too heavy, eat less and become thinner in a matter of weeks. But for the majority of would-be-slimmers the process is more complicated.

The first thing to work out is *why* you have put on weight, and if you over-eat, *why* you do. Knowing the reason, or reasons, is at least a third of the way to finding a solution. Ask yourself whether you fit into any of the categories described on pages 49–50. Are you pregnant and eating for two? Do you finish the family's left-overs? Do you eat as much as your husband? Have you been eating sandwiches, sausage rolls and chocolate bars for lunch on a regular basis? Do you eat when you are unhappy or bored?

Once you have pinpointed the cause, or causes, of your over-indulgence you should be able to work out a plan to help get you back into better eating habits. But the plan will only work if it is logical, appropriate to your needs and, above all else, if you want it

to work. There is no sense in deciding to fast for a week (see below) because, apart from the fact that it would be dangerous unless you were under medical supervision, you would have to be almost superhuman to stick to your decision. A will of iron and a week abstaining from food would certainly result in a large weight-loss, but once you resumed your normal eating habits the weight would go straight back on. It is generally true to say that the quicker the weight-loss the faster the subsequent gain, which is largely why most crash diets do not bring permanent results. However, crash diets can be useful if followed for a couple of days for a particular reason, such as a special party, in preparation for Christmas so that you can tuck in without feeling guilty, or afterwards to shed the surplus gathered quickly before it settles and becomes much more difficult to get rid of.

If you are very over-weight and start to diet you will tend to lose the first few pounds relatively quickly, but thereafter the loss will be smaller. This can be discouraging and is often the point at which dieters give up. But you must remember that it has probably taken you a long time to put all that extra flesh on and you cannot get rid of it all overnight. Tell yourself that although results are not spectacular, a weight-loss of say 2½ lb (1.11 kg) a week is far better in the long run than a quick, larger loss. A month may seem an eternity when you are trying to lose weight, so set yourself a series of targets, perhaps to lose 7 lb (3.17 kg) by the end of one month and then a further 5 lb (2.25 kg) by the end of the next. You will probably be pleasantly surprised to find that you have lost more; it is always better to aim for less than you secretly wish for. Use other tricks to help you to stick to the diet. Weigh yourself once a week, in the morning, and mark up your weight-loss on a chart; buy yourself something, or get a shop to reserve it for you, that you really like but which is a size too small; get a friend to take a picture of you at the start of the diet, then at monthly intervals until the photograph reflects the way you want to look. Buy a sack of potatoes weighing the amount you wish to lose and, when you weaken, pick it up to remind yourself of the extra weight you are dragging around with you every day. Remember also that many women tend to gain some weight before a period, so don't get discouraged if you do not appear to be losing weight at this time. Above all, keep telling yourself that a slimmer you will be a healthier, better-looking version of the present you.

Your attitude to food and eating at this time is crucial. It takes time to re-educate yourself into sensible eating habits, to acclimatize to less sugary, starchy foods and to smaller intakes, but remember that just as you were once used to large helpings of fattening foods and thought you could not do without them, the day *will* dawn when you wonder how you could ever have eaten like that. It is amazing how a stomach and appetite programmed to enjoy lots of rich food can literally be re-programmed to expect and want fresh fruit, vegetables, wholemeal bread and other 'healthy' foods instead – as thousands of success-ful dieters would testify. Few people who give up sugar in tea or coffee during a diet ever go back to it; the taste becomes almost repellent. The whole point of a diet is to get rid of surplus fat and bring you back to your natural weight, which is one that you can maintain thereafter with a normal, well-balanced, healthy eating programme.

Finally, it is worth remembering that one, two, or even three failures do not mean that you will never succeed. Motivation and a determination to be healthier and better looking are the key, but if you still find it very hard to diet it may be worth consulting your doctor, or joining a group such as Weight Watchers. The cost of enrolling alone can act as a spur to succeed, but more important you can draw on the support and the shared successes (or failures) of others who have found it just as difficult to lose weight as you. Over-eating is often an addiction, just as smoking, gambling and drinking can be, and there is no shame in admitting that you are an addict, particularly when you do so in the company of others.

WAYS OF DIETING

The sort of diet that you opt for in your quest to become slimmer and fitter will depend on your tastes and should take your life-style into account. You should try to find a diet that is viable, that is not beyond the limits of your budget, will power or circum-stances, and that is not boring.

Fasting

Fasting, or eating nothing at all, is by definition the most basic 'diet' of all. It has been practised for centuries in the East as a way of purifying not only the body but also the spirit. Fasting for longer than a day should not be under-taken without first consulting a doctor. Although most people would not suffer from abstaining for several days, provided they drank plenty of water, someone suffering from an undiagnosed complaint might.

Ideally, if you are going to fast you should do so in calm, relaxed surroundings. Trying to carry out your normal routine, whether as a housewife or working girl, without the aid of food and drink would defeat the object of the fast and probably make you weak and dizzy, feelings which often accompany fasting anyway. On a strict fast you are only allowed unlimited quantities of water – in fact you must drink lots, at least 1⅔ pt (1 litre) a day. Inevitably you will lose weight on a fast, but this is not the main object of the exercise. Those who believe in fasting maintain that it also enables the body to rid itself of accumulations of toxins; skin, eyes and hair all benefit, as well as the digestive system. Many people find that their mind actually benefits as well; after a fast they are able to think more clearly, are less agitated, and find life easier to handle.

Those who take fasting seriously believe that a minimum fast lasts three days. On the third day, they claim, most of the toxins are released from the body through urine, faecal matter, sweat and breath. Accompanying odours, though not pleasant for a bystander, are actually interpreted as good signs, demonstrating that toxins are being shed.

Some people find it easier to fast in the company of a friend. You should make sure, as far as you can, that you will not be interrupted, that you can rest, sleep, walk, listen to music, have a bath, or whatever takes your fancy, in peace. If you do feel giddy or nauseated, lie down and rest, or sleep. The first twelve hours will be the most difficult: hunger pangs and the desire for sweet drinks may tempt you to break the fast, but resist them if you can; after twelve hours you will find it becomes progressively easier. When you break your fast do so gently, perhaps eating just fruit or salad and wholemeal bread at first and building up gradually. If you go from nothing to a three-course meal your digestive system will quite justifiably protest vigorously.

Health farms

If you have the time and money you can invest in a visit to a health farm. Here you will be weighed, measured, medically examined and then prescribed a diet, a series of exercises and other treatments, such as underwater massage or steam baths, appropriate to your needs. Health farms are not cheap, but some dieters find them well worth the expense because surroundings tend to be pleasant, dieting and exercise are supervised, and you find yourself in the company of others who are also seeking their slimmer, healthier selves.

CRASH DIET
Loss: Approximately 8-10 lb (3.62-4.53 kg) in ten days

For a quick weight-loss to boost morale, try this crash diet. You must not stay on it for longer than ten days. If you want to lose more weight, go on to one of the long-term diets.

Daily allowance
1 cup skim milk
1 tablespoon wheatgerm
no sugar at all

DAY ONE
breakfast
½ grapefruit, 2 slices ham
coffee or tea with milk from allowance
lunch
poached egg on spinach
dinner
grilled steak, 2 tomatoes, 2 oz (56 g) cheese, stick of celery or green salad
black coffee

DAY TWO
breakfast
½ grapefruit, 1 boiled egg
coffee or tea with milk from allowance
lunch
2 rashers lean bacon, 2 grilled tomatoes
dinner
grilled fish (not oily),
2 oz (56 g) cheese, 1 apple
black coffee

DAY THREE
breakfast
1 apple, 2 rashers lean bacon
coffee or tea with milk from allowance
lunch
2 hard boiled eggs, 2 tomatoes
dinner
grilled steak with watercress
black coffee

DAY FOUR
breakfast
½ grapefruit, 1 boiled egg
coffee or tea with milk from allowance
lunch
2 slices ham, 2 tomatoes or celery
dinner
veal chop, spinach, 1 peach
black coffee

DAY FIVE
breakfast
½ grapefruit, 2 slices ham
coffee or tea with milk from allowance
lunch
consommé, small carton fat-free yoghurt or cottage cheese
dinner
grilled chicken, 2 grilled tomatoes, green salad
black coffee

DAY SIX
breakfast
½ grapefruit, 1 boiled egg
coffee or tea with milk from allowance
lunch
2 slices roast beef, hot or cold, with horseradish, 2 tomatoes or celery
dinner
grilled fish (not oily), spinach, 1 orange
black coffee

DAY SEVEN
breakfast
½ grapefruit, 2 slices ham
coffee or tea with milk from allowance
lunch
small carton fat-free yoghurt or cottage cheese, 1 apple
dinner
lean lamb chop, green beans, 1 grilled tomato
black coffee

DAY EIGHT
breakfast
½ grapefruit, 1 boiled egg
coffee or tea with milk from allowance
lunch
cold chicken and watercress
dinner
grilled liver and bacon, green beans, 2 tomatoes, 2 oz (56 g) cheese, 1 apple
black coffee

DAY NINE
breakfast
½ grapefruit, 2 rashers lean bacon
coffee or tea with milk from allowance
lunch
2 oz (56 g) cheese, green salad
dinner
grilled steak, 2 grilled tomatoes, 2 oz (56 g) cheese, stick of celery
black coffee

DAY TEN
breakfast
½ grapefruit, 1 boiled egg
coffee or tea with milk from allowance
lunch
1 small carton fat-free yoghurt or cottage cheese, 2 tomatoes
dinner
1 veal chop, green salad, 2 oz (56 g) cheese, 1 apple
black coffee

CALORIE-COUNTING DIET
Loss: Approximately 12-14 lb (5.44-6.35 kg) in one month

This is a basic diet of only 1,000 Calories a day, with the emphasis on fresh fruit and vegetables. It is a perfectly healthy diet to stay on for several weeks, so it is good for a steady weight-loss.

With your evening meal, in place of the steak, you could have a medium portion of grilled or baked white fish, lean roast beef or a veal chop. Once a week have braised or grilled liver. You can drink as much tea or coffee as you like, as long as the milk allowance is not exceeded. No sugar is allowed; if you must sweeten, use a sugar substitute. The fruit portions below are all estimated at fifty Calories. If you cook any of the fruit, sweeten only with a sugar substitute.

1 medium apple · 4 fresh apricots
1 small banana
4 oz (112 g) cherries
16 grapes · 2 grapefruit
1 large orange · 1 large peach
¼ pt (150 ml) fresh orange juice or unsweetened frozen juice
4 oz (112 g) fresh pineapple
1 large pear · 3 plums
7 oz (196 g) raspberries or strawberries
3 small tangerines
Do not put a dressing on your salad, but squeeze fresh lemon juice over it if you wish. Any fat for cooking should come from your daily allowance.

Daily allowance
½ pt (300 ml) skim milk
3 slices wholemeal bread
½ oz (14 g) low calorie margarine
raw vegetables (as many as you like) for nibbling

Calorie counting
You put on weight if you eat more calories than you need to maintain your body according to its various requirements. All foods contain calories, but some contain more than others. Since the calorific values of all foods are now known, it is logical to work out how many calories you need to keep your weight constant and to cut your intake down if you are trying to lose weight. The speed at which your body uses up calories depends on your metabolism, and everybody's metabolic rate is different. 'Slow metabolism' is a common excuse for being fat, but it is rare to find anyone who cannot lose weight by reducing their daily intake to 1,000 Calories, and most people, even slow metabolizers, can lose on 1,500 a day. If we do not balance our

intake of calories against our energy expenditure, the surplus calories we take in are turned into body fat and stored for future use. So to have become fat we must have taken in too many calories and to lose weight we must force the body to draw on its fat reserves. This it will do, suffering no ill-effects so long as it is still getting enough vitamins and minerals. It would be easy to keep to 1,000 Calories a day if you ate only salad stuffs, which are extremely low in calories, but to stay healthy you must include a good portion of protein foods such as meat, fish, eggs or cheese. The easiest way to keep a check is to carry a small book of calorie counts with you always. Pocket-size calorie counters are readily available from shops or your doctor and although it is virtually

impossible to be absolutely accurate about the number of calories you are consuming, for example you can't very well ask for your chop or vegetables to be weighed if you are eating out in a restaurant, if you are honest you can keep a fairly accurate check. The advantages of dieting by counting calories include the fact that you can vary your diet; if you are desperate for a piece of cake or a sweet drink you can see at a glance how many calories these contain and how many you have left for your daily requirement. You can also, whether you like it or not, know when you are cheating, by doing a little simple arithmetic. The disadvantages are that counting calories is a fiddly, time-consuming business; the method also does little to re-educate you into a generally

better way of eating, if you keep substituting heavy or sweet foods for nutritionally better protein or vitamin-dense foods. It is up to you to decide whether calorie counting is something that you can do easily and constantly whilst you are dieting. If it works, that is to say if you lose weight, stick with it. Otherwise look for an alternative method.
Low carbohydrate diet
Carbohydrates have long been regarded as the enemies of slimmers. Potatoes, bread, cakes, confectionery, pastry and especially sugar are all high in calories and by drastically cutting down your intake of carbohydrates you will certainly lose weight. Carbohydrate foods are not necessarily more fattening than other foods, but if you cut out bread, puddings, cakes and so on,

breakfast
fresh lemon juice with water,
½ grapefruit,
1 boiled or poached egg,
1 slice plain or
toasted wholemeal bread with
margarine from allowance
lunch
fresh lemon juice with water,
4 oz (112 g) cottage cheese with large
portion salad, 1 slice wholemeal
bread with margarine
from allowance
tea
50 Calorie fruit portion
dinner
fresh lemon juice with water,
½ grapefruit, medium-size lean
grilled steak, 1 slice wholemeal
bread, large portion green vegetables,
50 Calorie fruit portion

CARBOHYDRATE-COUNTING DIET

Loss: Approximately 12-14 lb (5.44-6.35 kg) in two months

If you find counting calories complicated, try working on carbohydrate units instead. By cutting down drastically on bread, cakes and biscuits your carbohydrate intake is automatically reduced, although you should eat some wholemeal bread every day. Eat reasonable amounts of protein foods, meat, poultry, cheese, eggs and fish, as they have no carbohydrate unit value; cook where possible without using any oil and avoid frying. Eat a minimum of butter or margarine and, if you must sweeten, use a sugar substitute. Try to drink ½ pt (300 ml) milk daily, in tea or coffee if you wish. Start off by working out a menu of fifteen carbohydrate units a day. If you wish to speed up your weight-loss you can reduce the number to twelve, but do not follow this indefinitely; fifteen units is a better long-term level. Two one-day menus at fifteen units are suggested here. Work out some alternatives using the unit list below.

MENU ONE
½ pt (300 ml) milk (3)
breakfast
grilled bacon and tomatoes (0),
1 slice of toast and butter (3)
lunch
omelette (0), large green salad (0)
1 slice wholemeal bread and butter (3),
1 fresh pear (2)
dinner
grilled gammon rasher (0). 2 oz
(56 g) boiled potatoes (2), Brussels
sprouts (0), portion fresh pineapple (2)

Total: 15 carbohydrate units

MENU TWO
½ pt (300 ml) milk (3)
breakfast
1 small glass tomato juice (1), grilled
bacon and egg (0), 1 slice wholemeal
toast and butter (3)
lunch
roast chicken (0), 3 oz (76 g) boiled
potatoes (3), spinach (0), medium
portion carrots (1),
medium portion stewed apricots (1)
dinner
2 starch-reduced crispbreads and
butter (1), average portion cheese (0),
orange (2)

Total: 15 carbohydrate units

No carbohydrate units
rhubarb · tomatoes
onions · button onions · green
peppers · French beans · green beans
Brussels sprouts · spinach ·
mushrooms · cauliflower · broccoli
spears · lettuce · celery · cucumber ·
kippers · sardines · cod · lamb · steak ·
gammon · bacon · chicken · ham ·
liver · eggs · cheese

One carbohydrate unit
grapefruit · stewed apricots (1 portion)
orange or tomato juice (1 glass)
carrots (1 portion) · 1 oz (28 g) potatoes
2 starch-reduced crispbreads with
butter or margarine

Two carbohydrate units
melon (1 slice) · apple · stewed prunes
(1 portion) · pear · pineapple
(1 portion) · orange (medium) · sweet
corn (1 small portion) · peas (1 small
portion) · small carton
natural yoghurt

Three carbohydrate units
½ pt (300 ml) milk
1 slice wholemeal bread with butter
or margarine
dry wine (1 glass)
pork sausages (2)

Four carbohydrate units
1 oz (28 g) boiled rice

you will automatically cut out the things you normally eat with them, such as butter, margarine, custard and cream. The end result is that total food consumption is reduced. Although they provide a source of energy, most carbohydrates are also of less ultimate nutritional value than proteins or fats, and so it makes sense to eliminate or reduce your intake of such foods. If you are dieting by means of calorie control, it is easy to see that high carbohydrate or sugary foods contain so many calories that to stay within your prescribed daily calorie intake you can eat far fewer of these than you can of low carbohydrate foods. Nevertheless, it should be remembered that it *is* possible to eat a certain amount of carbohydrate and still lose weight. Potatoes baked in their jackets and seasoned with salt and pepper,

wholemeal bread and marrow fat peas are all mostly carbohydrate, but in addition they contain vitamins, proteins and, in the first two, valuable roughage. They are also 'filling' and give you the sensation of having eaten something of real substance.

STARTING A DIET

Most diets are started in spring or early summer, for obvious reasons. When the sun comes out, the weather gets milder, layers of winter woollies can be discarded, and your shape immediately becomes more noticeable. What you may have been able to hide under chunky sweaters will show far more in a lightweight spring suit or dress. Also, the summer holidays loom and you may start worrying about how you will look on the beach. Of course, it doesn't

have to be spring when you decide that you want to let out a slimmer, fitter you – you can start a 'spring-clean' diet at any time of year – but psychologically it is easier to make an effort when everything around you is being re-born.

Before you embark on any diet, strip off and take stock of what you see in a full-length mirror, in daylight. Don't cheat by holding in slack tummy muscles or looking at yourself in subdued light. Weigh and measure yourself and decide on your new target weight and size, but be realistic in this. Work out a basic and realistic exercise routine; aim to swim or jog or play tennis or squash energetically, if only for an hour each week.

Choose a diet which you feel you can follow and which will

help you to lose the amount of weight you have set as your target at approximately the rate you wish. Bear in mind that the faster you lose weight the faster it goes on again afterwards and that no two people lose weight at the same speed, so there are no guarantees whatever the claims made for particular diets. Having chosen your diet, give away to friends any food on your shelves which might distract you from your programme – let them get fat, you do not need the temptation – then stock up with the foods you will be needing. Plan your diary so that you don't run into a spate of parties or dinners just when you are beginning to lose weight; you don't want to bore everyone with your diet. It is also wise to consult your doctor before you embark on the diet.

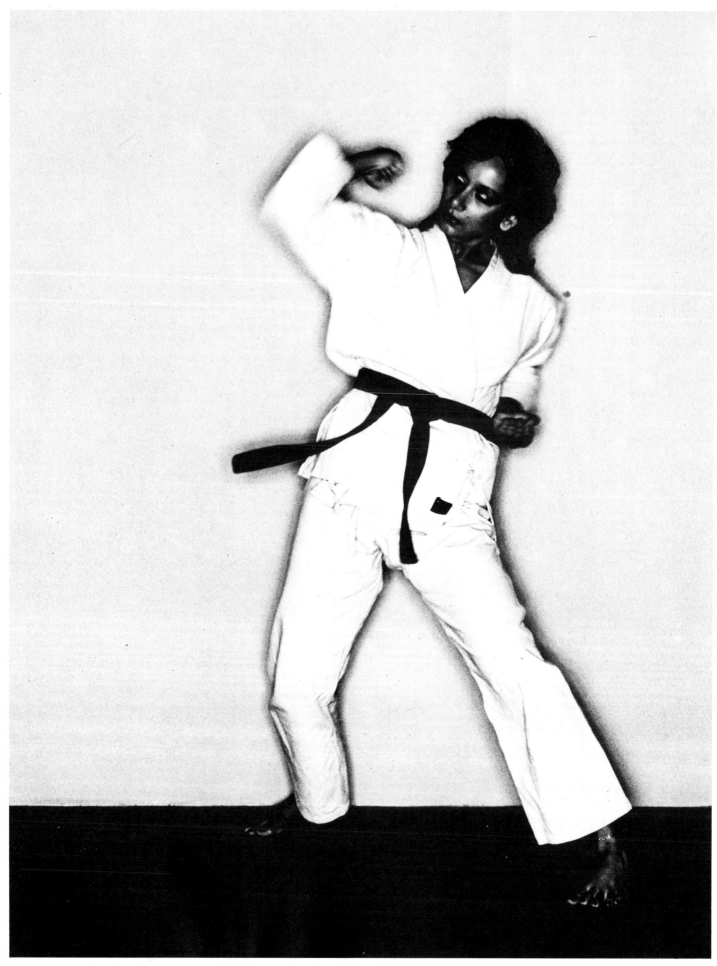

A Supple Body

Almost all of us have suffered from the same introduction to exercise. As little girls, running, skipping and jumping were fine. But the punishment of being sent on to a damp hockey pitch in shorts which left our knees exposed was not. Netball, tennis or basketball were all right for those who were good at them, but the gym could be hell on earth for the girl who collapsed every time she attempted a handstand. Sport seemed to represent the worst aspect of the competitive element in school life, something you gave up as soon as possible. It has taken women a long time to accept the idea that exercise is not just something for those who excel, nor is it only for men who work in offices and eat large business lunches. It is for working women too, even though they are exhausted from trying to do ten jobs at once, and for mothers who may feel fatigued and weary at the end of the day but have not really exercised themselves physically. Today, the notion that exercise can be something other than punishment, that keeping fit means that a woman looks better and feels healthier, is beginning to catch on. Women are going to yoga or keep-fit classes, and are taking up tennis, swimming, jogging or golf. Physical fitness is at last becoming an integral part of the life of a modern woman.

There are few things more exhilarating than the elation you feel after a good work-out. The lungs inhale deeply, the heart is pumping strongly, the skin tingles and feels rejuvenated, and the eyes sparkle. The whole secret is to find a form of exercise that you will like enough to keep up. It is a small step at first, but an enormous leap forwards once you have taken it. Exercise becomes not a drudge, burden or chore, but an addiction. You cannot lose interest in something you positively enjoy. Take a look at children playing in the park and remember that you were once like that. You are the same person, living in the same body, and the likelihood is that you still have the same zest and energy somewhere inside you. Don't wait until you have persuaded a friend to take up a sport or class with you; the chances are that she won't want to do the same as you and you will end up doing nothing. Decide on what you want to take up, or at least try, and get started; you will find plenty of other enthusiasts when you get there. It may take months to get your body back to a good standard of fitness if you have let yourself go, so the sooner you start the sooner you will see the benefits. You may not lose much weight, but you will certainly become trimmer as your muscles regain their elasticity, your posture will improve, and your body will become both stronger and more supple.

POSTURE

The human skeleton was designed originally for a four-legged creature, and man has been struggling to live with this rather ill-fitting structure ever since he, or she, first decided to stand up and use the front feet to reach for a more interesting life. More than 60 per cent of the body is composed of muscle and bone, so if we are to be healthy and move freely without aches and pains it is vital to keep these two components in good order. Our tall, jointed frame would not remain erect if it were not held in the correct position by the many pairs or groups of muscles which work together and against each other to maintain our upright stance. So, if we let our muscles go slack, the structure will be weakened and will start to curve, putting pressure on all the wrong places.

How we stand, sit and hold ourselves are of prime importance. Bad posture, wrong balance and incorrect weight distribution lead to tension in the neck, shoulders and spine, and more serious back problems such as curvature of the spine or disc displacement. The weight of the body is distributed equally on three points of the foot: the heel, the base of the big toe, and the base of the little toe. If the feet become flat, i.e. the arches which provide the spring between these points drop, weight will not be carried properly and you will certainly suffer; try the foot exercise on page 64, which will help to strengthen your feet. You also throw your balance out when you wear high heels. These shorten the back leg muscles, throw the head forwards, round the shoulders, and hollow the back. The tension that this causes through the spine and the muscles will cause neck pains and headaches, unless you vary the height of your heels and walk with bare feet when you can.

Balance in the body also comes from gravity. Your centre of gravity will be properly positioned if your head, shoulders, back and pelvis are positioned correctly. Check your posture regularly against the photographs on page 61 to see that you are holding yourself in the right way and you will soon find that good posture becomes a natural reflex.

When you are standing correctly, with weight evenly distributed, a line drawn vertically down from just behind the ear should touch the centre of the ankle bone; if the line falls in front, the muscles of the neck and spine will be under stress to support the head, and if the line falls behind the ankle bone, you are probably curving your back and putting the lower vertebrae under considerable stress. If the shoulders slant, the head is held to one side, or the pelvis is tilted forwards or backwards, your balance and weight distribution will be wrong. Standing, the crown of the head should be the highest point, not the forehead. You should be able to bend by flexing knees and hips, with minimal spinal effort.

Your stomach and back muscles work as a team. People with strong abdominal muscles will almost always have strong backs as well; weak abdominal muscles will give rise to back disorders. To make sure that your stomach muscles are being used correctly, hold yourself upright from the diaphragm, pulling the stomach muscles upwards towards the diaphragm, not in towards the lower back.

During pregnancy, a woman's centre of gravity will move forwards and her back will curve more to carry the extra weight. If her abdominal muscles are strong and help with the extra load, there should be no permanent damage, but she should remember to hold herself as straight as possible at all times. The obese experience a similar dysfunction of gravity and weight distribution. If they do not diet, and the condition lasts for several years, the spine may be damaged irreparably. Diet and strong abdominal muscles are the only way to avoid permanent damage.

Back pain can be agony, and even mild back pain can cause misery. It is difficult to understand why it is treated as a rather comic disorder; there is nothing funny about it to those who suffer. The people most vulnerable to back pain are those who drive a great deal, mothers with small children and heavy shopping baskets, people with sedentary jobs such as telephonists and secretaries, and those who stand for many hours at a time, such as shop assistants.

Caring for your back
The following tips should help to keep your back straight and strong and avoid the misery of backache.

1 When sitting, the spine should be supported by a good chair or specially-fitted seat support. Sit up straight, don't slump, and sit well back in your chair. Avoid deep, squashy armchairs and ones which are so deep that you have to perch on the edge. When driving a car or sitting at a typewriter, consciously try to hold the spine upright, with shoulders straight, not hunched forwards. Your knees should be higher than the hip joints so that your feet help to balance you and so that you will be able to stand by bending forwards from the sitting position, straightening the knees.
2 When lifting heavy weights from the ground, bend at the knees and hips to a squatting position, taking the strain of the lift in the leg muscles. Do not bend over taking the strain in your back. If carrying heavy parcels or shopping baskets, distribute them evenly in both hands and carry as close to the body as possible. Remember that whether right or left handed you will automatically favour that hand, so make a point of using the other as much as you can.
3 Always sleep on a firm to very firm mattress. A soft one will allow your spine to sag and bend.

MUSCLES

There are almost six hundred muscles in the body, comprising approximately 35 per cent of a woman's body weight. Those muscles which stimulate the body functions, for example pumping blood through the veins and food through the digestive system, cannot be consciously controlled and are called involuntary muscles; the rest, the voluntary muscles, we can and should control. All muscles need regular use, which means exercise, if they are to maintain strength and elasticity. If they are not used, muscles decrease in size, attract excess fat around them, sag, bulge and turn into flab. Diet alone cannot get rid of flab, but exercise can, and in a surprisingly short space of time if done regularly. Muscle fibre also decreases in size as you grow older, particularly if you have been inactive, and the hunched, shrivelled look of old age is a result of this. One of the best ways to prevent ageing, or at least to slow down its advance, is to exercise the muscles regularly, particularly those which help to maintain good posture.

Stomach muscles, unfortunately, have come to mean little more than modern woman's preoccupation with the flatness of her stomach, although women naturally have slightly protruding tummies and a concave one is rather unattractive. Strong stomach muscles are important, however, because they control the whole pelvic area, particularly vital during pregnancy, and work with the back to maintain correct posture and prevent back problems. If your stomach muscles are flabby, you would certainly be wise to strengthen them with exercise. Tennis, swimming, netball, basketball and badminton are especially beneficial.

While many women worry about the size and shape of their hips and thighs, they are often wary of exercise which they feel may develop arm or leg muscles to unfeminine proportions. It would take an excessive or disproportionate amount of exercise to build the look of a weight-lifter, but strong leg and arm muscles are an obvious advantage. Well-exercised arm muscles are less likely to turn into unsightly flab in middle age and strong legs are certainly going to do a better job of carrying us around without tiring. Swimming and cycling are the obvious choices to strengthen leg muscles, while the muscles of the shoulders, arms, chest and upper back all work together and will benefit from any sport which exercises the top part of the body, such as tennis, badminton, swimming, squash or archery. If you exercise regularly in this way you may develop your muscles to a certain extent, and it is worth remembering that large muscles burn up more calories than small muscles even when at rest, and strong muscles help to pump more blood into the heart.

The heart is the most important muscular organ in the body. It is about the size of a man's fist and weighs around 14 oz (395 g). Like every other muscle, the heart needs exercise to function efficiently and should be given extra training to cope with strenuous activity. When we undertake energetic physical exercise, the large muscle groups send more blood to the heart so forcing it to work harder to pump out the extra volume, thus increasing its efficiency.

Any exercise that helps the heart does so in three ways: it strengthens the muscular contractions of the heart and the

ENERGY EXPENDITURE

The chart below shows the energy expenditure for different activities and sports. The calories used per hour are based on those generally achieved by an averagely motivated person, and are therefore lower than the output that might be incurred by a well-trained and fit young person.

Around the home

EXERCISE/SPORT	ENERGY USED Calories per hour	BENEFITS	DISADVANTAGES
Light housework	120–300	Although not necessarily strenuous, these activities maintain a degree of mobility and muscle strength, but should be supplemented by a regular exercise routine to achieve real physical fitness.	People with back problems or heart conditions should take great care when bending, pushing or lifting, whether working in the home or pursuing a more strenuous form of exercise.
Hard housework	400–600		
Cleaning windows	240–300		
Making beds	400		
Mopping floors	240–300		
Washing dishes	100		
Gardening	250–450		

Water sports

Canoeing	220–315	Improves heart-lung efficiency and strength in top half of body.	
Rowing	220–315	Promotes mobility and good for muscles, heart and lungs.	
Sailing	125–220	Most water sports, with the exception of swimming, are light to moderate in energy expenditure and maintain or promote mobility, muscle strength and heart-lung efficiency.	
Surfing	220–315		
Swimming	395–475	Excellent for heart and lungs, mobility of major joints and muscular strength. Splashing about is not enough, though; to get maximum benefit, swim regularly for at least ten minutes.	For the unfit, the breathing pattern in front crawl can put extra strain on heart and cold dips can be bad for blood-pressure.
Water skiing	220–315	Does not contribute much to mobility or heart-lung efficiency, but may improve leg muscles.	

Acrobatic sports

Ballet exercises	300–360	Promote agility, co-ordination and muscle strength.	
Dancing	250–350	Aids co-ordination, flexibility and suppleness. Disco dancing can be good for body muscles, especially stomach, if you really move from centre.	
Diving	220–315	Acrobatic exercises are generally light or moderate in energy expenditure and are good primarily for flexibility and co-ordination.	
Gymnastics	220–315		
Trampolining	315–395		
Skipping	250–350	Good for flexibility and arm and shoulder muscles. Improves heart-lung efficiency if kept up for twenty minutes and done regularly.	Can be strenuous if not taken slowly at first. If you are in late thirties or forties, take plenty of rests at first.

Team games

Baseball	220–315	Improves mobility, strength, heart and lungs.	Competitive activities involving teams probably have a higher injury rate than lone sports. Most ball games involve sporadic bursts of intense exertion and periods of relative inactivity which makes great demands on the body, particularly heart and lungs. So make sure you are fit enough to undertake strenuous activities and build up gradually to peak level.
Basketball	315–395	Better for mobility than strength, but good for heart and lungs.	
Cricket	125–220	Maintains degree of mobility and muscle strength.	
Soccer	395–475	Improves mobility and maintains leg muscles; good for heart and lungs.	
Hockey	315–395	Both hockey and lacrosse are good for strength, mobility and heart-lung efficiency.	
Lacrosse	315–395		
Handball	475–1,000 +	Like squash, provides good all-round benefit if played for thirty minutes or more.	Although team games are social sports, and thus more enjoyable for the gregarious than lone sports, they have the drawback of your having to fit in with other people's availability.
Volleyball	220–315	Best for mobility, but also maintains strength and stimulates heart and lungs.	

Locomotive sports

EXERCISE/SPORT	ENERGY USED Calories per hour	BENEFITS	DISADVANTAGES
Strolling	120	Daily walks, increasing in length and pace, are not taxing but maintain a degree of mobility and muscle strength.	
Walking	150		
Walking briskly	450	Walking briskly is more beneficial, especially up hills and stairs.	
Walking briskly uphill	850		
Climbing	395–475	Beneficial for muscle strength, mobility and heart-lung efficiency.	Make sure you have proper equipment and are reasonably fit before you start.
Jogging	485	Ideal for leg muscles and excellent for heart and lungs. Try to limber up before setting off.	Does not help trunk or flexibility. Start slowly and build up gradually to peak level; there is a danger of heart strain if taken too fast or you are over-weight.
Running	800	Builds up leg muscles and heart-lung efficiency.	Like jogging, can be dangerous if you try to do too much too quickly. Work up slowly to total fitness.
Cycling	315–395	Very good exercise, improving leg muscles and heart-lung efficiency if you take in some stiff hills or sprint stretches.	Does not exercise chest or shoulders.
Skating	315–395	Beneficial for mobility, leg muscles, heart and lungs if done continuously.	
Skiing	475–1,000 +	One of the best sports for all-round fitness. Excellent for mobility; increases strength of shoulders, arms, legs and ankles; good for heart and lungs.	Has high accident rate because many people are unprepared for it physically. Combined stress of altitude, cold and exercise may be too great for some. Tends to be seasonal and spasmodic.

Racquet games

Badminton	220–315	Vigorous, continuous play benefits heart and lungs.	Remember, in all racquet games, that if you are unfit sudden exertion can jar a muscle or strain the heart. If in doubt about your fitness, seek medical advice.
Table tennis	150–250	Vigorous play can improve heart and lungs and helps co-ordination and mobility.	
Squash	475–1,000 +	Most physically demanding of racquet games. Should be played regularly to give all-round benefit.	Needs initial training. Often very competitive and may increase stress and tension. Over-exertion in hot room may be dangerous for the unhealthy.
Tennis	315–395	Can be of all-round benefit if played for thirty minutes or more with an attempt to keep moving. Twisting and bending help mobility.	Benefits in heart-lung efficiency, mobility and leg muscles depend on frequency, duration and intensity of game. Tends to be seasonal and spasmodic.

Target sports

Archery	125–220	Archery works on the arm, shoulder and chest muscles, but other target sports provide little muscular exercise.	Most sports which involve marksmanship are light in terms of energy expenditure and not sufficiently taxing to help heart and lung efficiency or promote all-round fitness.
Billiards	125–220		
Bowls	125–220		
Croquet	125–220		
Rifle shooting	125–220		
Ten-pin bowling	125–220		
Golf	240–350	Walking provides the main physical exercise, so golf conditions leg muscles if played regularly. Twisting movement while driving ball can be good for waistline.	The swing increases mobility only in shoulders and is not vigorous enough to improve heart-lung efficiency. Blood-pressure can rise in cold weather. The sport is often competitive and frustrating, so not relaxing.

Combat sports

Fencing	315–395	Improves mobility and muscle strength.	All strenuous activity carries a degree of risk in the form of strain or some kind of accident. These risks can sometimes be reduced if you wear the proper clothing and use recommended equipment.
Judo	315–395	Both judo and karate improve mobility, strength, heart and lungs.	
Karate	315–395		

strong flow of blood helps keep the fatty deposits which build up in the arteries in check: it improves the co-ordination of all the muscles that are pumping the blood; and the strong flow keeps all the capillaries open as well as the main arteries, thus helping circulation. However, you need to exercise strongly for approximately twenty minutes before you begin to achieve any worthwhile effect.

Almost any exercise which benefits the heart will benefit the lungs at the same time, improving their capacity to inhale oxygen and increasing the essential supply of oxygen to the heart. When you run, skip or play tennis until your face is flushed and you are out of breath, it means that your heart and lungs have probably had a good work-out too.

Most people breathe too fast and shallow. Deep breathing increases your lung capacity and stamina. Breathe in slowly until your chest lifts up and expands sideways. The diaphragm moves down to allow the lungs room to expand. Poor breathing pushes the diaphragm down about $\frac{1}{2}$ in (1.25 cm). Deep breathing more than quadruples this. Breathe out releasing air slowly from diaphragm upwards.

CHOOSING AN EXERCISE ROUTINE

You don't have to reach Olympic standards or beat your fourteen-year-old daughter running down the street, you don't have to progress week by week so that your standard visibly improves, just as you don't have to play to win. You are not competing against anyone else, you are exercising to improve your muscle tone, to become stronger and more supple, to balance your calorie intake, to improve your heart and lung efficiency, and to become a healthier person, so you can set your own standards. The important thing is to find a routine which you will enjoy enough to follow regularly.

Exercise is not only for the already fit; invalids or the disabled should not feel excluded and often those with bad backs, heart complaints or nervous disorders, or those who are over-weight or pregnant, are the very people who need exercise most. However, if you suffer from any illness, disability, back or heart problem, always see a doctor before taking up exercise. You should also consult your doctor if you haven't undertaken any sport or exercise for more than five years.

With the help of your doctor and the suggestions here and overleaf, you should be able to find a form of exercise which will suit your lifestyle. An exercise or dance class, for example, or a regular daily exercise routine, will help to improve your posture and strengthen your back, but if you have a weak back you obviously shouldn't go in for weight-lifting.

Most doctors now agree that regular monitored exercise is the best way of countering heart disease. Heart patients are no longer treated as more delicate than lilies. Of course, exercise must be done under medical supervision, taking it easy at first and gradually building up strength, remembering that while the correct exercise will benefit a weak heart, inappropriate exercise may damage even the most healthy one.

Before you decide on an exercise routine or sport, consider the demands of your lifestyle. Exercise must be taken regularly if it is to be beneficial, so you must choose something which slots well into your living pattern. Consider, for example, the time you have available. Running, jogging, skipping or indoor static cycling can be done at any time for ten minutes, thirty minutes or more; while organized sports or team sports tend to be more time consuming and restrictive, because you have to fit in with other people's programmes.

Cost and convenience also need to be considered. Tennis, for example, may involve driving miles to a court, paying fees, searching for a partner and arranging schedules, all of which can discourage you. The cost of a static bicycle may also be prohibitive, but you can run for free or swim at little cost in the local pool.

Your capabilities must also be taken into account. It is no good arranging to play squash with the local club star if you know that you are not that good. The humiliation could put you off for ever.

Age, health and physical condition will also influence your choice. The older you are, the less rigorous the activity should be. If you are over thirty-five, you should have your blood-pressure tested before you start exercising. If you are over fifty, and have been inactive for a long time, get into training by walking regularly. If over sixty, perhaps you should keep to walking, swimming or easy cycling.

Remember that you will only keep up an exercise you enjoy, so give a new activity a trial of a month or two – it takes time to get into it. Then, if you are not enjoying it, try something else. If you cannot bear the thought of anything 'sporty', just concentrate on brisk walking or climbing twenty-five stairs at a comfortable pace every day; run for buses and never take lifts or escalators although even these activities should be worked up to gradually.

METHODS OF EXERCISE

Home exercise routine
The main benefit of a home exercise routine is that it can be varied to suit your needs and is, hopefully, enjoyable to do. Such routines are usually chosen by women who are mainly interested in improving their posture or figure. If the routine is done regularly, as a daily habit, it will improve mobility and flexibility, but the exercises are often not sufficiently vigorous to improve heart and lung efficiency. Combine these exercises with regular swimming, jogging, tennis or cycling and you will have an ideal routine.

Callisthenics
Callisthenics originated in Sweden in the nineteenth century. Fitness as a quality in itself was rarely considered, even 150 years ago, but the Swedish landowners were worried at the sight of the slouching, sagging bodies of the peasants working in the fields, so they devised a set of exercises which would improve their bodies and counteract the effects of the work. In fact, callisthenics means the type of exercise you might do at home, perhaps as a daily routine, or in a keep-fit class: the movements build up strength and suppleness, and return the body to its proper shape. The Swedish idea, however, was based on a military regime, which you may not wish to emulate. Callisthenics alone do not lead to all-round fitness, as they do not improve the condition of the heart or lungs.

Aerobics
Aerobic is the name given to the type of exercise which does improve the heart, lungs and circulation. The term covers any exercises that make the heart pump faster than normal and make you breathe more deeply and rapidly, so that the lungs are used to maximum capacity. They include jogging, swimming, cycling, running, skiing, squash, rowing and horse-riding. Aerobic exercise does not necessarily tone up muscles all over the body, nor does it help suppleness.

Isometrics
Isometrics are a less popular form of exercise, concentrating on building up individual muscle fibres. The theory is based on the fact that in normal daily activity only 25 to 30 per cent of our muscle potential is used. Normal exercise to strengthen muscles, called isotonic exercise, creates its effect by lengthening and shortening the muscle fibres and is a fairly slow, gradual process. Isometric means 'same length', signifying that during exercising the muscles are in a state of static contraction, with no movement of the joints. It works by a brief exertion of the muscles against objects that cannot be moved, and strengthens the muscles to 100 per cent quite rapidly.

Isometrics can be done against an opposing fist, wall, table or door-frame. Each contraction lasts only six seconds, and fifteen exercises are sufficient to condition the entire body. A minimum of ninety seconds a day is enough. You can exercise, if you wish, while the car is stuck at traffic lights, by holding opposite sides of the steering wheel and pushing so that the hands press inwards, towards each other. Or do the same exercise on the sides of a typewriter. However, isometric routines should be combined with some other form of exercise, as they help neither suppleness nor stamina, and are best avoided by the over-weight and those with heart or blood problems.

Home exercise machines
These include rowing machines, chest expanders and static bicycles. The main disadvantage is their cost: most forms of exercise are free. No machine works miracles; all it can do is help you to exercise regularly, because it is at hand. Rowing machines build up muscle strength and flexibility in the upper arms and chest, and also improve heart-lung efficiency if they make you pant. But they do little for the leg muscles, despite the strain. Chest expanders exercise the same muscles and may do something for an under-developed bust, by strengthening the chest muscles underneath, but do not exercise the lower half of the body. Static bicycles give the same amount of exercise as cycling, without the dangers of roads and pollution, but can be dangerous if you over-tax yourself. Start slowly, with plenty of rests, and work up to a maximum rate, carefully following the instructions supplied. If you have room for one, they are not a bad investment.

Yoga
Yoga is very popular with women; some offices provide yoga classes in the lunch-hour and many local authorities run classes in the evening. The aim of yoga, which has been practised for centuries in the East, is to attain union between the human spirit and the universal spirit. It does not necessarily involve a series of painful body contortions, but aims to increase the body's suppleness and mobility and ultimately to achieve deep mental relaxation. At least twenty minutes should be set aside each day to practise yoga and, at first, students are recommended to attend classes to learn all the positions correctly.

CAN EXERCISE REDUCE WEIGHT?

The honest answer to this question is, on its own, no. However, controlled diet together with exercise is a much more positive answer than either one or the other on its own. The reason why exercise alone does not take off weight is connected with our metabolism, i.e. all the processes, changes and chemical reactions that take place in the body to maintain life. The release of energy is an essential part of metabolism and the rate at which energy is used is known as the basal metabolic rate. Two-thirds of our metabolic rate is taken up in the ordinary daily living processes such as breathing and digestion. This leaves only one-third to be accounted for by other exercise or activity, which means that it is practically impossible to get rid of large accumulations of stored food simply by exercising more. On average, we burn up 2,500 Calories a day. A brisk walk will use an extra five Calories or so a minute, so a daily thirty-minute walk would use 150–225 Calories, which might account for under 1 oz (28 g) of body fat. Since a piece of chocolate cake would add 180 Calories or a slice of apple pie 380, just exercising to lose weight would clearly be an uphill struggle. However, if you eat sensibly and still find that you put on weight, there is only one thing to do: increase your calorie expenditure with exercise, which will help to maintain a balance between the foodstuffs you enjoy eating and the lifestyle you have to adopt to allow you to eat them.

Exercise also helps to balance the cholesterol in the system. This is a harmless, natural substance and a necessary part of the body, but our way of life, with too much stress and too little exercise, causes it to be dangerous. When we are under stress, whether from job frustration, persistent noise, or anger in a traffic jam, cholesterol is one of the substances released into the bloodstream to supply the muscles with energy to cope with the required reaction. Inside our modern bodies we are basically primitive beings. If we still lived in the jungle, the day-to-day stresses might involve coming face to face with a tiger or a threatening spear. In those circumstances, we would either flee or fight, both of which would use the energy provided. Face to face with our boss, or having an argument on the telephone, the body releases the same energy propellants, but we do not move. Thus the cholesterol and other substances produced to deal with the emergency are not burned up and accumulate in the body, sometimes to a potentially dangerous level.

Cholesterol is released by two emergency-responsive hormones,* adrenalin and noradrenalin. The latter is sometimes known as the 'kick' hormone and it is this which is activated when we are aggressive, competitive or under stress. One of the few times it is put into action harmlessly is during vigorous physical exercise, when we can burn up the cholesterol released.

EXERCISE DURING AND AFTER PREGNANCY

The time in her life when a woman most needs to be fit is during pregnancy. She may not be entering a race, but childbirth is certainly a time of great physical exertion. A body that is strong and flexible works more efficiently, tires less easily and gets back into shape more quickly afterwards, too. You do not need any special strength or stamina to get through labour, but all stages of pregnancy – before, during and after the birth – pass more easily and safely if you are fit.

A pregnant woman is not ill and should not be treated, or treat herself, as such. In primitive societies, a woman often worked in the fields until her baby was due, took a couple of hours off for the birth, and then returned to work. Although this is certainly not desirable, even in Western society pregnant women are now encouraged to live as normally as possible. If you are a healthy, active person and are used to enjoying a particular sport, carry on with it for as long as you can without straining yourself, obviously avoiding very strenuous sports such as squash or potentially hazardous ones like skating, where a hard fall could be dangerous. If in doubt, consult your doctor. Walking and swimming are ideal exercise; gentle jogging, running, bicycling or tennis are also good, but modify your exercise by taking them more easily. You won't have the same stamina as before you were pregnant, so do not expect to achieve as much. Remember that your body is already expending a great deal of energy building and maintaining the baby. Don't push yourself beyond what is comfortable, you are bound to get out of breath and tire more quickly, and always rest afterwards. Don't take up a sport if you are not used to it, that would be foolish; if you want to start to exercise, keep to walking but don't overdo it.

Your posture and breathing need special attention during pregnancy. Here are a few exercises which will help you to strengthen certain muscles, give you the knowledge and control which are so vital during childbirth, and ensure that you regain your figure quickly afterwards. Practise them regularly during pregnancy and immediately after the birth. After six weeks, you can start on the daily exercise routine

on page 60, taking it easily at first and building up carefully.

Posture

Stand and sit as straight and tall as you can. When sitting, make sure your back is supported and if you can put your feet up so much the better. While you have your feet up, bend and stretch your ankles and circle your feet in both directions several times. Standing, keep your weight evenly distributed on your feet; don't lean forwards on to the balls of your feet or sway back on to your heels, a particular temptation as pregnancy advances and your balance changes. Remember that strong abdominal muscles mean strong backs, so tuck your bottom in and make your tummy muscles do the work of supporting the extra weight.

Breathing

Good deep breathing and control of your breathing are invaluable during childbirth. Breathing exercises will help to increase your lung capacity and control and will also improve your circulation. Breathe in slowly and deeply until your lungs are full and you feel pressure on your diaphragm. Let the breath out slowly from the diaphragm upwards (see page 57).

Breasts

You may put on as much as 3 lb (1.3 kg) in extra weight in your breasts during pregnancy. Exercises to strengthen the pectoral muscles help to give your breasts support. Try numbers 5 and 10 in the exercise routine which begins on page 60.

Abdomen

Strong abdominal and pelvic floor muscles make for an easier delivery, so pay special attention to exercising them. Abdominal muscles also need strengthening during pregnancy to support the baby, preventing backache, and to help you to regain your figure more easily after the birth. Lie on your back with knees bent and hands by your sides. Tighten muscles in buttocks and abdomen until waist and small of the back press flat on to the floor and bottom of spine lifts. Hold for a count of five, then slowly relax to original position.

Pelvic floor

The weight of the baby pressing on the pelvic floor can put the muscles here under great strain and weaken them. Luckily, pelvic floor strengthening exercises are the sort you can do at any time, lying down, sitting up, waiting at traffic lights, or in the bath. However, first of all, it takes some practice to isolate the muscles of the urinary tract, vagina and rectum, all of which need strengthening. Try stopping the flow of urine in the middle of passing water, close your vaginal muscles around an imaginary penis, and clench rectal muscles

as though trying to stop a motion. When you recognize the three sets of muscles, tighten first the urinary sphincter, then the vagina, then the rectal muscles, hold all together for a count of ten, then relax and repeat. Do this as often as you can.

LEARNING TO RELAX

Stress and its partner tension are conditions of the world in which we live, the result of too much noise, too much speed, too much pressure. The reasons why we get tense vary, but the root cause can nearly always be traced to some imbalance in our lives. Fear, anxiety, and pressures of work and home all contribute to a state of tension, and unless we find ways of coping with the situation it can cause both mental and physical pain and distress.

Tension manifests itself in a number of familiar ways: irritability, deep frowning, hunching our shoulders, biting our nails, fiddling with our hands or our hair; headaches, backaches and just about every other ache you can think of may all be symptoms of tension. As we try to wrestle with whatever problems beset us, the brain sends messages to our nervous system telling it that all is not well and we exhibit real and visible signs that this is so.

Headaches and backaches are possibly the most common manifestations of tension. Both may, however, have some physiological cause: your back may actually be aching because you are consistently putting it to bad use, assuming a posture which it does not like, or you may even be suffering from something more serious like a slipped disc. And your head may ache because you have eyestrain or sinusitis or you are suffering from an excess of alcohol, nicotine or sun, or even because you have an infected tooth. But if your doctor cannot find any physiological reason for your aches, the chances are that some form of tension is responsible. Sleep, as any migraine sufferer will know, is the best immediate cure for a headache, but it isn't always possible. Fresh air or head rolling exercises (see pages 62–64) to ease the knotted muscles may also help. Drugs can bring temporary relief, but if the cause is underlying tension then a real cure will only be effected by eradicating the source of the tension and by learning to relax both mind and muscle.

If the problem causing the tension is something straight-forward like a difficult day at work or with the children, an argument, a frustrating shopping expedition or a deadline only just met, then simply taking a hot bath, a catnap in a dark room, a quiet drink with your feet up or listening to your

favourite record could do the trick. Laughter, too, if it is the real belly kind, can remove a feeling of tension as any comedian or politician knows. But the most effective way of relaxing is through contrast activity: simply doing something very different from what you have just been doing. If you are surrounded by people and noise, seek quiet and solitude for a while; if you have been by yourself for a long time, be gregarious; if you have been sitting a lot, run around the block or go for a bicycle ride; if you have been physically very active, lie down in a quiet, dark room. Variety is often the key to relaxation.

If tension is acute but momentary, taking a few really slow, deep breaths will help. Rapid, shallow breathing is usually a sign of stress. Not for nothing has the command 'take a deep breath' been issued before or during times of sudden tension: the extra oxygen released into the bloodstream and brain has a direct, if temporary, calming effect. If, however, feeling tensed up is a regular feature of your life, then mastering a good relaxation technique is vital.

One of the best methods of relaxing is based on the 'tense a muscle, let it go' technique. Very often we are simply unaware that our muscles are tense. Screwing up your face, clenching your fists, flexing your thighs, and then letting each area literally 'flop' will make you familiar with the difference between a tensed and a relaxed muscle and hence a tense and relaxed body. Lie down in a quiet room and, starting from the muscles in the head and working systematically down the body, tense and relax each muscle in turn and then the whole body. Once learned, this technique can be employed at any time, provided you have ten minutes to spare and a quiet place in which to do the exercise. Massage is also a useful aid to relaxation. The muscles in the neck and shoulders are particularly susceptible to tension and may have become permanently tense or 'knotted'. It is quite possible to learn how to massage these and other areas of the body. You will find instructions on pages 77–85. There are also exercises incorporated into the daily exercise programme on pages 60–75 which will help stop muscles knotting up.

Finally, if in spite of all the tricks and techniques you employ tension continues to grip you, then you must go right back and seek out the cause. Look into yourself as honestly as you can; try to discover what it is that you are really worried, frightened, anxious about, *even if you don't want to know the answer*, and resolve to do something positive about it.

Your daily exercise routine

As long as you are prepared to work for it, and make exercise part of your way of life, you can have a young and supple body long after others have given up bikinis and started easing themselves creakily in and out of armchairs. There is no need to resign yourself to getting stiff with age, or to losing your figure after childbirth.

The exercise routine mapped out on the following pages was designed by Lotte Berk, who has probably done more to save the shape of women than any other person. Her exercises are based on ballet and yoga movements and sound orthopaedic principles, and are especially geared to meet the needs of busy, modern women.

Getting the most from your exercise routine

1 Make up your mind that you are going to exercise every day. It is pointless to spend half an hour on the routine one day and then skip it for a week; by the time you come back to your exercises, your muscles will be as stiff as they were when you started and your work will have been in vain. Set aside a particular time of day for your routine, perhaps in the early morning, evening or before you go to bed; it doesn't matter what time you choose as long as it isn't after a heavy meal and you make it a regular habit. If you do not keep to your routine regularly, the exercises will do no good and the habit is too easily broken; it is far better to do just ten minutes a day, if that is all you can manage, than half an hour one day and nothing the next.

2 Get comfortable. Change into a one-piece swimsuit or leotard; this will help you to feel smooth and slender, and changing adds a ritual element which will make the exercise habit easier to keep. Work on a carpeted floor and have a small cushion handy in case you need it. If you can make space to have a mirror and a really firm ballet bar fixed at hip height, it will make some of the exercises easier and again add to the ritual of your regular exercising time. If you cannot manage a ballet bar,

organize a chair which is steady, the right height, and always available, but try to work near a full-length mirror.

3 Learn the exercises carefully, reading them through and studying the photographs until you understand them completely, and then try them out in front of a mirror to check that you are holding the right position. Make sure that you know them thoroughly, so that you don't have to break off and refer back to the book once you start your routine; this will break the rhythm of the exercises, which have been designed to flow smoothly from one to another. You may find that music with a good, strong beat helps you to keep the movement going.

4 Learn the special 'roll-in'

movement before you start exercising (see below and page 68). Many of the exercises are based on this movement; if you get it right, it will ensure that your back is not strained in any way.

5 Always start your exercise time with the warm-up routine which begins below. This will loosen up the whole body, get the circulation pumping, and warm up cold, stiff muscles which might otherwise tear. Check your posture (see opposite) front, back and side, make sure that you are holding yourself straight, not hunching shoulders or curving back, that your weight is evenly distributed and shoulders level.

6 When you first start exercising, you are bound to feel stiff and aching because you will be using muscles which have been

neglected, but your back should not hurt. If it does, you have been doing an exercise wrongly so check and check again. Build on your exercises gradually, adding more exercises and more repeats as your muscles get stronger. Never push yourself faster than your muscles can cope with. A steady build-up will ensure that you do not strain yourself. Take note of what each exercise is designed to accomplish. If it is meant to strengthen stomach muscles, then see that these are the ones that are working. It may be easier to take the strain somewhere else, but you will do yourself no good and possibly some harm.

7 Be patient. Don't expect results overnight and give up if you don't get them. If your muscles are out of condition, it may take several weeks before you see the difference, so persevere.

Note: These exercises are strong and rigorous, particularly if you are out of condition. Follow all the instructions carefully, particularly those for the 'roll-in' exercise. The exercises are not suitable for a pregnant woman unless she is really fit and they are not designed to be done as immediate postnatal exercises. However, from six weeks after the birth a mother can start on the exercises, gradually building up as her muscles strengthen. She will soon have her figure back in trim.

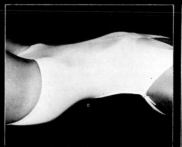

Lie on back on carpet, knees bent, arms stretched back above head. Spine will be slightly arched off floor, enough to slide hand under.

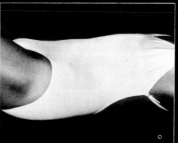

'Roll-in' pelvis by pushing spine flat against carpet until bottom lifts slightly off floor. Inner thigh muscles should appear to 'jump out'.

WARM-UP ROUTINE

These warm-up exercises are the most essential part of your daily exercise programme. They boost the circulation and, most important, warm up the muscles. Warm muscles are flexible, cold ones can strain and tear, so always start your exercise session here. The warm-up exercises are designed to exercise every bit of your body,

relaxing and toning up the muscles. They should be practised until they can be done as a continuous programme without breaking the flow. Once you have mastered these exercises, you can add others to tone up specific parts of the body. If your time is very limited just do this group, but do them without fail every day.

1 The first warm-up exercise stretches your spine and gets the circulation going as you sweep up and down in a continuous, supple, graceful, flowing rhythm.

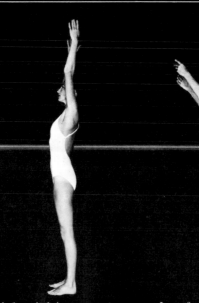

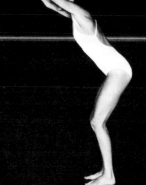

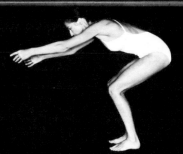

With feet slightly apart, raise arms and stretch spine up through whole body until you feel much taller.

Lean forwards, bending your knees slightly and starting to swing your arms loosely forwards too.

Bend your knees further and sweep arms down, stretching them loosely forwards as they go.

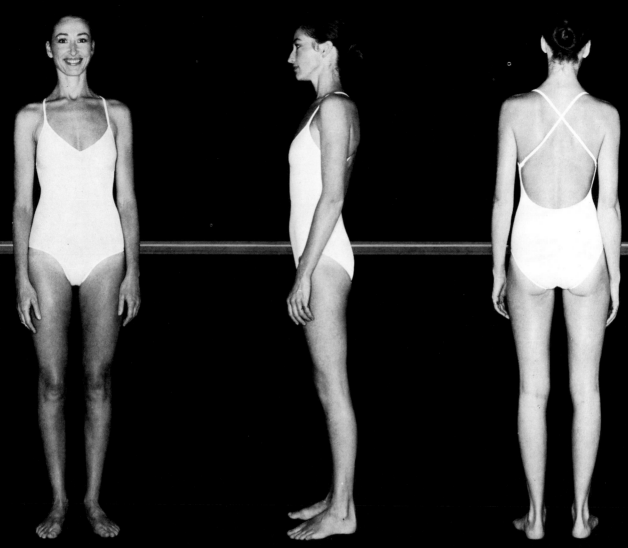

Good posture gives you a better figure instantly; the way you carry your body influences its shape and health. Faulty posture causes figure faults and aches, pains, tension and fatigue. Check posture every day in the mirror before you start on your exercise routine to avoid slipping into bad habits. Holding the correct posture should soon become completely natural.

The crown of the head should be at the highest point, not the forehead, and shoulders should be absolutely level. Many people get into the habit of always carrying things with one or other hand and shoulders eventually tilt. When standing with feet evenly spaced, neither tight together nor wide apart, legs straight, your weight should be evenly distributed.

Standing sideways, you should be able to see that a line taken from just behind the ear will pass just behind the hip joint to the centre of the ankle bone. Keep your weight evenly balanced in the centre of your feet; do not lean forwards on to the balls of your feet or backwards so that your heels and the muscles at the back of your legs take the strain.

Your back should be straight and the spine vertical. If you have a habit of sitting awkwardly, throwing your body to one side, or always carry loads on one side, you may find your spine is curving. Your back should not be hunched, with rounded shoulders, nor should it curve inwards, tilting pelvis forwards and putting excessive strain on lower vertebrae.

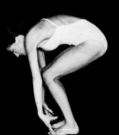 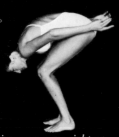 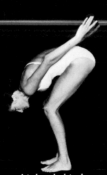 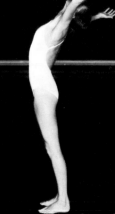

Continue to bend, letting hands sweep past your feet with arms, hands and fingers loose and relaxed.

Now swing your arms right up behind you, as you gradually straighten up at the knees.

Raise arms higher behind you, so head is pointing down and muscles down backs of legs feel stretched.

Swing arms down, forwards, up and back behind head, arms bent, in flowing movement. Repeat ten times.

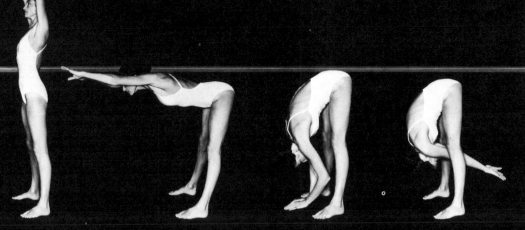

2 This bending exercise involves stretching and relaxing your body as it flows through a series of movements. However, you must remember to keep your legs straight all the time. If you are doing the exercise correctly, you should feel the muscles down the backs of your legs really pulling hard as you hold the parallel pose and then push through.

Stand with feet apart, arms raised, and stretch right up as in previous exercise. Bending forwards from

hips, push bottom out, arch spine, bring arms and trunk parallel to floor. Hold for a few seconds.

Relax to floor, legs straight. Push arms through legs and push, push hard. Swing up to starting position. Repeat five times.

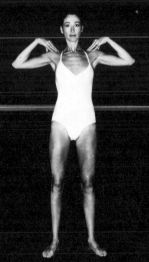 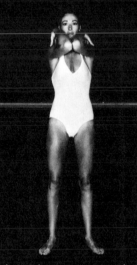 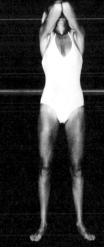

4 This exercise works on the shoulders and upper arms. Push your elbows as high and wide as you can, making them move in big circles. It is a marvellous exercise for relieving the aches and tensions that can build up in shoulders, so do it any time you feel stiff or aching.

Stand straight and tall, feet apart, and place finger tips lightly on your shoulders.

Make circling movement with your elbows, bringing them down, forwards and then together in front.

Raise elbows right up and circle backwards, down and back up to starting position. Repeat ten times.

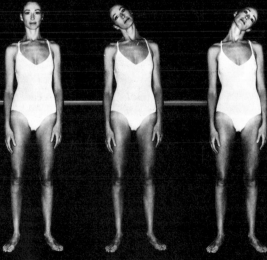

7 The way you carry your head has a great effect on your overall appearance. If your neck is supple and head held straight it will give you a graceful, youthful appearance. The following head and neck exercises work towards that end. They are an important part of the warm-up routine, but can be done at any time to release tension and stiffness in the neck.

8 This is another exercise which relaxes the neck, working particularly on the muscles at the front and back of the neck. It is very effective for firming up chin muscles and helping to keep a young jaw line.

Stand tall with head erect. Bend your neck over sideways, pushing ear down towards right shoulder.

Bring your head up and bend it over to left side. Straighten up and repeat exercise five times.

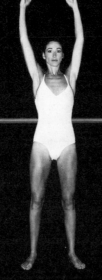
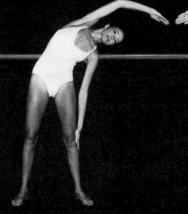
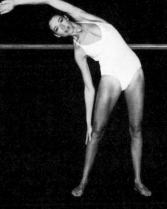

3 This exercise is particularly good for your waistline. As you bend over sideways you should really feel the pull on your waist. Remember never to lean forwards at all; keep arms, legs and body all in line. If possible, work at first in front of a mirror.

Stand with legs apart, arms raised, and stretch up tall really feeling your waist lift up and narrow.

With legs straight, swing right arm over head and slide left arm as far down left leg as you can reach.

Swing up and over to other side, reaching down. Straighten up. Repeat second and third movements ten times.

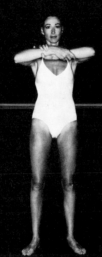
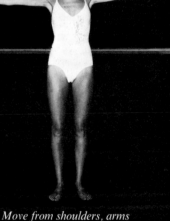

5 Few women are completely satisfied with the size or shape of their breasts. Exercise cannot do anything to change the size, but the muscles lying under and around the breasts can be lifted and tightened. This will keep breasts firm and lift a sagging bustline. Do this exercise in front of a mirror at first if possible. If you are doing it correctly, you should see your breasts jump up and down as you push.

Cross arms and grip inner wrists. Push hands hard against and up arms, as if pushing up sleeves. Repeat ten times.

6 This excellent exercise is specially for tightening the muscles in the upper arms to get rid of flab. It will also relax shoulders and tone up pectoral muscles.

Move from shoulders, arms stretched out hard, fists clenched. Make ten fast, tiny circles in backwards direction.

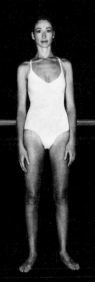
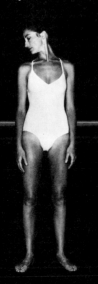
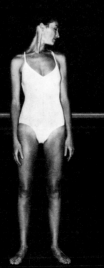
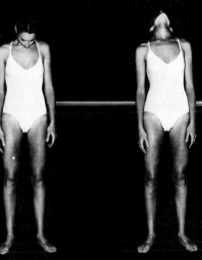

Stand up straight and tall, feet slightly apart and head held erect.

With shoulders still, turn your head to the right pushing round with chin; turn head to left and push again.

Let head fall forwards so that you can feel muscles down the back of your neck are stretched.

Drop head back, chin pointing right up, pulling muscles under throat. Straighten head, repeat five times. 63

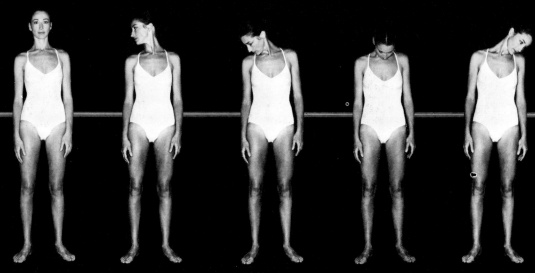

9 The continuous sweeping movement of this exercise relaxes the neck muscles and is useful for releasing the tensions that build up in this area, often causing headaches.

Stand straight and tall, head erect. Twist your head until you look over your right shoulder.

Now relax your neck, making your head feel heavy, and start to roll your head down and forwards.

Continue the movement, sweeping down and across your chest, lifting up towards your left shoulder.

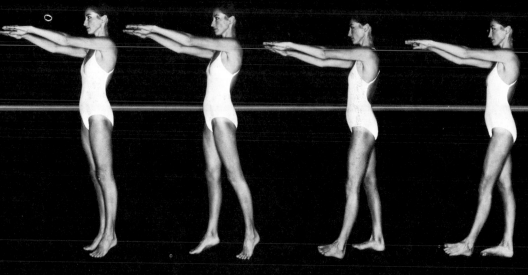

11 After a long day, your feet often feel the strain more than any other part of your body. Simply changing your shoes for a pair with a different heel height will do a lot to relax foot and calf muscles, but this walking and gripping exercise will tackle the problem far more thoroughly and will keep your muscles strong and supple. It will also strengthen the arches under your feet and help to prevent flat feet.

Stand straight, feet flat on ground, arms held out in front. Raise yourself up on toes as high as you can.

Take two steps forwards in this position, keeping as high on toes as you can without losing balance.

Then take two steps on your heels, toes lifted as high as possible, then two steps on the outside of feet.

13 This exercise strengthens your grasp and stretches and relaxes the muscles down the backs of your hands.

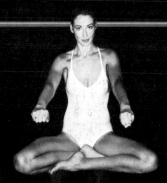

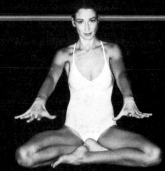

14 A finger-spreading exercise which helps to extend the span of your hands and keep your fingers supple.

Sit cross-legged, back straight, and hold arms out in front of you, fists clenched strongly.

Now unclench them quickly and firmly, spreading fingers as wide as you can. Repeat ten times.

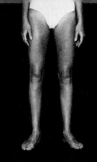

to be kept especially supple as they govern our expression and, with tension, lines form around mouth, eyes and forehead. This exercise may make you look rather grim, but it is excellent for the muscles in the neck and chin, for tightening the skin over the cheek-bones, and for lifting the breasts as it pulls up the whole network of muscles over the upper chest. If possible, do this exercise in front of a mirror and then spend a couple of minutes pulling other faces at yourself until you feel all your facial muscles relaxed.

Roll head back over left shoulder, lifting chin high, then reverse swing from left to right. Repeat five times.

Stand tall, looking straight ahead, and completely relax all the muscles in your face and neck.

Tighten face, chin and neck muscles, grimacing hard and pulling mouth down. Relax and repeat ten times.

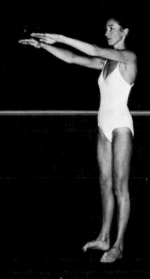

12 The following four exercises work to keep the hands supple and strong and help to protect them against stiffening and problems such as rheumatism and arthritis. This first exercise is particularly good for stretching the fingers\and knuckles and also the span between thumb and fore-finger.

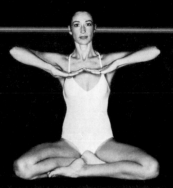

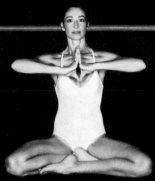

Stop and relax. Curl your toes under as though trying to grasp a pencil. Repeat cycle five times.

Sitting cross-legged, back straight, put finger tips together lifting elbows to make backs of hands curve.

Push thumbs down bringing arches together, stretching fingers. Push hands towards each other in bouncing movements.

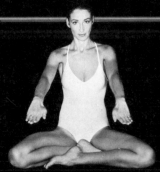

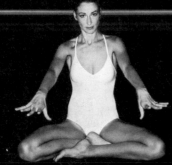

15 Try a finger-circling exercise to help keep the fingers supple and knuckle joints loose. It will also help to improve your co-ordination. It is very much harder than it looks.

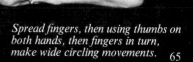

Sit cross-legged, back straight, arms out in front. Stretch hands, fingers together, until backs arch.

Now spread thumbs and fingers, opening as far and as wide as you can. Repeat quickly ten times.

Spread fingers, then using thumbs on both hands, then fingers in turn, make wide circling movements.

programme and continue them until the toning-up is done. You can then either keep them all going or just one or two from the group as you wish. Many of these exercises are graded from very simple to those suitable for advanced exercisers only. Take note and judge your capabilities so as not to risk strain, particularly of your back.

long time to reshape, so don't expect miracles after only a few weeks. But be persistent and results will come. Your legs will probably feel very stiff and sore when you first start, but don't take any days off to rest. Begin with the warm-up routine and go through the following exercises daily. Gradually your muscles will loosen, then start to firm up.

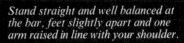

16 This first exercise stretches your calf and ankle muscles. If you get cramp, stamp your feet until it goes and then start again.

Stand straight and well balanced at the bar, feet slightly apart and one arm raised in line with your shoulder.

Raise yourself slowly up on to toes as high as you can, stretching calf and ankle muscles. Repeat ten times.

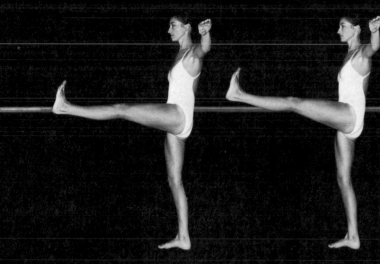

18 This is a tough three-in-one exercise, but it is the best all-round exercise to shape up your legs; it really makes the front thigh muscles work. Remember to keep your back absolutely straight throughout and take all the strain in your thigh muscles.

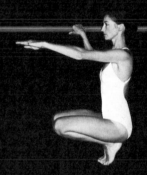

Keeping legs straight, turn toes up as hard as you can, really pulling toes towards you.

Do several little lifts, pulling leg higher, until thigh muscles really work. Repeat five times with both legs.

Sideways to bar, arm raised in front, squat on balls of feet, knees slightly apart, heels together. Do ten little bounces.

19 This exercise also works on the thigh muscles. The lower you can hold your starting position unsupported, the more effective the exercise will be. Remember that this is a thigh exercise and it is these muscles and your tummy muscles which must take the strain, never your back, although the exercise will help to keep your back supple.

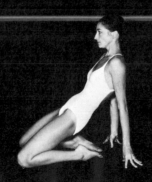
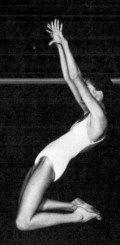
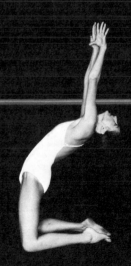

Kneel with knees slightly apart, toes almost together. Keeping body straight, lean back on finger tips.

Without moving upper part of body, thrust forwards from hips with pelvic bone, pushing arms forwards and up.

Follow movement through until your thighs, body and arms reach straight up and then over.

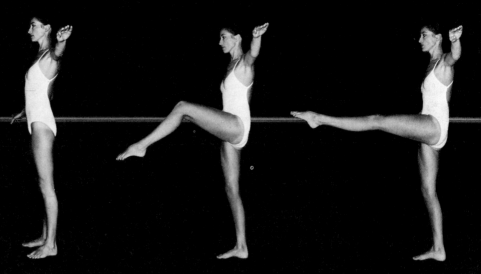

17 Here is the ideal exercise for toning up lazy thigh muscles. You should really feel them work when you pull your leg right up. It will be agony to begin with, but persevere.

Stand sideways to the bar, feet apart, back straight, left arm out at shoulder level, right hand supporting lightly.

With toes pointed, bend your left knee and lift knee as high as possible in front of you.

Now stretch your leg until it is really straight and point your toes as hard as you can.

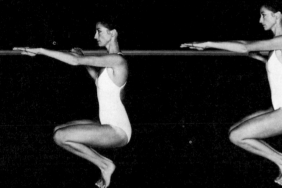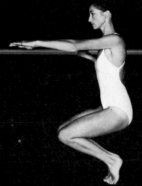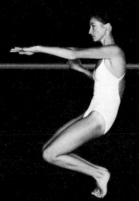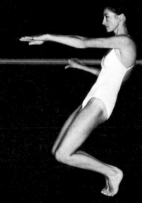

Keeping back straight, heels together, lift body a little off heels, open thighs wide and push, push knees open to count of ten.

Start again, squatting on heels, but this time up on toes. Lifting body up a little, hold, then a little more, hold again.

Without moving upper part of body, lift a little more and push pelvis forwards to make front thigh muscles really work.

Raise body higher again and push pelvis further forwards. Hold for count of three. Relax down. Repeat five times.

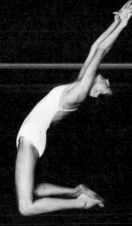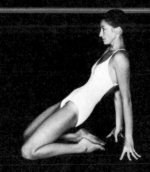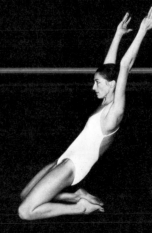

20 This is another rather difficult exercise and you may not be able to do it straightaway. If you find it too much for you, continue with the other exercises in the routine and come back to this one when you are stronger. When you do finally master it, you will know that you are on the way to getting your legs properly in trim. Again, it is very important to remember that it is always thighs and tummy which must take the strain, not the back.

Move arms through, arching back, still holding with thighs and tummy. Swing forwards to starting position. Repeat five times.

Kneel with knees apart, toes touching. Lean back in straight line, supported by finger tips.

Holding position, quickly raise arms. Don't let body drop back ; rely on thigh muscles for support.

21 This exercise, which strengthens thigh and stomach muscles, is a very good one for beginners with weak muscles. If you are very weak, you can start by walking against a wall. Beginners may only be able to do the small walking movements, but as you get stronger progress to bigger and bigger strides. You may feel an ache across your ribs at first; this is a good indication that lazy muscles are starting to work.

STOMACH

Even a thin person can have a flabby tummy because the stomach muscles are not used enough. These exercises work to firm and flatten the stomach and trim the waistline. They do wonders for a tummy loose after a crash diet. The first two are good for beginners or the over-weight, and

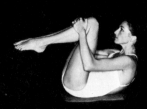 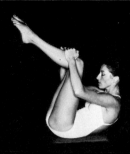 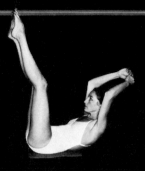

Lie on a carpet on your back, holding knees, toes pointed. Curl body to bring knees and head together.

Gradually unfold to raise your legs towards ceiling, always keeping spine pressed flat to floor.

With spine still flat, and holding with tummy and thigh muscles, lift legs higher and raise arms.

mothers can do them six weeks after childbirth to regain their figures. If you get menstrual cramps, these exercises practised regularly help relieve abdominal tension.

22 This exercise is the key to the whole routine. It teaches you to 'roll-in' the pelvis so that your spine rests flat on the floor. Practise this hard to strengthen your tummy muscles before starting the other exercises, to ensure that your back is not strained. If strain is felt, practise this exercise some more.

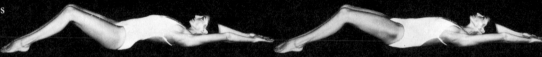

Lie on a carpet with knees bent. Your back will be just arched off floor so you can slide a hand under.

Now push spine flat against carpet, rolling pelvis in and pulling on tummy muscles; your bottom will

come slightly off floor. If you do the exercise correctly, inner thigh muscles will appear to jump out.

24 Beginners with weak stomach muscles may need to tuck their feet under the edge of a bed or sofa at first to do this exercise. As you get stronger, you should be able to support yourself.

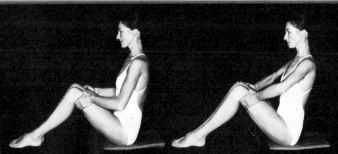 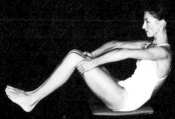

Sit on a carpet on floor, bend your knees and grip thighs, elbows bent, keeping spine straight.

Begin to push backwards by gradually 'rolling-in' pelvis, pulling with stomach muscles, elbows bent.

Move slowly backwards, gently pushing each vertebra into ground. Beginners may have to stop here.

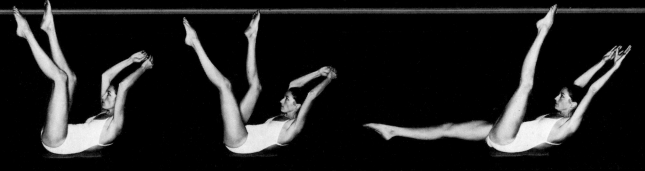

Now take tiny walking steps in the air, pulling arms and shoulders up, feeling strain in diaphragm area.

As you get stronger, continue, with waist and lower back still pressed to floor, gradually increasing length of step.

Now move on to really big walks. With arms stretched out, swing legs wide, still keeping spine on floor. If back starts to arch,

stop immediately, you will have lost the movement and may damage your back. Start exercise again.

23 This is another simple exercise for beginners to strengthen and tighten the tummy muscles. If you are weak, it is a temptation to strain from the neck when reaching up and this causes tension which you are trying to avoid. Shake your head, relax and start again, being sure to pull this time with the tummy muscles. You may ache a little across the shoulders at first, but this will go as muscles in the stomach get stronger and take the strain. Remember to 'roll-in' well so your back doesn't arch and strain.

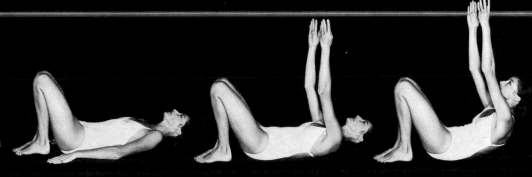

Lie on a carpet on your back. With feet flat on floor, bend knees and bring heels close to your bottom.

'Roll-in' pelvis, spine flat to floor as in previous exercise, and raise arms straight up to ceiling.

Stretch up, up, up, lifting head and shoulders off floor, hold, then relax. Do five repeats; fifty with practice.

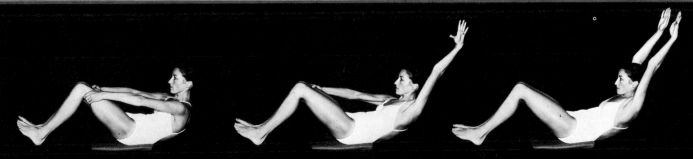

As you get stronger, you will be able to get lower on ground, arms almost straight, stomach still taking strain.

Keeping body still, lift one arm above head, pulling with other arm in little bounces to feel pull in diaphragm.

With practice, you will be able to raise both arms still keeping pelvis tucked in. If back arches, stop

immediately and start again. Sit up, stretch to ceiling and return to first position. Repeat five times.

69

25 This is an advanced exercise and should only be done when you can do all the other stomach exercises in the routine without strain. When you can complete this one successfully, your stomach muscles are really strong and firm. All beginners should see this as their goal. As you get better, do the exercise with legs wide apart and try to put your head on the floor between them.

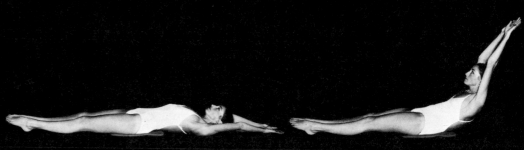

Stretch out on a carpet with legs together, arms straight behind head, spine flat on floor. 'Roll-in' pelvis.

Keep arms still and slowly lift your body off ground by using stomach and diaphragm muscles only.

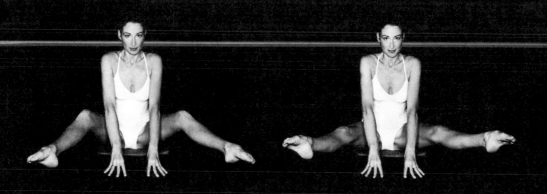

27 This exercise works on the stomach and thigh muscles, flattening the tummy and shaping the legs, but here the addition of the foot circling action relaxes feet and shapes up ankles.

Lean forwards on to your fingers and raise legs, taking strain in thighs, pointing your toes.

Stretch legs out hard, pointing toes as much as you can, hold, then lower to start position and repeat five times.

As you get stronger do second and third positions, bending and stretching, five times before lowering feet.

28 This is another thigh and tummy strengthening exercise. As you get stronger, make a wider and wider scissor movement so that eventually you are stretching your legs to their full capacity.

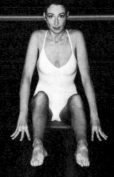
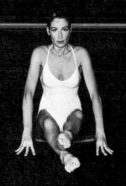
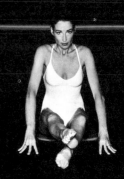

Sit straight, lower back against wall, knees bent, legs slightly apart, fingers on floor outside legs.

Lean on fingers and straighten legs, pointing toes. Cross legs at ankles with small scissor movement.

Open and re-cross the other way. Repeat movement at least ten times, making wider scissors if you can.

STOMACH AND THIGHS

This sequence of exercises is primarily designed to firm and strengthen the thighs, but also involves using the stomach muscles and so will tighten those, too. Once again it is a tough routine and you will doubtless feel sore and sorry at first. Don't give up or, worse still, cheat! Persevere and the exercises will produce great results. If you take a break between exercises, remember always to start again with knees bent as in first position in first exercise, right. This will prevent back strain.

26 The first exercise stretches and strengthens the thigh muscles and is excellent for calves and ankles too.

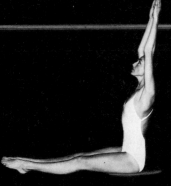

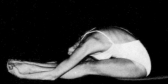

Sit up straight and stretch towards ceiling as hard as you can, then swing forwards, bending from hips.

Bending forwards, grasp feet and rest head on knees. Lie back curling spine into floor. Repeat five times.

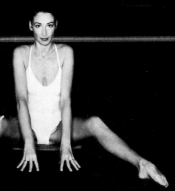

Sit on a carpet, lower back against wall. With legs apart, bend knees and place finger tips in front.

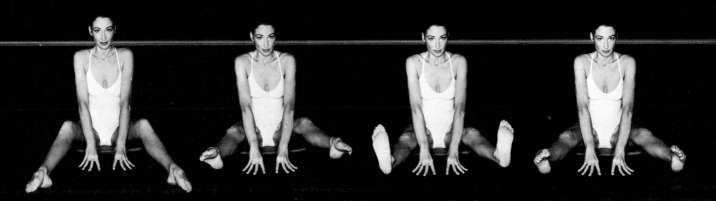

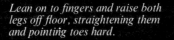

Sit against wall as before, legs open, knees bent and finger tips on floor in front of you.

Lean on to fingers and raise both legs off floor, straightening them and pointing toes hard.

Pull toes up and begin to circle feet, supporting yourself with fingers and stomach and thigh muscles.

Do complete circles with your feet, ten clockwise, ten anti-clockwise. Lower to starting position and relax.

BOTTOMS

If your job means sitting down for most of the day you are more than likely to develop a droopy bottom. So if you are worried that your backview is getting flabby and soft, these exercises are for you. They will tighten and 'lift' the cheeks of your bottom and gradually smooth away pads of fat that may have built up just below the waist.

29 This exercise tightens up buttocks. Do not expect to be able to raise your leg much in this position.

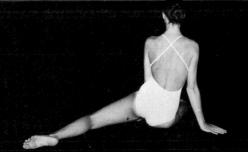

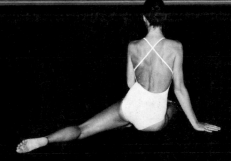

Sit on floor, right leg bent across in front of you, left leg stretched out to the side and slightly bent.

Lean slightly into left leg, roll left hip forwards and lift leg off floor. Lower; repeat five times each side.

30 All flabby bottoms will benefit from this exercise, which is also good for thigh muscles. It is important that the movement comes from the hip. If you are doing the exercise correctly you will only be able to raise your leg very little.

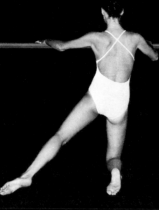

Kneel on right knee at bar and extend left leg diagonally behind you slightly bent. Lean into this leg.

31 This is a standing version of the two previous exercises and works on the bottom from a different angle, while also helping to tighten up thighs.

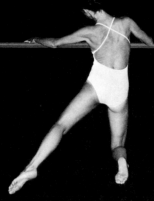

Without moving body, roll left hip forwards, raise and lower whole leg five times. Repeat with right leg.

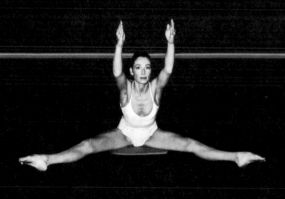

Keeping back straight, bend forwards from hips only, pointing toes hard and reaching forwards with hands.

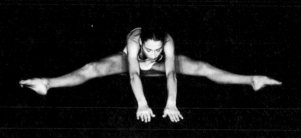

Stretch forwards, keeping legs straight and wide, still bending from hips. Place hands on floor in front of you.

33 This exercise first stretches and lifts the spine; the forward stretching movements work on the inner thigh muscles and loosen the hip joints. It is a tough exercise and the last stretching position, which pulls on muscles under the thighs, knees and calves, will probably take some practice.

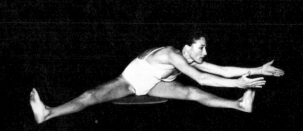

Sit on a carpet with legs wide apart, arms up to stretch spine, knees pressed to floor, toes pulled up.

Now swing across and stretch out towards your left foot, reaching out and keeping legs straight to feel pull.

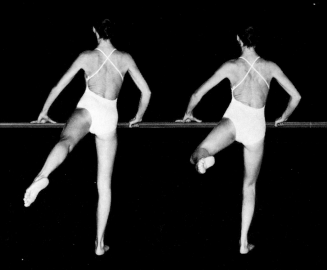

STRETCHING

Stretching exercises make your body supple and help you to move gracefully. As you grow older these exercises become increasingly important, because as you become less active your muscles start to contract and you can develop stiffness and muscular aches and

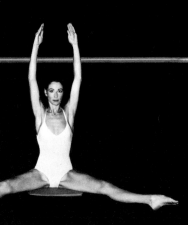

pains. Many of these problems can be prevented if you keep your muscles strong and supple. Do this stretching routine every day if you can, to finish your exercise session, and your whole body will benefit.

32 The first exercise is particularly good for stretching the inner thigh muscles and loosening the hip joints.

Stand facing bar, both legs straight, and raise left leg behind you leaning slightly into raised leg, body still.

Keeping left leg as high as possible, bend both legs; straighten and bend five times. Repeat with right leg.

Sit on a carpet with legs as wide apart as possible. Keep back straight and stretch upwards with arms.

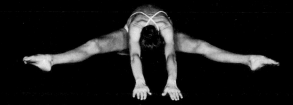

Gently slide palms along floor as far away as possible, feeling muscles in inner thigh really stretch.

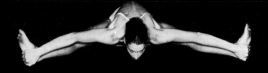

Stretch arms out and clasp under feet. Pull, pull, pull and try to touch floor with chin. Sit up and relax.

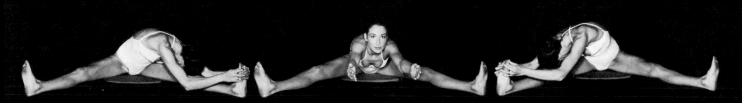

Lean over, clasp your foot and pull, trying to get your head as low as possible on to your knee.

Swing round and stretch right out in front of you, keeping back and legs straight, still bending from hips.

Stretch over right foot, then clasp foot, pulling head down. Straighten up; repeat five times.

34 Try this exercise to stretch the lower half of your body as before, but here the sideways bends and twists should really pull hard at the waist, stretching and slimming, keeping middle supple.

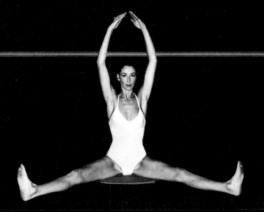 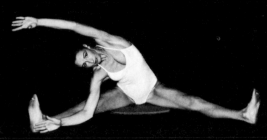

Sit as before, back straight, arms reaching up to stretch spine, legs as wide apart as possible, toes pulled up.

Lean over to right foot, resting elbow on floor in front of knee. Bring arm right over until you feel waist pulling.

35 This exercise looks impossible but it isn't at all, once you have learned to control your balance. To begin with it is safest to do the exercise in the middle of the room, just in case you topple over backwards. If you can master it, the exercise will really stretch and shape up legs.

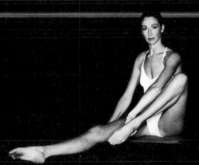 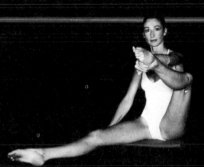

Sit on a carpet, back straight, legs straight and slightly apart. Hold left instep in left hand, toes pointed.

Lift leg as high as you possibly can, pulling up with your hand.

36 As you grow older the muscles on your instep can shorten and contract, causing a shuffling rather than a graceful walk. The way to prevent this is to keep the muscles well stretched and supple, which is what this exercise does. You will find that as your feet become more supple you will be able to raise your knees much higher.

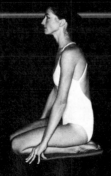 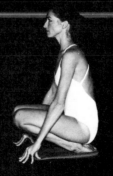 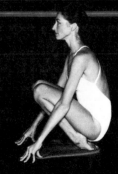

Kneel with knees together and sit back on your heels. Lean slightly forwards and rest on finger tips.

Taking weight on fingers and instep raise knees. Hold for count of three, lower, repeat ten times.

Gradually, as muscles stretch and loosen up, lift knees a little higher, until you can get them right up.

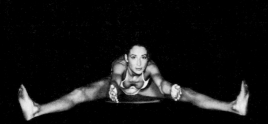

Bending forwards from hips make a low sweep across, keeping back straight and reaching as far forwards as you can.

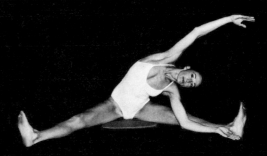

Swing over until left elbow rests on floor by knee, arm reaching over pulling waist. Sit up and repeat five times.

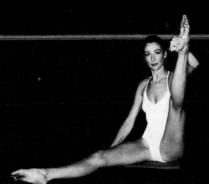

Now straighten leg, pushing knee down with hand if necessary. Bend and straighten five times. Relax and repeat with other leg.

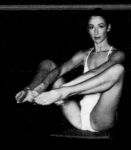

Clasp both insteps and lift legs up slowly, taking time to find your natural balance.

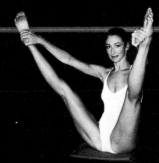

Raise and straighten both legs and hold. Try to bend and straighten legs five times, keeping back perfectly straight. Relax.

EXERCISES TO RELIEVE TENSION

Unless you are very lucky, and lead an unusually stress-free life, tension will inevitably build up in muscles during the day.

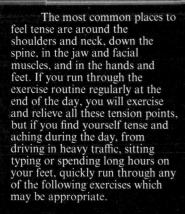

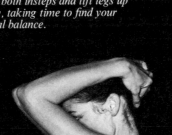

To relieve a headache, clasp one hand over the other and place both on back of head at base of skull.

Tucking chin in, firmly pull head forwards with several small tugs. Relax and repeat.

The most common places to feel tense are around the shoulders and neck, down the spine, in the jaw and facial muscles, and in the hands and feet. If you run through the exercise routine regularly at the end of the day, you will exercise and relieve all these tension points, but if you find yourself tense and aching during the day, from driving in heavy traffic, sitting typing or spending long hours on your feet, quickly run through any of the following exercises which may be appropriate.

Neck and shoulders. Any of the head circling exercises, nos 8-9. Elbow circling. Exercise no 4. Hands. Hand clasping and spreading exercises, nos 12-15. Feet. Toe and heel walking, no 11. Face and jaw. Jaw stretching exercise, no 10. The following facial exercises may also help.
1 With head upright, try to touch nose with tongue. Repeat five times.
2 Open mouth as wide as you can, as though screaming, opening eyes at the same time, hold for count of three. Relax and repeat five times.
3 Give big false smile, keeping mouth closed.
4 Blow out cheeks as though blowing up a difficult balloon.

Back. Try this exercise, based on sound orthopaedic principles, to relieve backache. Lie on a carpet on your back, bend knees and stretch arms back above head. Roll-in pelvis, pushing spine hard against floor so that bottom lifts slightly. Hold for count of three. Relax and repeat until aches and pains ease.

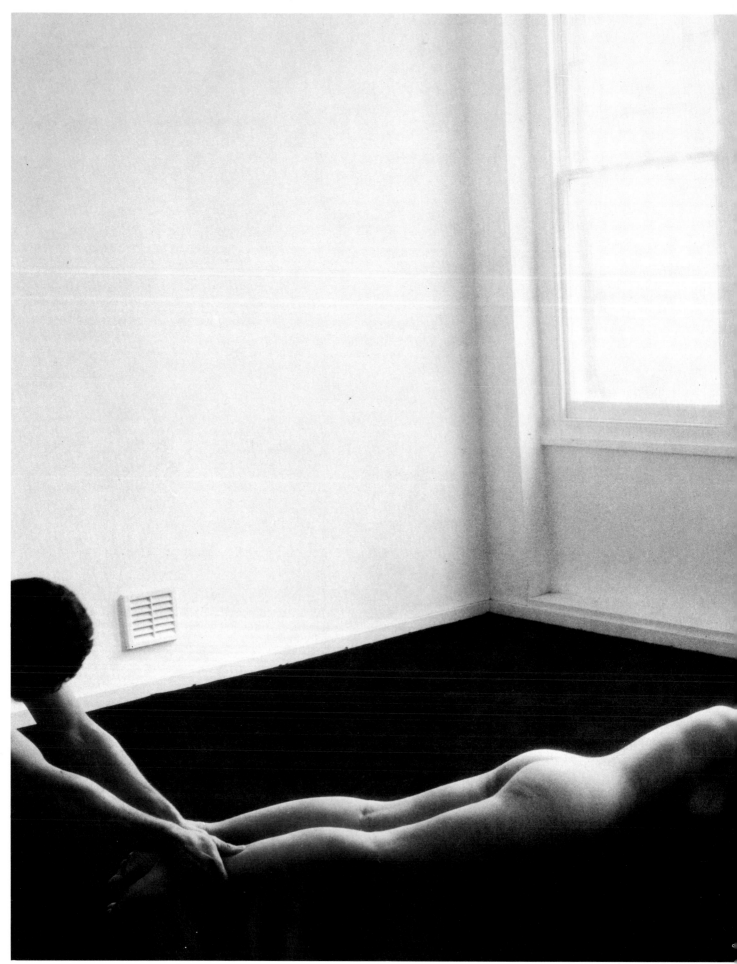

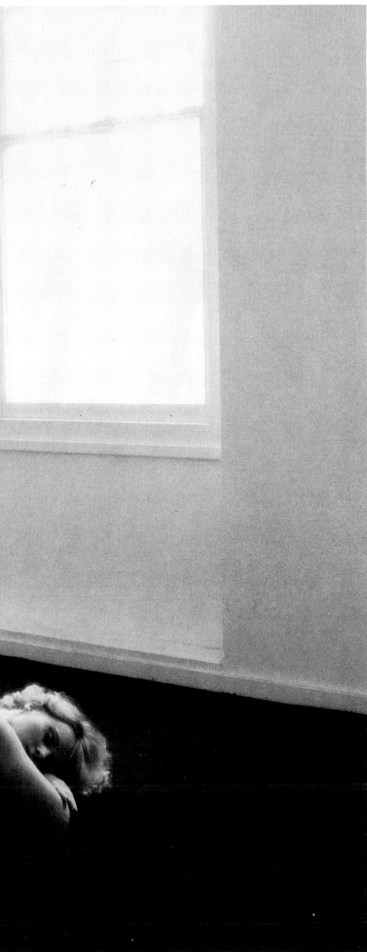

Massage

Massage is a non-addictive tranquillizer with absolutely no harmful side-effects. It relieves aches, pains and tensions and unknots the tangled muscles at the end of the day, and as the body relaxes so does the mind. It seems strange that something so beneficial should still be considered slightly shocking, permissible for athletes or for medicinal purposes but a little suspect if you enjoy it. Perhaps it has something to do with the rather dingy associations with dubious massage parlours, but massage is something which we all ought to learn how to do. There is no strange mystique involved, no laying on of hands, but a simple, warm extension of human care and touch.

On the following pages you will not find a full professional massage, but a series of easily learned massage movements that everyone can do, more than adequate to ease aching necks, shoulders, backs and heads after a hard day with the children, driving through traffic or working under pressure. They will also reduce bulges and tone up muscles and skin left flabby after a diet, when it is no longer padded out by fat. Although there are some parts of the body which it is quite impossible to reach, you can give yourself a perfectly satisfactory massage. Try to get into the habit of massaging face, hands and feet every day; even if you cannot go through the full routine, it will keep your joints supple and ache-free and facial massage, see pages 140 and 141, will not only make you feel better but look better too, since drawn muscles lift as you relieve strain and tension.

HOW TO MASSAGE

Work in a warm, well-ventilated room and ask the person you are going to massage to lie on a firm bed or a mattress on a table or the floor. Be sure that you are working at the right height. You must be comfortable; if you are bending too low over someone your back will get tired and ache, which will spoil the flow of the massage movements. If you are working on the floor, kneel down beside the mattress and you will be able to put your whole body into the massage. Wear comfortable clothes and either low heels or, better still, work in bare feet. Obviously, if you are massaging yourself, take off all your clothes and get really comfortable. Remove any jewellery that you are wearing or from the person you are massaging

if it is likely to snag or scratch and, although your finger nails don't need to be short, make sure they have no rough edges. Both you and your subject should be properly relaxed before you start work – deep breathing or music may help. If you are not relaxed, your movements will feel stiff and jerky to the person under your hands; if you are relaxed, your subject will be able to relax, too.

Warm and loosen your hands by rubbing them together and shaking them. Put on oil to ensure that they move smoothly without dragging the skin; a little light vegetable oil will do.

Use your whole body when you massage, not just your hands and wrists, or you will tire very quickly and the massage will be taut and jerky. If you work with your whole body it gives a stronger, but less rigid, pressure which is less likely to hurt. Use a strong pressure, the person you are massaging will soon tell you if it is too strong; light massage will only tickle and irritate and cause more tension, which defeats the object of the exercise. Keep your hands relaxed and supple so that they can adapt to the size, scale and contours of the body they are working on. Really <u>feel</u> the body, don't just touch it. A good massage flows from one movement to the next, with hands in continuous contact with the body. Never move hands jerkily or lift them suddenly or you will lose the flow and irritate your subject. Massage should both soothe and stimulate, so change the movements to give a variation of pace and pressure and glide imperceptibly from one movement to the next, touching with rhythmic continuity. To get from one place to another, fill in with basic stroking and circling so there are no abrupt changes. Practise your technique with a friend and criticize each other until you get the right flow and strength to your movements. You will find it tiring work, but well worth the effort once you have mastered it.

Warning: Never massage
- yourself or anyone else on a full stomach
- the stomach of a pregnant woman
- any varicose veins*
- any part of the body you know to be weak or injured
- anyone undergoing medical treatment
- anyone with a temperature
- a cardiac patient
- skin that is infected or inflamed, scarred or bruised.

Stop if any pain is experienced. The rule to remember is 'When in doubt, don't massage.'

BASIC MASSAGE MOVEMENTS

Variety is the key to good massage: variety of movement and variety of pace, strength and size of movement. Below is a list of the most useful massage movements. Try to learn and use them all, for a thorough, satisfying and really effective result.

Stroking and circling. This movement is exactly what the name implies. Keep your hands easy and relaxed and just stroke up the limb or the body towards the heart. When the movement is done gently, it soothes and relaxes; when done firmly, it stimulates the blood flow. Use it first of all to apply oil to the part of the body to be massaged; then work varying the rhythm, size and strength of the strokes. Move from large, flowing, basic strokes, using the whole hand in sweeping, flowing movements, to smaller circles with alternating hands, or stronger movements using both hands placed one on top of the other, or stroke with flats of hands in opposing directions, criss-crossing strongly over the body.

Kneading. Pretend you are kneading bread; pick up flesh and squeeze it. It is like pinching but a larger movement using the whole hand, pressing the fat between the fingers and the palm of the hand and thumb. Used properly it stretches and relaxes tight, contracted muscles. It also improves circulation and helps to eliminate fatigue. If it is strong and deep it is an effective aid to spot reducing.

Piano-playing. This movement is exactly as it sounds. It involves firm pressure with the fingers, running backwards and forwards across tense muscles as though you were picking out a tune or playing scales.

Pinching. This movement is the same as kneading, but using thumb and forefingers only.

Rotary movements. Using thumb or finger tips, these are small circling movements using a rather firm pressure.

Hacking, pounding, clapping or cupping. All of these are brief, brisk, rhythmic, bouncy movements applied with alternate hands to stimulate the flow of blood to the surface and help to break down fat. Hacking is done with the sides of the hands, with fingers straight but loose and relaxed. Try the movement on a table to gauge the strength you should use; if it doesn't hurt you, it shouldn't hurt the person you are massaging either. Pounding means using the side or flat of the fist, either loosely or more firmly clenched. Cupping or clapping is putting a cupped hand downwards on the flesh to give a loud clapping sound. Vary the speed and strength of all these movements, but do not use on any area where there are broken veins.*

Wringing and squeezing. Work with both hands, imagining that you are wringing out a cloth. Pick up the fat, twist and squeeze it. This movement is especially good for shifting the surplus fat that collects on thighs and upper arms and around waist.

MASSAGE MOVEMENTS TO LIFT A HEADACHE

Here are four invaluable methods of lifting a headache. Unfortunately, you cannot do them on yourself, so teach them to your husband or a friend so that you too can get relief. Massage is far better for you than taking aspirin, and much more pleasant. The movements should be done in a quiet, darkened room.

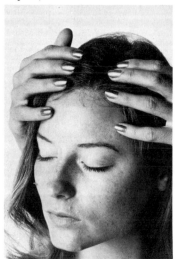

1 Place both hands on the top of the head and stroke the hair and head lightly with outspread finger tips. Bring the hands down to the end of the hair, flick them off and begin again, this time from the front of the head. Repeat both movements for several minutes.

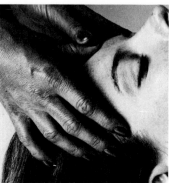

2 Place thumbs on top of each other and press down firmly, making a series of small pressures from the bridge of the nose, up across the centre of the forehead, continuing in a line over the head and down to the base of the skull.

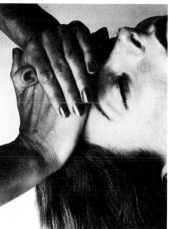

3 Cup hands one over the other and press down firmly on the forehead, release and press down again. Repeat several times.

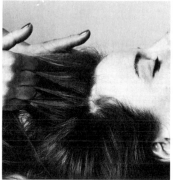

4 Run your fingers through the hair, pulling it gently but firmly towards you.

MASSAGING THE BACK

Most tension is felt up and down the spine, in and around the shoulders and the nape of the neck, and at the base of the spine. Thus the most important part of massage is the back. Once this is relaxed, all tautness gone and knotted muscles smoothed, the person you are massaging will be well on the way to feeling completely relaxed all over.

Back massage movements
The directions of movement for a back massage are shown on the photograph opposite. They mostly form circles and triangles. Circles sweep right up from the base of the spine to circle the shoulder blades. Smaller circular movements can be done on the buttocks and shoulder blades separately. Circles also move up from the buttocks, out across the pelvis, up the back and over the shoulders. Small rotary thumb movements follow the arrowed lines up both sides of the spine, from the top of the buttocks up towards the waist, from the top of the spine out to the shoulders, and up the back of the neck on to the skull. Supplement these movements with lots of circling and stroking, as shown on page 81, kneading, wringing and pummelling any bulges of surplus fat.

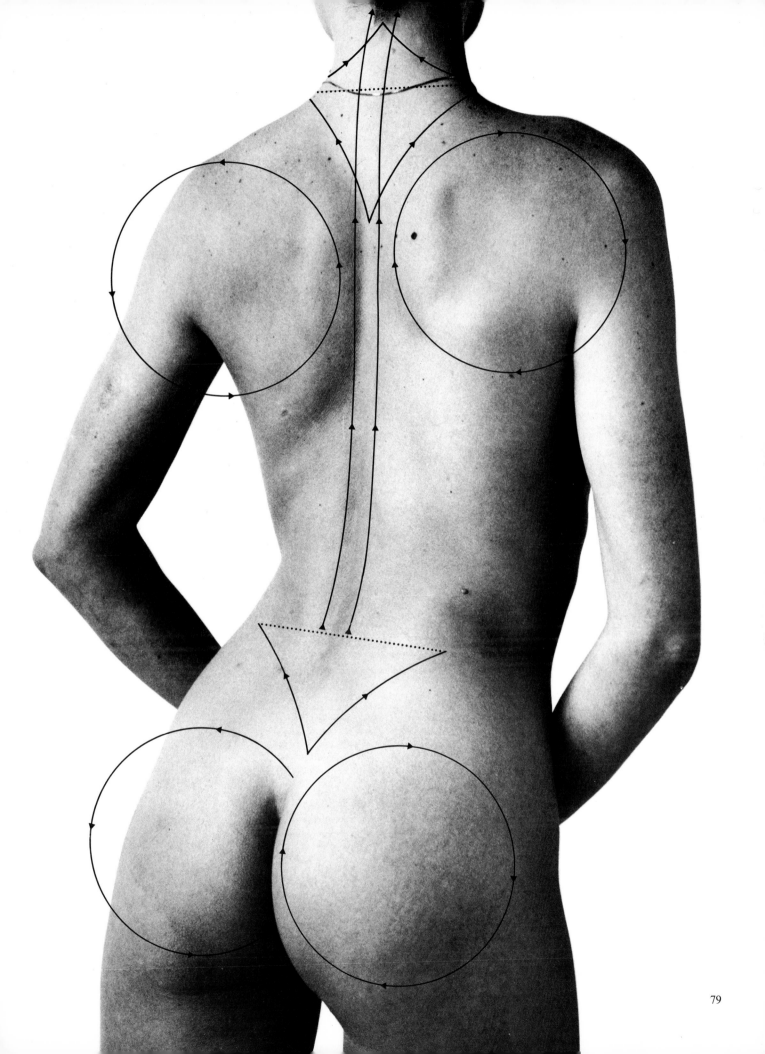

Massaging someone else should be hard work, but also a warm and satisfying experience. You must use your whole body to give strength and flow to the various movements, so wear comfortable clothes and kick your shoes off. Always warm and oil your hands first. Changes of pace and pressure are the secrets of good massage. Keep your hands in continuous contact with the body.

This first section shows how to massage from the soles of the feet, up the back of the legs to the bottom. Try to keep the movements continuous and always press too hard rather than too softly – you will soon be told if it hurts! Work slowly up the body massaging each foot and leg in ·turn and letting your hands respond to the contours of the body you are massaging.

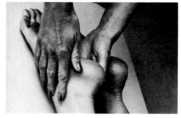

With finger tips, stroke with circular movements around foot and ankle.

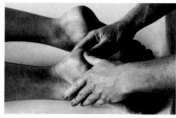

Make strong, small rotary thumb movements along sole of foot.

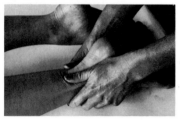

Small rotary movements to release tension around Achilles heel tendon.

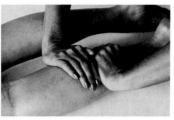

With both hands together, press and push up back of calf and stroke down.

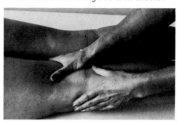

Stroke firmly up and round leg from behind knee to top of thigh.

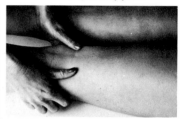

Small rotary thumb movements up centre back of leg; stroke to finish.

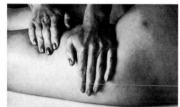

With flat hands, knead thigh by firmly criss-crossing across flesh.

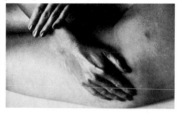

Press one hand on the other to give more pressure; circle firmly on thigh.

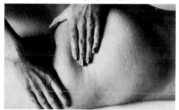

Using both hands, wring and squeeze surplus flesh at top of thigh.

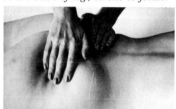

Knead and wring flesh where fat builds up at top of buttocks.

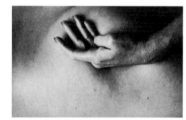

Circle hands round and round deeply into hollow cheeks of buttocks.

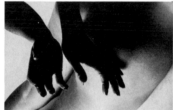

Make firm hacking movements with sides of hands on bottom and thighs.

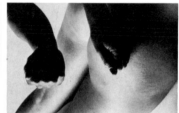

Repeat last movement but this time pound with clenched fists.

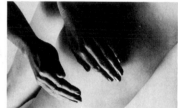

Cup hands and clap them up and down on bottom and thighs.

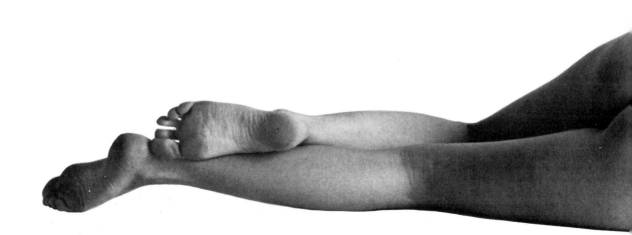

80

The back is one of the main areas in which tension builds up and a good masseuse can relieve back-ache and relax the body. The movements in this section are made up of wide sweeping motions and small rotating ones (see directional massage chart, page 79). Work up the back, concentrate on tense muscles in the neck, and finish with long relaxing strokes down the back again.

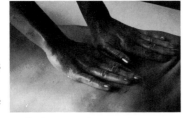
Make large, circling, stroking movements over back working up and out.

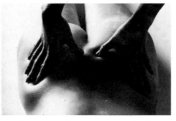
Find small indentation at top of buttocks and rotate with thumbs.

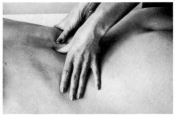
Small rotating movements with thumbs together at base of spine.

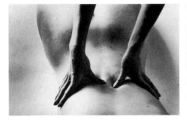
Continue small rotating thumb movements up either side of spine.

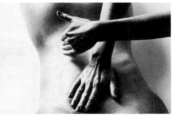
Make circular movements over whole of back, alternating hands.

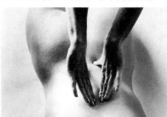
Thumb and fingers spread, apply springy pressure either side of spine.

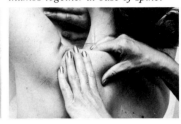
Knead and wring firmly round shoulder muscles and base of neck.

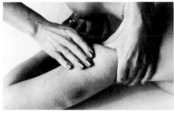
Squeeze and wring around front of shoulder, loosening muscles.

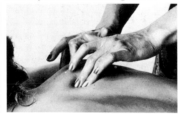
Make firm piano-playing movements across shoulder muscles.

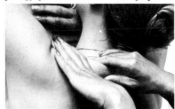
Squeeze and knead knotted muscles around base of neck and shoulder.

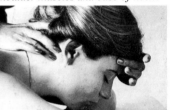
Firm, rhythmic, circular movements with finger tips up neck and skull.

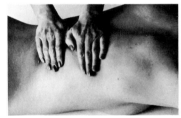
Work up and down back criss-crossing firmly with flat of hands.

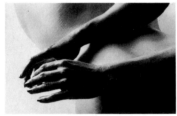
Rest lower arms together across back and gently stretch them apart.

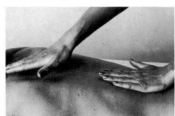
With alternate hands, stroke firmly and rhythmically right down back.

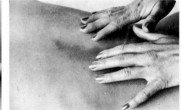
Draw finger tips lightly down whole of back in final relaxing movement.

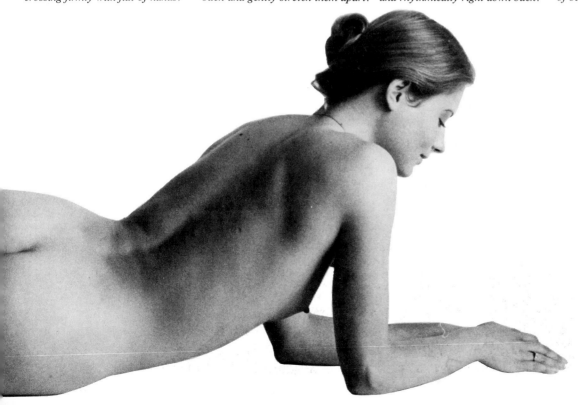

Massaging the head, neck and face can bring relief from tension, headaches and eyestrain and relieve congestion. Start by taking a strong line with knotted neck muscles and work gently upwards. Obviously, when working on the face itself your hands need to be well oiled as the skin is very delicate, but remember to make sure they are wiped clean before working behind the hair line!

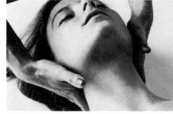

Place hands well behind neck and stroke firmly upwards on each side.

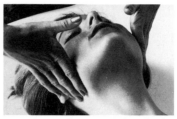

Continue stroking gently but firmly, bringing hands along to jaw line.

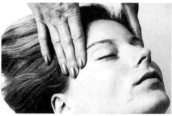

Press finger tips on temples and make small rotating movements.

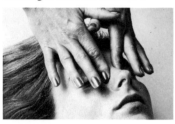

With oiled finger tips, lightly make circles around eyes and brow bone.

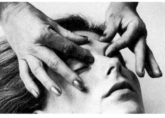

With thumb and forefinger, pinch firmly along line of brow.

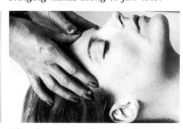

Thumbs on top of one another, press in a line up centre of forehead.

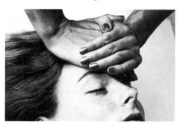

Cupping hands one over other, press down and relax on forehead.

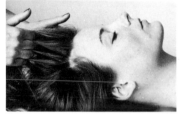

Draw fingers through hair and pull gently up and towards you.

This section deals with massaging the stomach and abdomen. As this is a particularly delicate part of the body it should be treated extremely carefully; it is one area where pressure should not be applied too hard. Massage round the breasts, never over them, and never massage the stomach of a pregnant woman. However, massage in this area can make you feel wonderfully fit and trim.

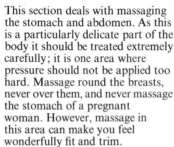

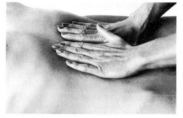

Hands flat, make sweeping circular movements up lower abdomen.

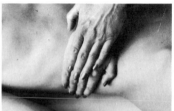

Press and pull across body with two hands, then criss-cross.

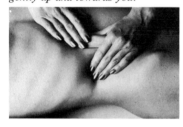

With firm fingers, pinch your way across waist and abdomen.

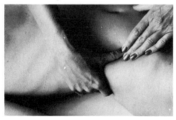

Working from sides of waist with both hands, knead and wring bulges.

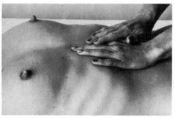

Make sweeping circular movements up centre of chest and round breasts.

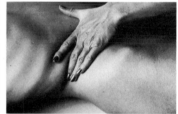

With hands round under waist, stroke up firmly, lifting and pulling.

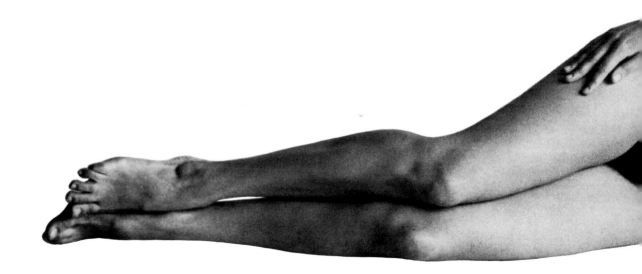

82

This section deals with massaging arms and hands. Massage of the hands is very similar to that of the feet and is equally effective. On the hands, the areas concentrated on are palm, fingers and wrist. On the arms, the upper arm is the part most prone to fat and rough skin and massage can do much to help in this area. Stroking movements should move up the arm.

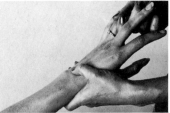

Firmly stroke sides, pull, flex and rotate fingers; massage between each.

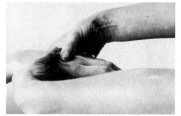

Using thumbs, make small, firm rotary movements over knuckles.

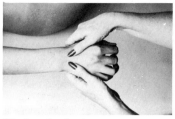

Work up back of hand with firm circling movements.

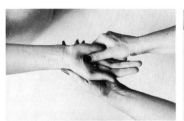

Turn hand over and make small rotary thumb pressures in palm.

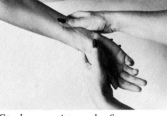

Stroke up wrist; make firm rotary thumb movements round wrist bones.

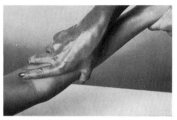

Work up lower arm, stroking and circling in upward direction.

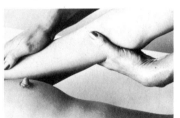

Stroke firmly up and round upper arm, knead and pinch the fat areas.

Massaging the feet and legs is very relaxing for the body. You need to take a firm grip on the feet, otherwise the feeling can be unbearably ticklish. Work along the foot and up the leg in continuous movements, stroking and kneading and applying pressure with the thumbs where necessary. Grip heel and toes and pull up and down and circle round to relax ankle.

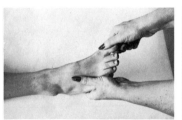

Pull each toe, press and rotate joints, small rotary movements between toes.

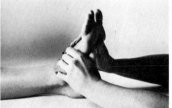

Press with rotary thumb movements, especially on ball of foot.

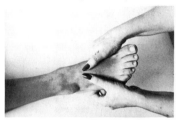

Circular thumb movements on top of foot, stroking firmly underneath.

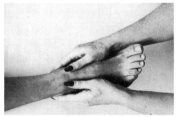

With finger tips, circle behind ankle and round Achilles tendon.

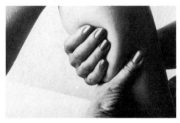

Knead up back of calf and circle in long upward strokes.

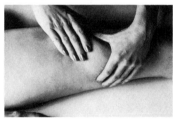

Knead and wring around knee; make rotating movements with thumb.

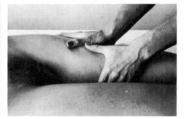

Wring and knead top and inside of thigh, firmly stroke up and round.

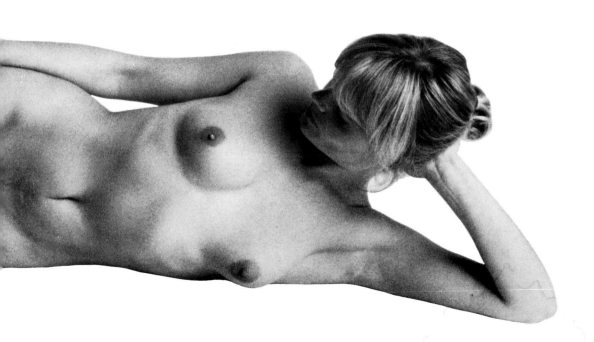

Although self-massage is never quite thorough enough to be completely reviving, you can reach most parts of the body where tension builds up. Strip off in a warm room, shake and rub hands to loosen and warm them. Apply a little light oil so that hands move smoothly over the body without dragging. Use wringing, kneading, pounding and hacking movements to break down excess fat.

This first massage sequence concentrates on the sides of the body, from neck to feet, taking in upper arms, thighs, knees, calves and feet. Work slowly down one side and then the other, breathing deeply to help your whole body relax. Spend a lot of time working around the neck and feet as these are the areas most affected by a long, tiring day, and massage here can be particularly beneficial.

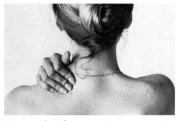
Rotary thumb movements across top of chest; reach over, knead shoulder.

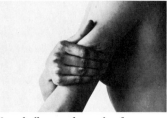
Knead elbow and muscle of upper arm; stroke up from wrist.

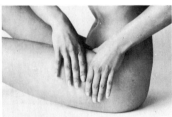
Wring, pinch and knead thigh. Also try hacking, cupping and pounding.

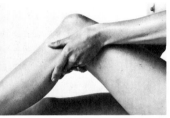
Stroke whole leg under and over with long, firm, upward movements.

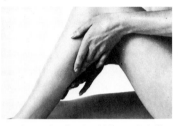
Stroke up back of calf from Achilles tendon and knead muscle firmly.

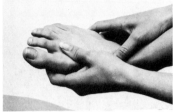
Make rotary thumb movements on top of foot and firmly stroke ankle.

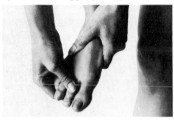
Pull, stroke and rotate toes. Make rotary movements between each.

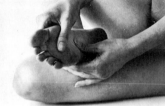
Press and relax with thumb, making rotary movements along sole of foot.

These exercises concentrate on the hands, which are often neglected. They teach you to massage the hand, palm, fingers and wrist. It is surprising how much tension can build up in your hands and massage here can help to relax your whole body. Massage before a manicure and always at night, rubbing your hands with cream or oil first. Make circling movements with wrists first to loosen up.

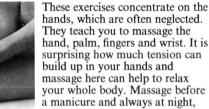

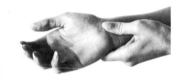
Stroke wrists and make small rotary thumb movements around bone.

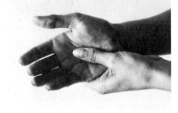
Stroke palm; press and make rotary movements all over with thumb.

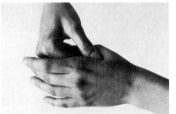
Knead between thumb and fingers with small circling movements.

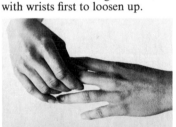
Stroke, pull, flex and rotate each finger; rub knuckles and joints.

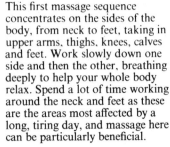

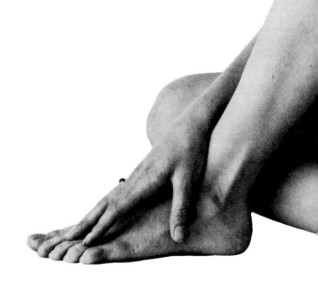

This section shows how to massage the neck and back of the head, marvellous for relieving headaches, and the back, hips and bottom. The back is one of the most difficult areas to massage yourself; you can only really get to grips with the lower area at the base of the spine. Nevertheless, massage here will relieve backache. Do these exercises sitting cross-legged comfortably on the floor.

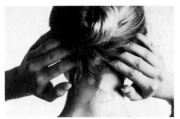

Using finger tips, make small firm rotary movements up back of skull.

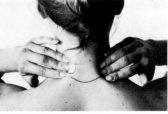

Work down neck making similar rotary movements with finger tips.

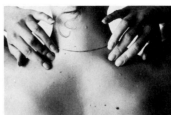

Make firm piano-playing movements out along each shoulder.

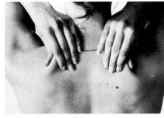

Reach as far down your back as you can, knead and pinch surplus flesh.

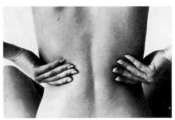

Circular movements with finger tips either side of spine; knead waistline.

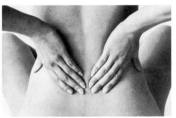

Start at base of spine and make rotary movements working upwards.

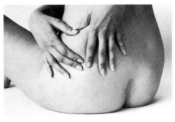

Knead and wring pads of fat which form around hip.

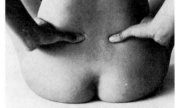

Place thumbs in two indentations near base of spine and rotate.

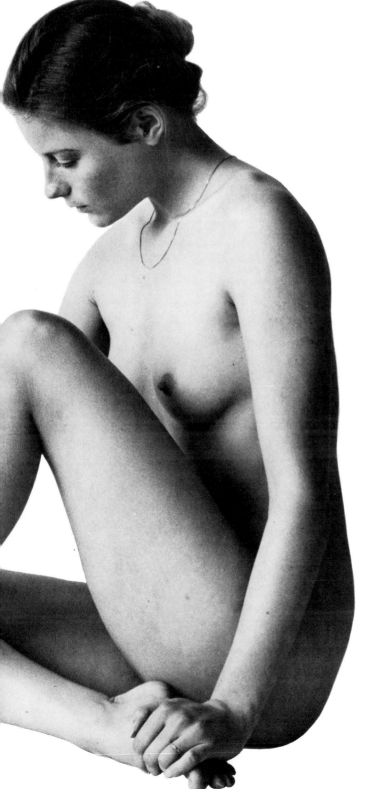

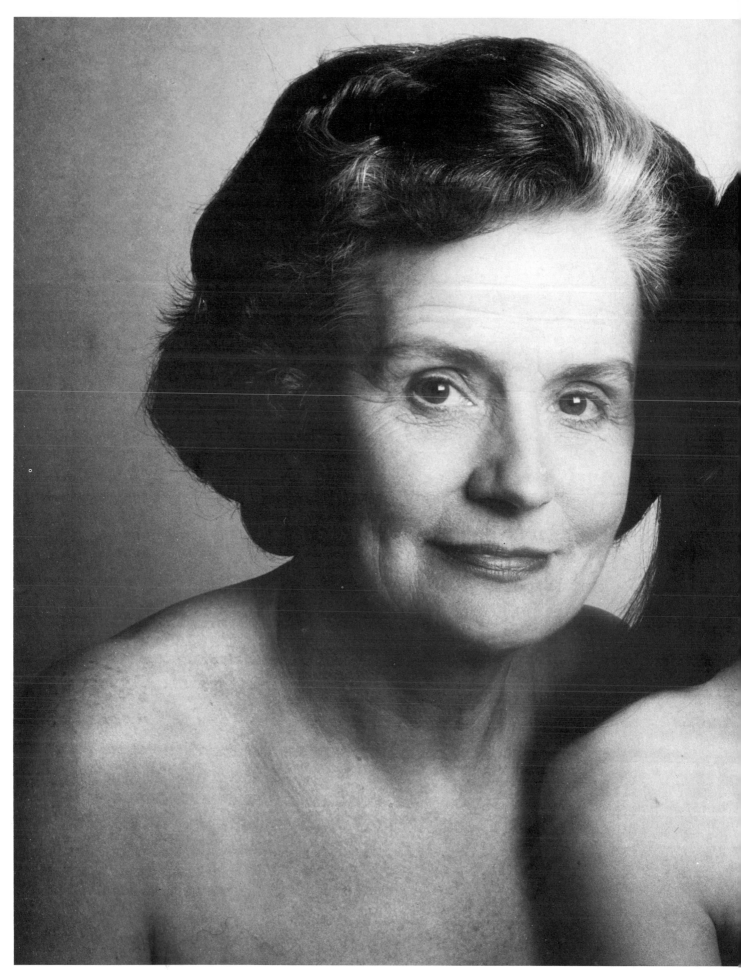

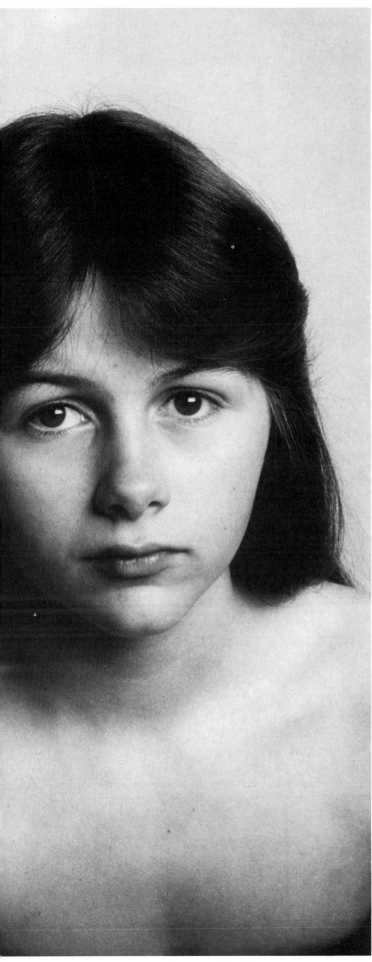

A Woman's Body

In the rush and confusion of modern life, we tend to go for appearances first and to let other things slide. We hope that by smoothing on a face, keeping our figures trim and hair clean and well cut, and dressing in a style that suits us, we will create an image to present to the world which reflects what we want to reveal of ourselves. Learning how to make the best of yourself is what this book is all about, but it is not just how you look to others which matters; how you feel inside about yourself also counts. If you feel quite happy inside your skin, then the confidence this gives you will irradiate your external appearance, no matter what the calendar says about your age or the mirror tells you about your shortcomings as regards conventional standards of beauty. But if the reverse is true for you, if you are puzzled or uneasy, possibly even a little fearful about what happens inside your body, particularly below the navel, then those feelings will also be betrayed on your face and in your bearing.

Understanding how your body works is an important key to understanding yourself, yet many women shudder at the idea of intimate acquaintance with their bodily functions. Bad enough having to cope with the physical demands made on you just because you are a woman – menstruation, pregnancy, menopause to name a few – without dwelling on the intimate details. Morbid, say some; hypochondria, say others; not quite nice, murmur the extra-delicate. But can you afford to risk your health and well-being by joining the 'shut your eyes and hope for the best' set?

Body knowledge obviously cannot tell you everything about yourself. To be aware of yourself as a whole person you also need to understand how you tick emotionally and mentally, and that is a lifelong process. However, more clues than you may imagine are embodied in your physical constitution, your state of health and the way you care for yourself.

What follows is a guide to the way a woman's body develops from the first signs of puberty through to menopause and beyond; how it functions reproductively and sexually; and how to cope with changes brought about by the circumstances of your life, your personal needs, your health and your age. The purpose of this section is to give you all the information you require in order to be the mistress and not the slave of your body. Confident and well-informed, you will then be in a strong position to talk to your doctor on equal terms at the many times during your life when you may need to consult him or her.

THE ADOLESCENT

Adolescence is probably the most difficult period of life for anyone to go through. Boy or girl, the body is changing faster at this time than the developing mind can understand or the emotions control. For girls it is additionally complicated by the obvious changes in their appearance. Swelling breasts which appear too early and too big, or too late and too small, can cause profound misery and embarrassment. Even the most balanced girl will be plunged into depths of depression at times because she despairs of ever conforming to the ideal standard of beauty being beamed at her from all quarters – television advertisements, magazine articles, newspaper pin-ups and the like.

A girl's physical development draws attention to herself at a time when she is struggling with the internal conflict of moving from childhood into adulthood, and all the uncertainty, loss of security and fear of independence that that brings with it. Without realizing it, she is going through a profound identity crisis and there is nothing steadfast she can hold on to, not even her appearance, because that too is changing. In this confusing, disturbing time, what she needs above all else is support and understanding, even when she seems most hostile.

The best person to give her that help is her mother, yet it is a lamentable fact that many mothers still do not prepare their daughters for the experience of puberty and, in particular, for menstruation. They may put it off because they want to protect their child's innocence or fear to introduce ideas for which they consider she is not ready, or they foresee being forced into explanations about sex in general which they don't regard as appropriate for a girl of her age.

But if you listen to a young child asking about where he or she comes from, or the purpose of different parts of the body, you will realize that it is never the child who introduces shame and embarrassment into the discussion. When such questions are answered simply and directly, the child's curiosity is quickly satisfied and often the answer as quickly forgotten. But if the adult reveals dismay or disapproval, then those feelings are instantly communicated to the child, who won't cease wondering, but may stop asking. The body becomes an object of guilt and mystery.

Sexual jealousy – usually unrecognized, invariably unadmitted – is another reason why many mothers shirk informing their daughters. It can happen both ways. A mother sees her child growing into womanhood and inevitably the contrast between her daughter's firm young body and her own, perhaps grown slack and over-weight, becomes more marked. She sees her daughter's smooth, full face and recalls with a pang her own vanished youthful bloom. This can be especially bitter to the woman whose looks have always been of paramount importance to her because she has relied on them to bring her love, security and admiration.

A daughter may be jealous of her mother, and this is the more common case, in a different way, particularly if she has been taught that looks are all-important for success. She will notice the signs of age in her mother, perhaps repeatedly remark on them to her and to others, but silently she will be envying her mother's apparent self-confidence and sexual assurance, her ability to hold her own with any man who comes within her radius.

Fortunately, this is not a universal problem among mothers and daughters, but we are all guilty of forgetting or minimizing the pains of growing up. The crushes that many adolescent girls have – on an older girl, a teacher or a pop star – are also very typical of the age. While it may be tiresome to have to listen to endless eulogies about the beloved idol and to see your daughter alternating between wild enthusiasm and deep despondency, depending on how the 'love affair' is going, while treating you and the rest of the family with indifference or scorn

because 'you can't understand', console yourself with the thought that it is harmless and it will pass.

As an adult who is surely not so old that she cannot remember her own youthful crazes, it is up to you to steer a sensible, sympathetic course through your daughter's emotional storms. Above all, try not to over-react, either by unkind teasing or showing anger. She is not going to turn into a lesbian or a groupie overnight, but she may well become sullen and withdrawn for a while.

You may also find that you have to cope with your husband's jealousy when she starts going out with boyfriends. Many fathers find it very difficult to accept other male interest in their 'little girl'. They feel, quite unreasonably, rejected and threatened and may react by becoming absurdly possessive and strict. Again, it will rest on you to be a wise 'middlewoman' because, no matter what gestures of independence your daughter may make, inwardly she still wants to feel that you and her home are havens to which she can always return.

The best way a mother can help her daughter through this bewildering period in her life is by telling her, fully and frankly, what to expect, not just as it happens or, worse still, afterwards, but long beforehand. For instance, as part of explaining how a baby is made, it is the most natural thing in the world to introduce information about the woman's special reproductive functions.

A very young girl will only be able to absorb a limited amount of information, told in the simplest language, but as she gets older and provided that she has not been warned off asking, her questions will become more sophisticated and require more detailed answers. Not to explain to her well in advance about the changes she will experience in her own body is cruel as well as misguided, and the mother who repeats the mistakes of her own mother has no excuse.

However, unless you yourself fully understand what happens both within and without the female body during puberty and maturity, you are not going to make a very good job of explaining it to your daughter. Conversely, by helping her to grow up and accept her sexuality you will, at the same time, be helping yourself to a deeper, richer understanding of your own mature sexuality.

Physical changes in puberty
Contrary to popular belief, it is not the first menstruation which signals a girl's entrance into puberty, but interior changes in her hormonal balance which will have started two or three years earlier. After the first period it may then take another two or three

years for a girl to establish her menstrual cycle and become a regularly ovulating woman, capable of conceiving and producing a baby.

Thus the whole process of change during puberty lasts approximately five years. Possibly as early as eight or nine a girl's menstrual clock is wound up and started by a small gland* at the base of the brain called the hypothalamus.* This begins secreting substances called 'releasing factors', which travel to the pituitary gland,* situated immediately below the hypothalamus; this gland in its turn releases a hormone* called follicle stimulating hormone (FSH).* FSH travels to the ovaries where it stimulates the growth of certain follicles or sacs containing the eggs (ova). As these follicles swell and enlarge, they produce a new hormone called oestrogen* which is gradually released into the bloodstream.

Oestrogen is a vital hormone for women at all ages. Its first effects are to change a girl's appearance. Externally her breasts will begin to bud, her outer sex organs (the vulva) will enlarge and pubic hair will grow on the mons veneris, the pubic bone above her genitals. Her face will become fuller, she will grow taller, and her body will lose its boyish straightness and become curved and rounded; in addition to breasts, she will develop a waist and hips.

At the same time, oestrogen will be effecting changes within her body. The vaginal walls will thicken, the womb or uterus* will enlarge and its lining, the endometrium,* will also thicken. It is only when these changes have occurred that she is ready for her first menstruation.

MENSTRUATION

For reasons which are not fully understood but probably have much to do with better nourishment and higher standards of living, the average age of first menstruation has been coming down steadily for the last one hundred years at the rate of approximately three months every ten years. Today in the Western world the average age is twelve-and-a-half, but any time between the ages of nine and sixteen is regarded as normal. About 5 per cent of girls start somewhere between sixteen and eighteen; this does not indicate any abnormality. After the age of eighteen, however, if menstruation has still not started and there are no other signs of sexual maturation, such as pubic hair or developing breasts, it is important to consult a doctor.

There are various reasons why some girls experience delayed menstruation. The least serious

and most usual is that an individual girl's biological timetable may run slower than average and the evidence for this will be borne out by her generally slower rate of growth. Some girls suffer from glandular disturbances or hormonal imbalances; for others it may be that chronic illness or emotional problems, resulting in a nervous disorder like anorexia nervosa,* either prevent menstruation from ever starting or stop it after it has appeared for several cycles. Where any such cause is suspected, specialist medical help must be sought.

Early periods may be light, irregular and painless and it is quite likely that the girl is not ovulating. Ovulation* is the release of a mature egg from one or other of the ovaries, usually alternately. A few women know when they are ovulating because they feel a sharp pain, mittelschmerz, across the lower abdomen. Sometimes the cervical mucus is streaked with a little blood.

For ovulation to take place there has to be further action by another hormone called luteinizing hormone (LH).* This is stimulated by the rising level of oestrogen which inhibits the production of FSH. As FSH falls off the hypothalamus instructs the pituitary gland to release LH, which stimulates one egg follicle to swell and burst, thereby releasing the egg, previously matured by FSH, to travel down the Fallopian tube.* The ruptured follicle, now known as the corpus luteum, continues to produce oestrogen and a second hormone, progesterone,* which prepares a special lining for the uterus to receive the hopefully fertilized egg. If, as usually happens, fertilization does not occur, the levels of oestrogen and progesterone both fall off, the thickened lining is sloughed off the uterine wall and the resulting bleeding discharge is the menstrual period.

In the final stages of puberty a girl develops underarm hair, her breasts grow bigger and her pubic hair thickens. In most cases her periods will settle into a regular cyclic pattern.

She has now reached sexual maturity, and after the age of eighteen she is unlikely to grow any taller or develop further in any other direction. It is an interesting fact that girls who start puberty earlier tend to go through all the stages of transition faster.

However well-prepared a girl may be for these dramatic physical changes in herself, the reality can still be hard to accept. Inevitably, she will find that periods and everything associated with them – pads, tampons, bleeding and possibly pain – restrict her freedom of action and temporarily reduce her energy. The prospect of thirty to forty years of the same ahead can be very daunting, so she needs time and understanding to become adjusted to her new condition. It is therefore very important that mothers, teachers or anyone concerned with the care of young girls should be sympathetically aware of the psychological conflicts that menstruation can induce, without making them over-anxious or over-careful. Some girls will be unlucky and suffer painful cramps, or nausea and headaches, others will hardly notice their periods, but all should be encouraged to lead a normal, active life whatever the time of the month. Swimming, bathing, hair-washing can all go on as usual.

When you tell your daughter about menstruation you will obviously give her a packet of sanitary towels so that she is properly prepared. However, she will soon hear from her friends, if not from you or from advertisements, about the advantages of tampons – easy to use, no menstrual smell, less messy and invisible – and she will want to try them.

Unless she has an exceptionally tight vagina or an imperforate hymen which covers her entire vaginal opening, both rare conditions, there is absolutely no reason why she should not use tampons, and there are several good reasons why she should. Convenience and comfort are obvious, but, just as important, she will learn to be at ease with her body and not mind touching herself. Studying the insertion diagram will give her a good basic idea of her anatomy. Tampons, incidentally, are also more hygienic than sanitary towels, which often slip backwards into the rectal area, picking up bacteria which cause infection if they are introduced into the vagina.

The menstrual cycle

A baby girl is born with anything from 40,000 to 400,000 immature ova stored inside her two ovaries, of which 400 at the most will be released as mature eggs ripe for fertilization during her reproductive life. The remainder end up as minute particles of scar tissue embedded in the ovary which, fully grown, is about the size of a small plum.

Although menstruation is such an intrinsic part of our lives, many women are confused about what is normal. The first thing to understand is that a normal menstrual cycle covers a wide range of variations, so each woman must learn to recognize her own biological timetable.

A twenty-eight-day cycle is merely the average. Longer and shorter cycles for the same woman within a year are perfectly normal. Some women never have a cycle

which lasts longer than twenty-one days and others never have one which is less than thirty-five days. Length of period and quantity of blood-loss also vary from woman to woman. Whereas one always has a very light flow which may last for only two days, another will have a heavy flow which may continue for five to eight days. The same woman may find that her period changes character as a

SPASMODIC DYSMENORRHOEA

CONGESTIVE DYSMENORRHOEA

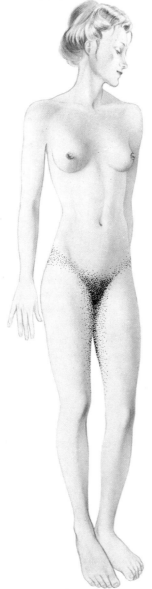

Spasmodic dysmenorrhoea affects women between the ages of fifteen and twenty-five, before they have had their first pregnancy.

Symptoms. Acute stomach pains and cramping often causing diarrhoea and vomiting. Cramps are in fact mini uterine contractions similar to labour pains. Shooting pains often extend down legs. Symptoms are at their worst on first day of period but can last two or three days. For further details and treatments, see pages 92–93.

Congestive dysmenorrhoea can affect women of all ages but gets worse with age and successive pregnancies.

Symptoms. Headaches, tension, depression, exhaustion, irritability, breasts tender and pains under arms. Stomach feels heavy and swollen with dull pains, constipation and nausea. Aching in back and joints, ankles swollen. Symptoms are often felt for a week before period starts but vanish quickly once it is under way.

result of the type of contraceptive that she is using, or after pregnancy or illness.

The best way of recognizing your personal pattern is by keeping a menstrual chart (see page 223). If you cannot be bothered with this because you are one of those lucky people for whom menstruation is a minor monthly incident, it is still important that you keep a calendar check of the first day of your

period in your diary. This is both for your own reference, so that you know when to expect your next period, and so that you will be able to tell the doctor should you have to visit him or her for any reason. Girls starting menstruation should be told how to do this by their mothers and the reasons for doing so should be explained. An astonishing number of women are vague about their dates or refer to themselves as 'always late' or 'always early' because their particular cycle falls outside the conventional twenty-eight-day cycle.

Generally speaking, a sexually mature, normally functioning woman ovulates once a month for approximately thirty-five years, releasing one egg each time. However, here again there are many normal exceptions to the rule. To produce more than one egg a month is not unusual, although it is unlikely to happen very often. And to have anovulatory cycles,* when no egg is produced, is also quite common, particularly in the first year or so of menstruation. It is nature's way of protecting a girl from too early a pregnancy before the rest of her body, and particularly her pelvic bone structure, is ready to carry a baby. Some women continue to have anovulatory cycles more often than not, and this is a major cause of female infertility. Others who have ovulated normally most of their lives may find that they are not doing so as they approach the menopause. Again, this could be the body's way of fending off an undesirable pregnancy when both the woman and her ova are getting too old.

If we had the choice, would we really prefer to do without menstruation? Although the monthly bleeding is often inconvenient and may bring with it problems of pain or concealment, most women, if questioned hard, would probably still opt for the reassurance of its arrival rather than otherwise. Remember how you felt when you were waiting anxiously for it to start because all the girls in your class who had 'come on' seemed enviably mature? Similarly, although many women profess to look forward to the time when the menopause will relieve them of the fuss and mess and discomfort, secretly they may be viewing the prospect with regret and dismay.

Menstruation is bound up with our deepest feelings about how we regard ourselves as women. Condemn it as conditioning if you like, but it exists, it is deep-rooted and it must be recognized. However, recent surveys have shown that women are beginning to change their attitude, and while many are reassured by its monthly appearance, others wish fervently

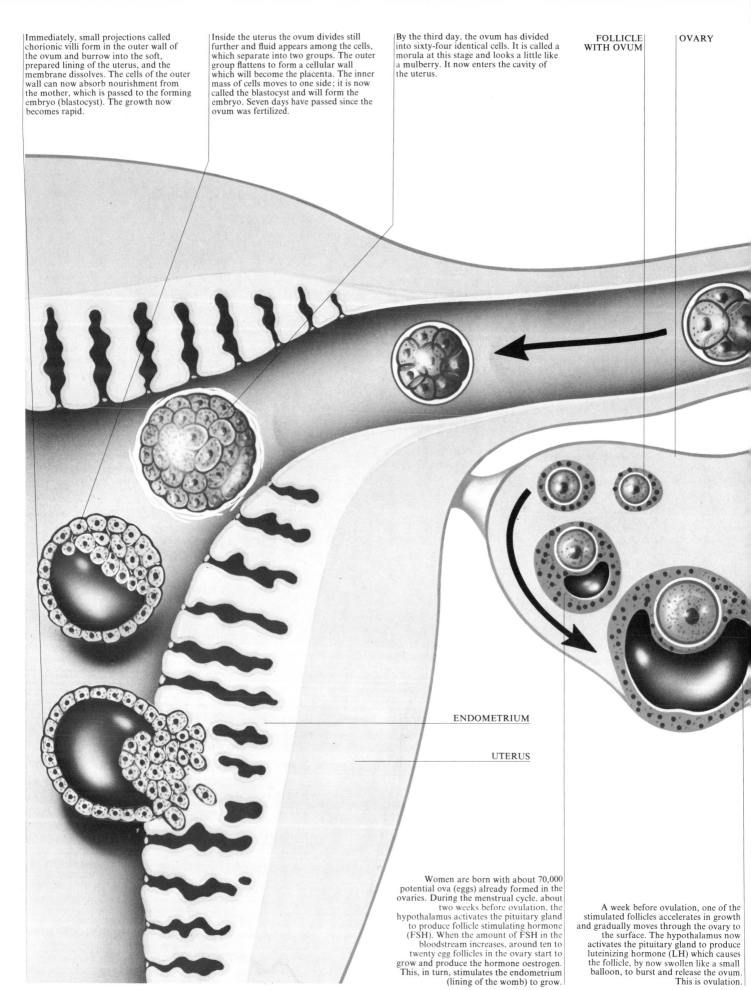

Immediately, small projections called chorionic villi form in the outer wall of the ovum and burrow into the soft, prepared lining of the uterus, and the membrane dissolves. The cells of the outer wall can now absorb nourishment from the mother, which is passed to the forming embryo (blastocyst). The growth now becomes rapid.

Inside the uterus the ovum divides still further and fluid appears among the cells, which separate into two groups. The outer group flattens to form a cellular wall which will become the placenta. The inner mass of cells moves to one side; it is now called the blastocyst and will form the embryo. Seven days have passed since the ovum was fertilized.

By the third day, the ovum has divided into sixty-four identical cells. It is called a morula at this stage and looks a little like a mulberry. It now enters the cavity of the uterus.

FOLLICLE WITH OVUM

OVARY

ENDOMETRIUM

UTERUS

Women are born with about 70,000 potential ova (eggs) already formed in the ovaries. During the menstrual cycle, about two weeks before ovulation, the hypothalamus activates the pituitary gland to produce follicle stimulating hormone (FSH). When the amount of FSH in the bloodstream increases, around ten to twenty egg follicles in the ovary start to grow and produce the hormone oestrogen. This, in turn, stimulates the endometrium (lining of the womb) to grow.

A week before ovulation, one of the stimulated follicles accelerates in growth and gradually moves through the ovary to the surface. The hypothalamus now activates the pituitary gland to produce luteinizing hormone (LH) which causes the follicle, by now swollen like a small balloon, to burst and release the ovum. This is ovulation.

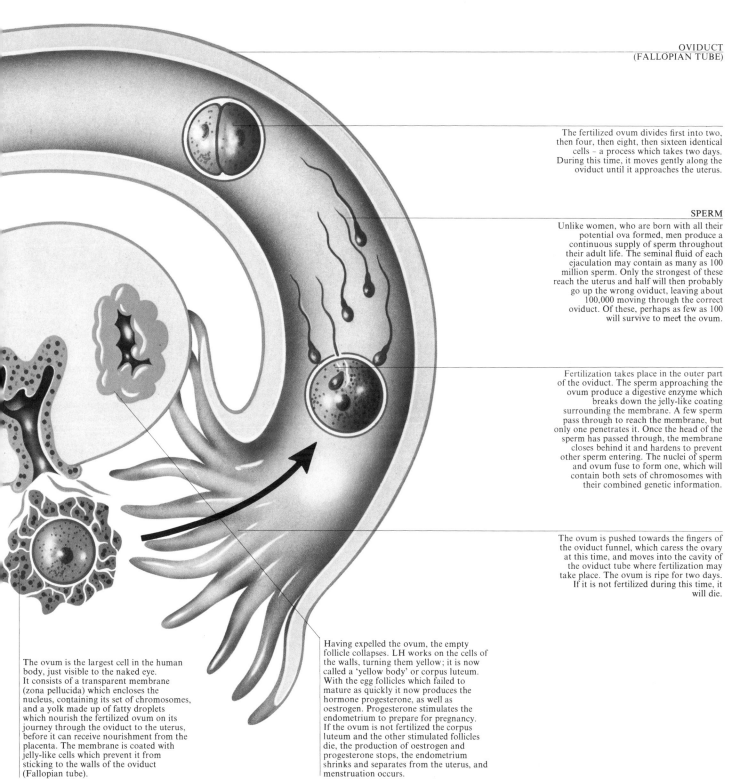

OVIDUCT
(FALLOPIAN TUBE)

The fertilized ovum divides first into two, then four, then eight, then sixteen identical cells – a process which takes two days. During this time, it moves gently along the oviduct until it approaches the uterus.

SPERM

Unlike women, who are born with all their potential ova formed, men produce a continuous supply of sperm throughout their adult life. The seminal fluid of each ejaculation may contain as many as 100 million sperm. Only the strongest of these reach the uterus and half will then probably go up the wrong oviduct, leaving about 100,000 moving through the correct oviduct. Of these, perhaps as few as 100 will survive to meet the ovum.

Fertilization takes place in the outer part of the oviduct. The sperm approaching the ovum produce a digestive enzyme which breaks down the jelly-like coating surrounding the membrane. A few sperm pass through to reach the membrane, but only one penetrates it. Once the head of the sperm has passed through, the membrane closes behind it and hardens to prevent other sperm entering. The nuclei of sperm and ovum fuse to form one, which will contain both sets of chromosomes with their combined genetic information.

The ovum is pushed towards the fingers of the oviduct funnel, which caress the ovary at this time, and moves into the cavity of the oviduct tube where fertilization may take place. The ovum is ripe for two days. If it is not fertilized during this time, it will die.

The ovum is the largest cell in the human body, just visible to the naked eye. It consists of a transparent membrane (zona pellucida) which encloses the nucleus, containing its set of chromosomes, and a yolk made up of fatty droplets which nourish the fertilized ovum on its journey through the oviduct to the uterus, before it can receive nourishment from the placenta. The membrane is coated with jelly-like cells which prevent it from sticking to the walls of the oviduct (Fallopian tube).

Having expelled the ovum, the empty follicle collapses. LH works on the cells of the walls, turning them yellow; it is now called a 'yellow body' or corpus luteum. With the egg follicles which failed to mature as quickly it now produces the hormone progesterone, as well as oestrogen. Progesterone stimulates the endometrium to prepare for pregnancy. If the ovum is not fertilized the corpus luteum and the other stimulated follicles die, the production of oestrogen and progesterone stops, the endometrium shrinks and separates from the uterus, and menstruation occurs.

that they could dispense with it entirely, provided that there was no risk to their health.

There are now two methods by which the nuisance aspect of menstruation can be diminished. One is hormone therapy along the lines of the Pill, which automatically regulates the menstrual cycle to twenty-eight days. The individual woman who wants either to delay or bring forward her period to prevent it interfering with an important event like her wedding or a holiday can be given hormone therapy to adjust it accordingly. This is also often done on a semi-permanent basis for women who are stricken by a physical handicap or illness which prevents them from ever becoming pregnant.

An alternative method for women who are worried by the consequences of prolonged hormone therapy is menstrual extraction, practised by women's self-help groups,* particularly in the United States. The menses are extracted on the first day of the period by a hand-operated syringe attached to tubing and a plastic cannula (tube) inserted through the undilated cervix. The procedure is similar to menstrual interception (see page 106), but at this stage it is not an early abortion. However, it is vitally important to use the right equipment, and to have sufficient training to know exactly what you are doing. Periods which drag on with minimal menstrual flow for several days can be effectively cut short by douching (see page 127).

Menstrual myths abound throughout the world, but basically all of them carry the same message: the menstruating woman is unclean, mischievous in intention, at best temporarily disabled from performing even the simplest household task, at worst positively evil and dangerous. We should beware of adopting a few new pseudo-scientific myths, such as the theory that there is no such thing as premenstrual tension or that menopausal symptoms are all in the mind, on the pretext that only neurotic women suffer menstrual distress.

Dr Katharina Dalton, who in more than twenty years of treating thousands of women for menstrual disorders has done more than anyone to throw light on this vexed question, believes that daughters are more likely to inherit their mothers' hormonal make-up, and consequently a tendency to experience similar menstrual problems, than their psychological attitudes. All the same, a mother with strong emotional or religious reasons for disliking menstruation or regarding it as unmentionable or dirty will almost certainly have a negative influence on her daughter's attitudes to her periods.

Menstrual problems
About 20 per cent of women encounter few if any difficulties with their periods, but among the remaining 80 per cent a variety of problems may be experienced. A few very unlucky women suffer acute menstrual distress for long intervals in their lives. The majority, because they think there is no cure and have been conditioned not to make a fuss, learn to put up with one or more of the less serious but recurring discomforts brought on by menstruation: cramps, dragging pain in the lower abdomen, backache, bloatedness, tender breasts, excessive or irregular blood-loss, swingeing headaches and unaccountable mood changes.

Many women are afraid to admit to menstrual problems because they fear that their jobs may be affected, although there is a good argument for saying that women are at least as well if not better suited to jobs requiring a stable, responsible personality just because they have learned to take monthly inconvenience, even pain, in their stride.

Fortunately, dysmenorrhoea (menstrual pain) need no longer be endured in silent misery, nor should a woman be made to feel inadequate or neurotic for admitting it. Providing that it is correctly diagnosed, it can nearly always be cured or certainly brought under control. In severe cases, this is usually achieved by some form of hormonal therapy.

Dr Katharina Dalton has isolated two distinct types of dysmenorrhoea:

Spasmodic dysmenorrhoea manifests itself in acute cramping pains in the lower abdomen which start with the period and may continue for two or three days. Sometimes the pains are so severe that a woman may be vomiting and feel quite unable to get up and about.

These pains are basically due to mini uterine contractions, but their exact cause is still a mystery. It could be the action of certain chemicals in the blood called prostaglandins,* or it could be an excess of progesterone over oestrogen, or a combination of these and other as yet undiscovered factors. Since spasmodic dysmenorrhoea mainly affects young women between the ages of fifteen and twenty-five and usually ends after the first pregnancy, Dr Dalton's theory that it is related to the size and muscular development of an untried uterus may also be relevant. Many women experience this type of menstrual pain only occasionally.

Whatever the causes, severe symptoms respond well to oestrogen therapy. The treatment must be followed for several months if it is to have any effect,

and the dosage has to be carefully monitored for the individual woman. If you don't want to conceive, then the answer is to take one of the combined birth-control pills containing variable proportions of oestrogen and progestogen, a synthetic version of progesterone. It may take a few months to find the right brand with the right dose of oestrogen for your individual needs, but most women find that the ultimate relief of pain is well worth the bother. If you *do* want to conceive, oestrogen therapy can only be administered after ovulation, and this treatment may take longer to be effective and also require larger doses. While having the treatment, you should be carefully noting on your menstrual chart the presence or absence of pain to help your doctor regulate the dosage. (For disadvantages of oestrogen, see page 123.)

Here are some tips for dealing with milder attacks of spasmodic dysmenorrhoea which don't warrant hormone therapy. As the attack starts, take a pain-killer such as paracetamol and, if you can, go to bed with a hot-water bottle, having had a warm bath and a hot drink. If it is the evening you could take a nightcap of brandy or whisky, but of course don't mix alcohol with a drug. Orgasm, whether self-induced or during intercourse, works marvellously well for women who are not inhibited by their menstrual flow. Good posture and stress-relieving and controlled breathing exercises also help (see page 55ff).

Congestive dysmenorrhoea afflicts women of all ages, but it tends to worsen as they get older, particularly with successive pregnancies. The name suggests the symptoms: in addition to the physical problems mentioned on page 89, many women feel at a psychologically low ebb for several days before their period starts. Often they become forgetful and unco-ordinated, or they may be overwhelmed by profound lethargy and depression or uncontrollable irritability. Few women suffering from congestive dysmenorrhoea are unlucky enough to suffer all these symptoms at the same time, but the symptoms do occur in clusters and they are now collectively called the premenstrual syndrome.

At long last the medical profession is taking this unpleasant condition seriously. Although the basic cause of premenstrual tension is still unknown, recent research has uncovered some of the precipitating factors. An inadequate amount of progesterone in the second half of the menstrual cycle is one; a lack of pyridoxine, Vitamin B6, which upsets the control mechanism in the hypo-thalamus and therefore the

hormonal balance, is another.

If the main symptom is fluid retention, causing an increase in weight – possibly as much as 7 lb (3.2 kg) – a distended stomach and swollen legs, wrists and ankles, then cutting down on your intake of salt towards the end of your menstrual cycle and taking diuretic pills which eliminate excess water may be sufficient. However, diuretics will not cure other problems such as depression or headaches; nor will tranquillizers, often prescribed by impatient doctors, do more than mask the symptoms.

There are two main forms of treatment available: progesterone therapy, administered either by injection or pessaries during the second half of the menstrual cycle, or a course of pyridoxine tablets, taken for approximately the same period. Dr Dalton favours the first and stresses that it is no good substituting the synthetic progestogen used in the Pill because in certain conditions it mimics oestrogen, with the result that the imbalance of oestrogen over progesterone is actually increased.

Pyridoxine is the preferred treatment for those women whose tests do not show a marked drop in progesterone, but the amount prescribed varies enormously. Some women get by with a very small dose, others need to have it stepped up. The advantage of this treatment is that it is easy to administer and has no side-effects.

If you think you suffer from premenstrual tension severe enough to require treatment, look at the premenstrual tension chart on page 223 and fill it in according to the instructions. In the section 'Other symptoms' you should note anything which you find recurs periodically, such as asthma, hay fever, muscle or joint pains, cold sores, boils, etc. Show it to your family doctor; if he seems unsympathetic, ask for a second opinion or a referral letter to an endocrinologist, a specialist in glandular problems.

A woman suffering from severe premenstrual tension must be treated, not only out of compassion for her – because her life can become quite literally a living hell – but also for the sake of her husband, her family, her workmates, her employer and society in general.

Dr Dalton's extensive research shows that the pre-menstrual syndrome can have disastrous effects. Half of all the crimes committed by women happen during the premenstruum, the four days preceding the period. Half the female suicides, half the cases of baby battering and other accidents to children also happen at this time. Schoolgirls are

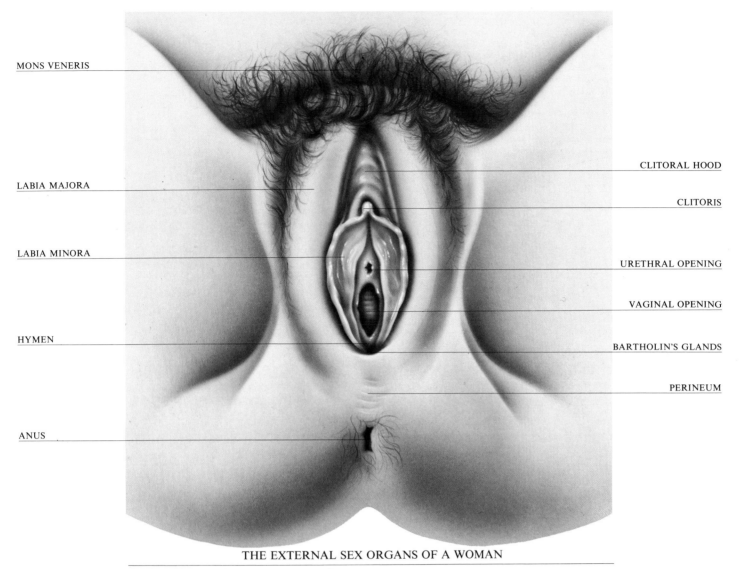

MONS VENERIS

LABIA MAJORA

LABIA MINORA

HYMEN

ANUS

CLITORAL HOOD

CLITORIS

URETHRAL OPENING

VAGINAL OPENING

BARTHOLIN'S GLANDS

PERINEUM

THE EXTERNAL SEX ORGANS OF A WOMAN

naughtier and do less well in their exams at this time; half the women admitted to hospital with infections or mental illness are in their premenstruum, and so it goes on. While we should beware of putting all our ills down to 'that time of the month', it does seem sensible to acknowledge that we are psychosomatic* creatures: our hormones do affect our emotions and vice versa.

Amenorrhoea

Amenorrhoea is the name given to failure to menstruate. It is called *primary* if a girl has not begun to menstruate by the age of eighteen and *secondary* if her periods cease, having been established, for reasons other than pregnancy. It means that a woman is not ovulating and it can be caused by a hormonal imbalance, glandular disturbance, stress, disease or a congenital defect. The most common cause is dieting and sudden loss of weight. Always see your doctor. Persistently heavy periods or prolonged bleeding can be symptoms of some serious uterine problem. It is always advisable to consult your doctor in these cases.

SELF-EXAMINATION

Some women find it very difficult to think about themselves sexually, and especially to know about their sexual and reproductive organs, where they are, how they function, etc. This is partly due to anatomy: even a woman's external organs are tucked away between her legs so that it is impossible to see them properly without a mirror. It is also because we have been brought up not to think too much about how our sexual organs function. Yet when it comes to dealing with such matters as contraception, pregnancy, childbirth – commonplace incidents in the lives of most women – it makes obvious sense that if you know what the doctor is talking about you are in a stronger position to make your own decisions.

External organs

First, have a look at your external organs. To do this easily, lie on your back on your bed and hold a mirror so that you can see what you are touching. The whole genital area is called the vulva. At the top is the mons veneris, a fleshy mound over the pubic bone which, from puberty, is covered

with pubic hair. Extending downwards and backwards from the mons veneris are the outer lips (labia majora) which are fleshy and change in size and shape quite considerably during a woman's life. They conceal and protect the inner lips (labia minora) which are much thinner and more sensitive. At the top end, below the mons veneris, these inner lips form a hood over the clitoris, a small pea-sized organ which is immensely sensitive as it is full of nerve endings. Below the clitoris there is a tiny opening called the urethra, through which a woman passes water. Below this is the vaginal entrance, on either side of which are the openings of the ducts of Bartholin's glands,* almost invisible to the naked eye.

Just inside the vaginal entrance, on either side, there are strong pubococcygeal muscles which give elastic tone to the vagina. By tightening them when you go to the lavatory you can stop the flow of urine. By keeping them in trim with the following simple exercise you will enhance your own sensation of orgasm and pleasurably stimulate your

partner's penis during intercourse. Relax and tighten them ten to fifteen times whenever you think about it at odd moments during the day, standing or sitting at work, waiting for a bus, watching television. Consciously feel them contract. This exercise is particularly important after childbirth (see also page 59).

The girl who has not had sexual intercourse may also see just inside her vaginal opening a thin membrane of skin surrounding the opening which is called the hymen. It usually ruptures quite easily on first penetration, causing minimal bleeding and pain if she has a gentle lover. Frequently the hymen breaks much earlier, especially if you are an active, sporty type. Horse-riding, for instance, is a common cause. However it happens, this banal physiological incident represents lost virginity over which, in the not-so-distant past, girls have been shamed and cast out of their parents' home, duels have been fought and lives and dowries lost.

The area of skin stretching from the vaginal opening backwards to the anus is called the

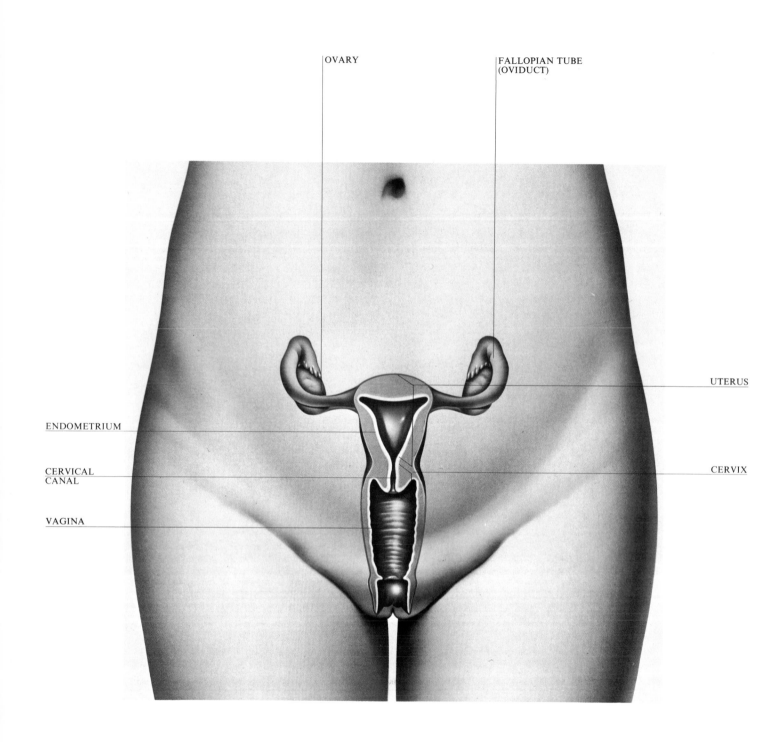

OVARY

FALLOPIAN TUBE
(OVIDUCT)

UTERUS

ENDOMETRIUM

CERVIX

CERVICAL
CANAL

VAGINA

THE INTERNAL SEX ORGANS OF A WOMAN

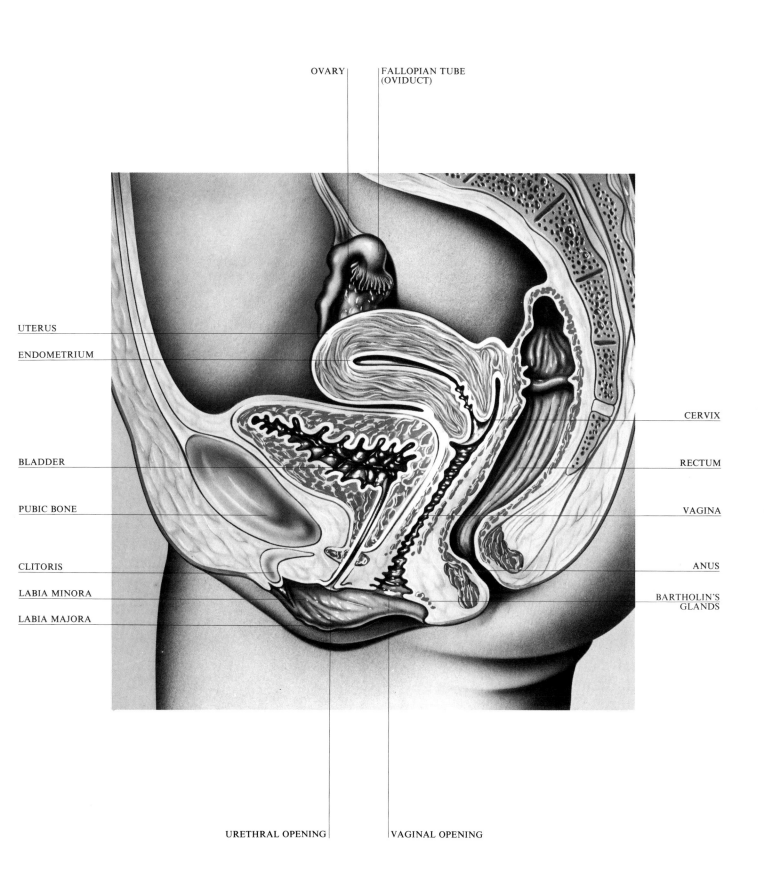

OVARY | FALLOPIAN TUBE (OVIDUCT)

UTERUS

ENDOMETRIUM

CERVIX

BLADDER

RECTUM

PUBIC BONE

VAGINA

CLITORIS

ANUS

LABIA MINORA

BARTHOLIN'S GLANDS

LABIA MAJORA

URETHRAL OPENING | VAGINAL OPENING

CROSS-SECTION SHOWING INTERNAL SEX ORGANS

perineum and it covers muscles and fibrous tissue. It is also highly susceptible to sexual stimulus.

That completes your external sex organs or genitals. If you have used tampons or masturbate you will be accustomed to inserting your fingers into your vagina and generally feel at ease with touching yourself.

Internal organs

Now you know what you look like on the outside, and every woman is as different in her genitals as in her face, let us move inwards. Many people think – wrongly – that the vagina is a rigid hole. In reality, it is a potential space enfolded by soft, nerveless and therefore insensitive tissue which stretches backwards at an angle of forty-five degrees to the cervix, the neck of the womb. The ideal way to inspect the inside of your vagina is by inserting a speculum* – the same instrument a doctor uses when doing an internal examination – which holds apart the vaginal walls.

By tilting a mirror and shining a light up your vagina you will be able to see your cervix. In the centre of this shiny pink knob you will see a tiny hole, or larger slit if you have had a child. This is called the os, and through this opening the menstrual blood passes, the sperm swim up into the uterus, and in childbirth a baby emerges.

Like the vagina, the cervix is capable of a considerable degree of dilatation and expansion. It is normal for it to change colour and consistency of mucous secretions during the menstrual cycle and pregnancy. The vagina secretes additional fluids during sexual arousal, making it easier for the penis to penetrate. This is called lubrication.

The uterus of a nulliparous woman, one who has not had a full-term pregnancy, looks somewhat like a small pear. It is an immensely strong, hollow, muscular organ, 3 in (7.5 cm) high, 2 in (5 cm) from side to side and 1 in (2.5 cm) from front to back. It is capable of expanding to hold a baby, together with the placenta and amniotic fluid* (see page 113), and yet after childbirth it retracts to its original size.

On either side at the top of the uterus are the Fallopian tubes, hollow tubes looking a bit like macaroni, through which run hair-like ducts about 4 in (10 cm) long and leading sideways towards the ovaries. Their fronded ends reach out towards the ovaries without touching them and their function is to entice the ovum, once it has ruptured its follicle and escaped from the ovary, and help its journey down towards the uterus and the waiting sperm. For information about uterine

disorders, refer to page 220.

ENJOYING SEX

Your body is not just a mechanical object like a car, which must be kept well-serviced, filled with oil and petrol, and have all the parts lubricated and replaced when necessary to keep it in good running order. It is also a vital source of pleasure and delight to yourself and to others. Inevitably, when we describe physical function we talk about *how* the system works and what to do when it breaks down, but we should also be thinking about what the system is *for*.

So far in this chapter we have been concentrating on the reproductive function of a woman's body, but many of the same organs that are used for producing children are also used for sexual pleasure. Our sexuality is an essential part of our personality. Most people are keenly interested in sex, women as much as men, but even today, when we live in an age of sexual enlightenment and freedom, many of us still find it difficult to reconcile our sexuality with the rest of our living.

We have won the right to speak openly about our sexual needs, but some of us still have not given ourselves the right to enjoy ourselves sexually. Much of this is due to the double sexual standard still operating and to the conditioning which says that 'nice girls don't . . .' If they do, then they are branded wrongly as nymphomaniacs.*

So often sex is thought of as forbidden fruit. Then, when it is tasted and found wanting, either because of ignorance or guilt, those two great passion-killers, a woman decides that sex is over-rated or matters more to a man than to her and, quite literally, turns off the whole thing. Hence the myth of the frigid woman. But no woman needs to be frigid, nor, if she is completely honest with herself, does she want to be. The woman who has lost interest in sex or says that she has never had much interest in it is deceiving herself and her lover. She has lost interest either because, at the physical level, she is not being stimulated properly or is afraid of being physically hurt, perhaps because of a previous experience, or at the psychological level, she is afraid of abandoning herself to her sexual feelings.

We each have our own level of sexual drive which depends on many factors – our age, experience, upbringing and temperament – but many women never allow themselves to discover their true sexual potential. The first thing to realize is that we hold the key to sexual pleasure within ourselves, in our own bodies and minds. It is no good waiting for the ideal,

romantic hero to sweep us off our feet and carry us away into an enchanted land of love and ecstasy.

The sexual woman is sensually aware of herself. She has learned for herself what gives her pleasure and she can show her lover how to please her and turn her on, just as he will teach her to please him. If a woman is in tune with her own body, if she feels happy inside her own skin, if she can relax and enjoy her own sexual pleasure, then not only will she find all these pleasures intensified in sexual intercourse, but she will also add immeasurably to her lover's pleasure and satisfaction.

Achieving orgasm

Arousal and orgasm – these are the two essential processes in sexual pleasure. Many women are worried because, although they recognize arousal in themselves, or the lack of it, they are not so sure whether they have ever had an orgasm. Here is a simple test. Judge yourself by the way you feel after you have had intercourse. If you feel lazy, contented, glowing, then you have had an orgasm. If you feel frustrated, irritated, let down, sad, then you have not. The experience of orgasm varies from woman to woman and can be quite different for the same woman on different occasions. Some experience it as a high peak of pleasure which fades away rapidly. Others come to the peak and then feel it rippling on and on for seconds, even minutes, maintaining them on a high plateau of pleasure.

In the section 'Self-examination' (page 93), we described how you can look at your sexual organs and identify the various parts, all of them designed for pleasure. Now we are going to suggest ways of using them for pleasure, to enjoy sexual intercourse or to masturbate. The woman who knows how to masturbate herself to climax need never again be unsatisfied. Furthermore, she will be able to teach her lover how to please her. If all this sounds a bit selfish, accept it for that. Two people making love *should* be mutually selfish, because by knowing what pleases them they will be turning on their lover and pleasing themselves at the same time.

To enjoy masturbation choose a time when you know you will be alone and undisturbed. Take the telephone off the hook. Make the atmosphere exciting and erotic for yourself in whatever way suits you best: dim the lights, play your favourite record, look at a sexy magazine. Undress slowly in front of a full-length mirror. Run your hands over your body. Feel the weight of your breasts. Enjoy the curve of your hips and bottom. Then lie on your bed or a soft carpet and enjoy touching

yourself, gradually letting your hands concentrate on the sexually sensitive areas of your body. These will be your breasts, your nipples and between your legs, but there may be other areas as well. Discover your erogenous zones. Heighten your sense of voluptuous well-being by massaging yourself with a body lotion or skin oil.

Now let your fingers circle and probe and delve gently between the folds of skin surrounding your vagina. As you begin to feel the lips swell and become moist, let your fingers respond to your feelings. Treat yourself lovingly and, as pleasure mounts, concentrate on producing more and more by rubbing or stroking or touching your clitoris in whatever way excites you most.

Let your imagination take you where it leads you and, as you become more aroused, abandon yourself to your favourite fantasy. You may think it strange, possibly a bit wicked, to be deliberately producing pleasure in yourself, especially if you have never before given yourself this permission. Dismiss this thought and any others which threaten your total self-absorption. Think only of yourself and your pleasure and luxuriate in it. As long as you feel good about what you are doing, then you can make your own rules.

When you feel yourself rising to the peak of your pleasure, let it carry you over the top. Lose yourself in your orgasm.

There are as many ways of masturbating as there are women. Once you have discovered how to bring yourself to orgasm, you can involve your lover and show him how easy it is to arouse you.

Some women find that although they are easily aroused and come easily if their clitoris is sufficiently stimulated, they still cannot get an orgasm through intercourse. If this is your problem, then experiment with positions which keep up a steady level of clitoral stimulation throughout intercourse.

One way of doing this is by making love in a position where the woman continues to feel pressure on her clitoris all the time that the man is thrusting. You, the woman, kneel over him in what is technically called the 'female superior position' and, as you both move together, you can press your clitoris against his pubic bone.

A development of this technique is that he stimulates your clitoris with his fingers at the same time as he is thrusting with his penis, either in this position or when you are lying side by side. As you both become more practised at doing this, he can withhold the clitoral stimulation for short periods to start with, gradually lengthening them until finally you are sufficiently aroused by the

For sex to be a really sensuous and satisfying experience a woman must be erotically aware of her body. The areas of the body most sensitive to sexual stimulation are called the erogenous zones. These are highly individual, varying considerably from one person to another. One woman may become sexually excited when being caressed on the neck or ear, another may have no response at all or feel positively repulsed by the sensation, so it is important that you and your lover are aware of your reactions and preferences. Almost every area of the body is erotic to someone; the most obvious, and most common, areas are of course the mouth, breasts, genital area and inner thighs. Stimulation of these sensuous zones is an important part of love play preceding sexual intercourse. However, a great deal of erotic pleasure is missed if caressing these sensitive areas of the body is considered only in the context of intercourse since it can provide a sexual sensation satisfying in itself. There are women who can achieve orgasm merely from having their ear lobes stroked.

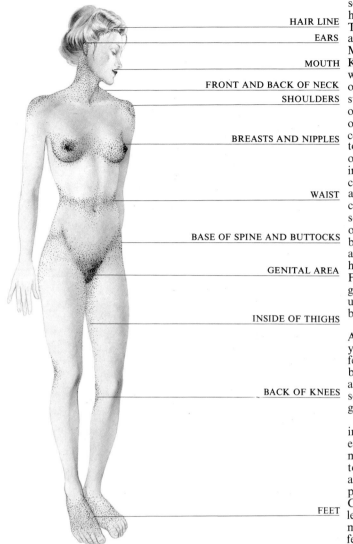

HAIR LINE
EARS
MOUTH
FRONT AND BACK OF NECK
SHOULDERS

BREASTS AND NIPPLES

WAIST

BASE OF SPINE AND BUTTOCKS

GENITAL AREA

INSIDE OF THIGHS

BACK OF KNEES

FEET

EROGENOUS ZONES

movement of his penis inside you not to need the clitoral stimulation any more. However, he should be ready to resume it at once if you signal that your arousal peak is slackening off, because it is very important that there should be no break in stimulation.

Another way of bringing yourself to orgasm, and one that your lover may also find very arousing, is for you to masturbate yourself when his penis is inside you. You can then bring yourself almost to the point of climax, at which moment he takes over and completes by bringing himself to climax and taking you with him.

Some women find that a vibrator helps them to reach orgasm faster. You can use it as a standby for times when you are on your own and want to pleasure yourself or as an additional aid in love-making. Battery or mains-electricity operated, vibrators

come in varying shapes and sizes – but the most popular one looks like a penis. These and many other aids to enhance or revitalize your love-making can be bought in sex shops or through mail order. Not so long ago sex aids were a matter for snicker and innuendo, but in today's more open and honest sexual climate it has become accepted that there is nothing perverted or nasty about using a 'mechanical' aid to heighten your experience of sexual pleasure, provided of course that it is not physically dangerous. It is much better to help yourself to orgasm in whatever way suits you best than to lie back and pretend that your partner has put you on cloud nine when in reality you have felt nothing and care less. Don't be taken in by the myth that says faking orgasm will preserve your marriage and protect your man from sexual

humiliation. In fact, your pretence is unfair and damaging to both of you; to him because it denies him the chance to explore and deepen his relationship with you on every level; to yourself because it denies you a valid and valuable human experience which it is possible for everyone to enjoy.

Mature, experienced lovers, who are at ease with their bodies and, therefore, with themselves, have realistic expectations about sex. They know that it will not necessarily be marvellous every time – a flash of bright stars, an explosion of glory. They know that sometimes they will feel tired or not in the mood, but that even so, it is good to be with a lover and perhaps do no more than caress and cuddle.

Because this is a book for women, we have concentrated on the female experience of sex; but the best sex is the sex shared, the

sexual communication a woman has with her lover, man or woman. There is still much to be discovered about human sexuality. Freud, Masters and Johnson, Shere Hite, Kinsey and the many other writers who have been opening the doors of our consciousness on this subject are all aware that we are only beginning to understand ourselves. One thing does seem certain: human beings may belong to one or other sex, but their range of sexual experience and inclination does not have to be confined within these strict dual and sometimes opposing, categories. We all of us contain something of the opposite sex in our make-up and for many people bisexual experience is a reality, not a fantasy. For others, homosexuality is the norm. Fortunately, there is today a genuine new tolerance and understanding of homosexuality, but we still have much to learn.

The lesbian relationship
A lesbian woman may spend many years denying her true sexual feelings because she has been brought up to believe that they are unnatural or disgusting, or something that she can control or grow out of.

There is not much difference in the way lesbian women love each other from the way that a man and a woman make love together, except that the absence of a penis makes the act of penetration less important. Contrary to heterosexual fantasies, lesbians do not wield vast dildos or make unbridled advances to every female that meet, but they do often find it easier to understand each other's needs, emotionally as well as sexually, perhaps because they experience the same sensations. The expression of love between two lesbians runs the whole gamut from gentle, undemanding caressing to wildly passionate, just as it does between a man and a woman. And as with any man or any woman, much depends on their mood, their state of arousal, their sense of well-being.

It is also a common mistake to think that because lesbians openly or covertly admit their sexual preference for their own sex, this means that all their encounters with women are necessarily lesbian. This is not so. Sexual attraction between women is as idiosyncratic and personal as it is between a man and a woman or between two men. Now that homosexuality is openly discussed and accepted, lesbians themselves are feeling less defensive and are, therefore, less likely to retreat into the familiar but misleading stereotypes. And there is no doubt that they can teach heterosexual women an enormous amount about how to accept and enjoy their female natures.

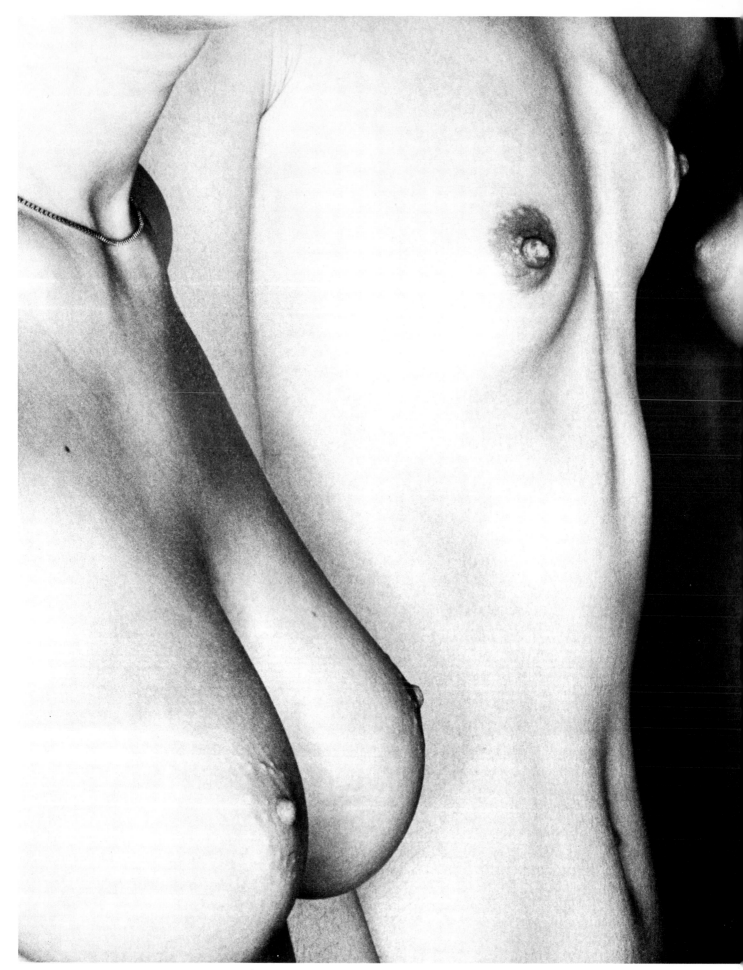

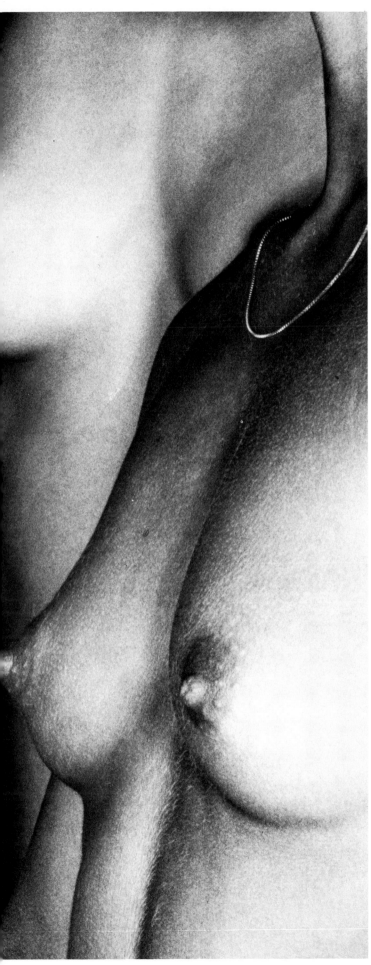

Breasts

A woman's breasts are a visible symbol of her femininity. Every little girl who waits impatiently for them to grow and compares herself despairingly or exultantly with her friends knows that. Other little girls dread their emergence for the same reason. They are embarrassed by these all too prominent signals that they are becoming women and they wonder how they are going to manage them. Like menstruation, breasts are often viewed by the young teenager as a constraint on her freedom, a symbol of bondage rather than independence.

Adult women are no less exempt from anxiety. They worry that their breasts are too big, too small, too low, too high or the wrong shape for the current criterion of beauty. What that standard is varies enormously in different societies and at different times. Compare the flat-chested Bright Young Things of the Twenties, who actually bound their breasts with bandages to make them look more boyish, with the pneumatic sweater girls of the Forties and Fifties, who prompted every fashion-conscious young woman to project whatever she had like twin ice-cream cones.

Tits, boobs, bristols, knockers . . . breasts go by as many names as they come in sizes. We undoubtedly live in a breast-crazed society which is avid to sell anything from cars to candy on the seductive curves of the female bosom. Only the focus has changed. Nudity has become as ordinary as applecake, surely a more appropriate description for today's bare-breasted pin-ups than the old-style leggy cheesecake. Nipples are in, cleavage has vanished.

An extraordinary streak of double-think persists in our culture. While a general preoccupation with the female body as an object of sexual gratification has become, if anything, more obsessive, women themselves have become much more relaxed and self-confident, and this new ease with their bodies is reflected in their appearance. Today the look is softer, more natural and often bra-less. Padding and boning have gone right out of fashion - is it too much to hope for ever? - together with corsets, roll-ons, waspies and all the other constrictive underpinnings into which women used to squeeze themselves in a painful effort to conform with the exaggerated outline of the moment. It is no accident that this development coincides with the revival of the women's movement. A liberated mind cannot function within a fettered body. Just as the New Woman at the turn of the century defiantly cast off her stays, so today her like-minded grand-daughters are discarding their bras.

All the same, a well-cut bra which holds rather than moulds the bosom is still advisable for all but the very young and firm. Without a bra, the full-bosomed woman will find her breasts drooping and eventually losing their shape, while the small-breasted woman who leads a normally active life will also find it uncomfortable to be swinging free all the time.

Breasts are practical as well as beautiful, and their size has little to do with their function. A small-breasted woman can feed her baby as adequately as her more amply endowed sister and, in later life, small breasts are probably an advantage because they are less prone to sagging. No one quite knows why they vary so much in size, but one factor may be the amount of hormonal stimulation they receive during puberty. There is also undoubtedly a strong genetic factor. Breasts are very elastic, enlarging quite considerably during pregnancy and lactation, and also during sexual arousal. Many women find their breasts change shape and size with age, or if they go on the Pill, and it is quite usual for a woman to have one breast larger than the other.

Some women have inverted nipples, rather like dimples, which may cause difficulty in breast-feeding. This condition can usually be put right by the use of a suction pump or, in more extreme cases, by surgery. However, women whose nipples normally stand out should go to the doctor if they notice that one or both nipples

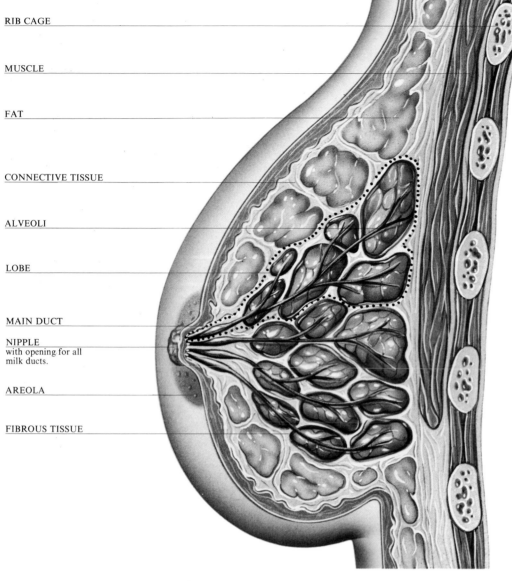

RIB CAGE

MUSCLE

FAT

CONNECTIVE TISSUE

ALVEOLI

LOBE

MAIN DUCT

NIPPLE
with opening for all
milk ducts.

AREOLA

FIBROUS TISSUE

STRUCTURE OF BREAST

have suddenly become inverted (see page 222). Much more rarely, a few women have extra nipples further down the rib cage or even under the armpits. If these are a cause of anxiety they can be removed by cosmetic surgery. A ring of hair growing around the nipples is quite common; again, if this is a cause of embarrassment or worry, the hair can be easily and permanently removed by electrolysis (see page 133).

Physiologically, the breasts are mammary glands* encased in fat, which is what gives them their shape. The milk-conveying ducts are contained in lobes, as many as fifteen to twenty-five in each breast, which are separated by fibrous tissues like the segments of an orange, and converge into a main duct behind the nipple. Contrary to what many women believe, breast-feeding does not ruin the shape of the breasts – provided an appropriate bra is worn. If the mother has the choice,

it is the best way to feed her baby, in terms of hygiene, nutrition and convenience.

The second important function of the breasts is to attract sexual interest, and during love-play they signal a woman's arousal. The nipples become erect, the breasts swell and often mottle, and the areola, the brown circle around the nipple, also swells and darkens, sometimes completely engulfing the nipple.

The breasts themselves contain no muscles but if you want to lift them, make them firmer and possibly slightly larger, see page 63 for some exercises which will strengthen the underlying pectoral muscles. Good posture also helps. If, however, you are seriously unhappy about their shape or size, then cosmetic surgery could be the answer. In the case of small breasts, silicone pads are inserted. This can also be done for some women after surgery for breast cancer. Where the breasts are too large,

the surgeon cuts out excess tissue. The dangers of silicone leaking out of the breasts into other parts of the body are a story of the past, and nowadays plastic surgery can be a safe and successful solution. In Britain, both augmentation and reduction of the breasts may be available on the National Health Service where it is clearly necessary for health reasons, which may be physical or psychological. Two obvious candidates would be the woman who suffers great discomfort, even handicap, from her outsize breasts and the flat-chested woman who feels unsexed and deeply unhappy because of her lack of feminine curves. However, it is not always easy to convince doctors that an operation is so desperately needed that you merit treatment (see page 207).

Perhaps now is the time to scotch some misery-making myths for ever. The size of a woman's breasts has absolutely nothing to do with her sexiness, her ability to

feed her baby, or, for that matter, her intellectual capacity. No two women's breasts are alike. One doctor said she had never yet met a woman who was satisfied with her hair, her periods or her breasts; but at least you can be sure that, whatever your breasts look like, they are unique.

The fear of breast cancer and mastectomy is a major one for many women. It is a good idea to check your breasts regularly, if only to allay this fear, and one way to do this is in the bath or shower: simply soap and smooth your breasts with your hands, so you become used to the feel of them and will notice any lump or change in shape. Though in most cases there is no cause for concern, always seek a doctor's advice if you are worried. Only one in five of the women who are referred by their doctors to a specialist turn out to have breast cancer; the remainder have cysts,* which can be cut out or aspirated (drawn out by suction), mastitis* and other benign conditions. One in seventeen women do get breast cancer, but their chances of survival are enormously increased the earlier the cancer is detected and treated, so do not let your fear of surgery stop you going to the doctor. The most vulnerable women are those with a family history of breast cancer.

Treatment is surgical, usually followed by drugs or radiotherapy. There are four types of operation, the choice of which depends on the size, nature and position of the lump, the surgeon's preference and, to a certain extent, the woman's.
They are:
1 Lumpectomy – lump alone removed.
2 Simple mastectomy – breast removed.
3 Modified radical mastectomy – breast and lymph nodes* under the arm removed.
4 Radical mastectomy (or Halsted after the surgeon who devised it) – breast, supporting pectoral muscle and all the lymph nodes removed. (This is rarely done in Britain now.)
Today there is a much better understanding of the physical and psychological problems facing a woman who has had a mastectomy. In both Britain and the United States there are volunteer organizations which counsel women about the practical difficulties they may encounter, such as finding the right bra, movements they should avoid and exercises to do. Women who have had the operation are becoming less reticent, and sharing their difficulties and experiences helps others to cope.

For a more detailed self-examination of your breasts, see page 222.

Birth Control

From the time a woman starts ovulating she is capable of becoming pregnant. Therefore the question of birth control – which method, when to start, who to consult – should arise before she has sexual intercourse for the first time. Studies of attitudes towards birth control reveal that many young women find it hard to initiate birth control because they feel that by choosing a method of contraception they are committing themselves to sexual intercourse for which they may not be emotionally ready. Nevertheless, it is obviously wise to think hard and seriously about it beforehand: abortion is not an easy way out of an unwanted pregnancy.
Social attitudes towards premarital intercourse have *changed greatly in the last twenty years and it is now the policy of Family Planning Clinics to accept anyone who seeks their advice and help without questioning their marital status. It is not only society at large which influences our thinking: much depends on the way we are brought up by our parents, whether or not sex education was part of the school curriculum, and if it was, how it was taught. Ideally, a couple in a stable relationship will make a joint decision about the best contraceptive for them, but an essential part of growing up is learning to take responsibility for your own mind, your own body and your own actions. Ultimately, the decision rests with the woman alone.*

You cannot make a wise and informed decision about which contraceptive to choose unless you are in full possession of all the known facts about the different methods, and this includes being aware of possible side-effects. Unfortunately, doctors are sometimes reluctant to discuss these because they assume too readily either that women won't understand the facts or that they will become unnecessarily over-anxious. Also, their enthusiasm for avoiding unwanted pregnancies at all costs sometimes over-rules consideration for the long-term effects on their patients' health.

'The ideal contraceptive should provide a sure means of preventing pregnancy, be reversible at will and allow normal sexual enjoyment by potentially fertile men and women with no danger to health,' say Mr Diggory and Dr McEwan* in their book, *Planning or Prevention?* No contraceptive now in existence fulfils all these criteria and it is for this reason that we suggest that you use the RSC Test when deciding which is the best method for you.

THE RSC TEST

R stands for Reliability: in other words, how good is the contraceptive at preventing fertilization?
S stands for Safety: does it have side-effects, and if so, what are they and how serious?
C stands for Convenience: does it suit your particular way of life? Is it personally acceptable to you? Is it easy to use? Also, bear in mind that your personal needs and circumstances will probably change during your reproductive life, so that what worked well for you at twenty may not be so good at forty, and what works for a married couple may not do so for a more casual relationship.

*Mr Diggory is Senior Gynaecologist to the Kingston Group of Hospitals. Dr McEwan is a family doctor and NHS Consultant in Family Planning at King's College Hospital.

INADEQUATE CONTRACEPTIVE METHODS

We will start by eliminating the unsatisfactory methods.
1 Withdrawal or coitus interruptus, whereby a man withdraws his penis before ejaculating, is still very widely practised but it does have two major disadvantages. Firstly, it interrupts love-making at a crucial moment, just as the man is reaching his climax, which he must then have outside the woman's vagina and this may deprive the woman of her orgasm unless either she or her partner continues afterwards to masturbate her to her own climax. Secondly, it doesn't always work, because sperm dropped on to the vulval area can sometimes still swim up the vagina.
2 Abstinence is neither practical nor desirable for most people.
3 Breast-feeding as a form of birth control is highly unreliable.
These 'natural' methods are inadvisable mainly because they are so unreliable, but there is also a 'man-made' contraceptive which women should be wary of for serious health reasons. The three-monthly injectable contraceptive has now been banned in the United States, but it is on limited trial in the United Kingdom and many other countries, mainly of the Third World. It produces very unpleasant side-effects in the form of menstrual pain and irregularity and definitely affects fertility. There are only two categories of women who may legally be given the three-monthly injectable Pill in Britain:
1 Women whose husbands have had vasectomies may be given it until it is certain that the man is sperm-free.
2 Women who have been inoculated against rubella may have it for a three-month period.

EFFECTIVE CONTRACEPTIVE METHODS

The four female methods of contraception are the Pill, the IUD (intra-uterine device), the diaphragm used with spermicide, and the mucothermic rhythm method. There is also one type of male preventive, the condom or sheath, and there is female and male sterilization. Spermicides in cream, foam or pessary form *must* be used in combination with the diaphragm and the condom: *never* rely on them as the sole method of contraception.

The Pill

There are two types, the *combined* and the *progestogen only*. Each, as the name implies, offers a different hormonal dose. Oestrogen* and progesterone* are two hormones* which a woman produces herself during the menstrual cycle. In the Pill they are produced in synthetic versions and have the following anti-fertilization effects:
– they prevent ovulation
– they prevent the uterine lining accepting a fertilized egg
– they thicken the cervical mucus, making a barrier against sperm.
a) The Combined Pill contains both hormones, is effective on all three counts and is therefore almost 100 per cent reliable, provided it is not forgotten. You start taking it on the fifth day of the cycle, counting the first day of your period as day one, then take it continuously for twenty-one days, followed by seven free days during which menstruation will occur. Should you forget to take the Pill one day you will still have contraceptive cover if you take it within twelve hours, but if the gap is longer, then you must use a second contraceptive while continuing to take the Pill.
b) The Progestogen Only Pill is taken at the same time every day throughout the full twenty-eight-day cycle. This means that it does not prevent ovulation but it does have the other two effects.

RSC Rating. The Pill rates higher than any other contraceptive, except sterilization, for Reliability and Convenience, but how Safe is it? There can be no complete answer to this until we have seen a whole generation of women live through their entire reproductive life on the Pill. Some women are symptom-free from the start; others find it takes a few cycles of feeling distinctly unwell before their bodies adjust to the artificial manipulation of their hormones; and some find that they develop side-effects, sooner or later, which become intolerable.

Here is a list of the most common side-effects and the action you should take if you notice one or more of them.
Side-effect. Severe leg or chest pains, blinding headaches, sudden complete or partial loss of vision, unexplained cough.
Action. Come off the Pill and see your doctor at once.
Side-effect. Depression, headaches, loss of libido, weight-gain, skin blotching, breast tenderness, pre-menstrual syndrome, thrush.*
Action. Unless the side-effects become intolerable, continue the Pill but make an early appointment to see your doctor, who should prescribe a different brand.
Side-effect. Irregular periods, breakthrough bleeding.
Action. See your doctor as soon as possible, but do not come off the Pill without using another contraceptive in its place.

There are also certain women who should either not go on the Pill at all or, if they do, should be extra careful about having regular medical checks.
Absolute contra-indications
1 The history or existence of deep venous thrombosis.
2 The history or existence of cancer of the breast or genital tract.
3 Confirmed liver malfunction.
Relative contra-indications.
1 Women of thirty-five and over who are over-weight and smoke more than twenty cigarettes a day are therefore already susceptible to raised blood-pressure.
2 Uterine fibroids* tend to grow larger under the influence of the combined Pill.

For women over forty, the progestogen only Pill is considered the safest.

It is advisable for anyone on the Pill to stop taking it one

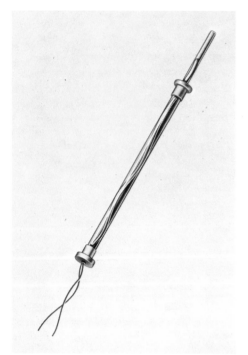

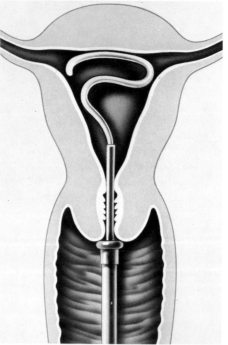

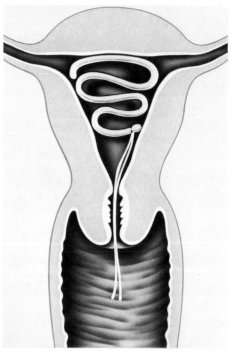

Most IUDs are easily inserted, the best time being at menstruation or after childbirth when cervix is relaxed. The vagina is opened with a speculum* and cervix cleaned with mild anti-septic to prevent germs entering uterus with IUD. The device, packed in a plastic insertion tube, is gently pushed through cervical canal.

Once tip of insertion tube reaches cavity of uterus, a plunger is pushed to expel device, which quickly regains its proper shape inside uterus. Insertion takes only a few minutes when done by a trained operator, but some women experience cramps and bleeding similar to a heavy period for two or three days.

Nylon threads attached to IUD are left hanging through cervix into vagina, so a woman can check regularly that device is in place. This is best done after menstruation. Periods may be heavy at first, but should revert to normal pattern after about three months. If heavy bleeding continues, try a different IUD.

month before an operation and resume not less than one month afterwards. You should also check with your doctor about the advisability of taking the Pill if at any time you are undergoing prolonged bed-rest.

It is worth knowing that there are times when the Pill may not be absolutely reliable. For instance, if you are taking a course of antibiotics or even a regular dose of aspirin you should back up the Pill with another contraceptive. The same applies when you start using it for the first time or switch to another brand: use a second contraceptive for a month. Finally, if you are having any medical treatment you should inform your doctor that you are taking the Pill – it is, after all, a form of medication.

While not wishing to sound negative about the Pill, there is no harm in sounding a note of caution about it to balance the exaggerated claims which continue to be made for it. Certainly its invention has enormously improved the lives of millions of women. It is good, but it is not perfect, and for some women it is definitely dangerous.

The intra-uterine device
In one form or other the IUD, or loop as it is also called, is the oldest known type of contra-ceptive. As its name suggests it is an object, nowadays made of plastic or copper, which is

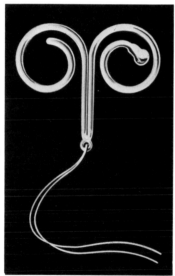

IUDs have been made in many shapes using polythene, an inert plastic which quickly regains its shape after stretching. The Lippes loop, top, is most popular. The Saf-T-Coil, above, is also in regular use. These devices are left in place indefinitely.

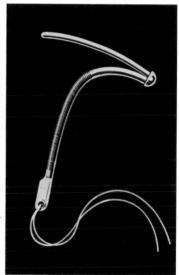

Smaller devices, easier to insert for a woman who has not had a child, are made more efficient by copper wire wound round stem, as in Copper 7 above, or by addition of progestogen. These devices become gradually less effective and are replaced at regular intervals.

inserted into a woman's uterus* through her vagina. This must be done by someone trained to fit IUDs, as then there is far less risk of complications such as rejection or a perforated uterus. In Britain, it is best to go to a Family Planning Clinic, where you can be certain that if you choose the IUD a trained doctor will insert it.

Types of IUD. The IUDs illustrated here are medically tested and approved. Do not accept any others. In particular, do not have a Dalkon Shield, which has been banned by the American FDA and the British FPA but may still be offered to women by a few out-of-touch doctors.

The Lippes loop and the Saf-T-Coil are for women who have had at least one full-term pregnancy. The Copper Seven and very similar Copper-T are for women who have not had a pregnancy and are so called because copper wire, wound round the stem, is released in minute quantities, enhancing the efficiency of the small polythene device.

No one has yet proved exactly how the IUD works contraceptively, but it alters the lining of the uterus, making it hostile to implantation, and the polythene inactivates the sperm.

Insertion. Doctors prefer to insert the IUD while a woman is menstruating because doing it at this time ensures that the woman is not pregnant, which is very important as it is now no longer considered wise to leave an IUD *in situ* if a pregnancy is confirmed. However, the best time to insert an IUD is when the woman wants it, and often that means immediately rather than waiting for her period. A few doctors are now inserting what they call post-coital IUDs within forty-eight hours of unprotected intercourse where a woman does not want to become pregnant. It is too early to say whether this is an effective method. A good time to fit an IUD may be

THE MUCOTHERMIC METHOD

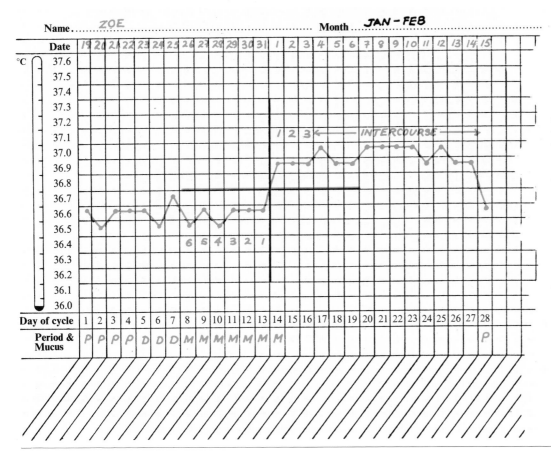

Name.... ZOE .... Month .... JAN – FEB

Using the mucothermic method, a woman calculates when it is safe to have intercourse by recording her temperature and mucus in the vagina. At ovulation, temperature rises sharply and stays up until start of next period. Left is the mucothermic chart of Zoë, who started her period on 19th January, the first day of her cycle. It lasted four days, marked P on the chart, followed by three days when vagina felt dry and intercourse was safe. As ovulation approaches, cervical mucus becomes thin and can be felt at entrance to vagina. Zoë marked M on her chart on the days her vagina felt wet. As soon as this occurs intercourse should stop. On 1st February, Zoë's temperature rose sharply, signalling that ovulation had taken place. Her temperature stayed at the higher level until 15th February, when next period started and temperature fell. A woman must refrain from intercourse while her temperature is at the higher level for three consecutive days, above the six temperatures before the rise. It was safe for Zoë to have intercourse again from 4th February. This is easy to see if you draw a cross on the chart at the point when temperature rises. The three raised temperatures will be in top right-hand corner, the six lower ones in bottom left.

at the postnatal visit, six weeks after the birth, whether the delivery was normal or by Caesarian section.*

Inserting an IUD is not usually a painful operation but some women experience quite severe cramps and sometimes heavy bleeding for twenty-four hours or longer. Surveys show that if women are able to get over the first three months and are prepared to put up with other drawbacks, such as heavier and more prolonged periods, then they are likely to stick with the IUD as a method of contraception.

Replacement. The copper bearing IUDs are changed every two or three years because in that time a calcified deposit tends to accumulate which may be counter-effective. Other devices are left in place indefinitely, providing there are no problems. A woman must, however, regularly check for herself that it is still in position, as it is not unknown for IUDs to slip out of the uterus and the woman be none the wiser. You do this by feeling for the nylon string which hangs down inside your vagina, and the easiest place to do this is in the bath, once a month after your period.

RSC Rating. After the Pill, the IUD is the most Reliable form of contraceptive – only about 2 per cent failure rate. In some respects it is safer than the Pill in

that it does not produce as many known side-effects, but some that it does produce can be quite serious. Apart from the heavier periods, low backache and cramps which may cause a good deal of discomfort, it is also possible that an IUD increases the chances of lighting up an existing pelvic infection. A low-lying infection in the uterus can flare into active life quite unexpectedly and infect the Fallopian tubes,* causing salpingitis* and a risk of infertility. Also, IUDs do not prevent the possibility of ectopic pregnancy.* Women who conceive normally with an IUD inserted are more likely to miscarry, but if the baby is carried to full term there is no increased risk of abnormality. The IUD is usually removed at the beginning of pregnancy.

Contra-indications
1 Women who have recently had an infection of either the uterus or the Fallopian tubes.
2 Women who have very heavy periods.
3 Women who have cysts,* fibroids or a cervical erosion.*
4 Women who have just given birth naturally or by Caesarian section or had an abortion: they should wait for six weeks to make sure there are no complications.

The IUD scores best on Convenience because once in, and providing that it gives no trouble, it requires no further attention or

thought from the woman, except for her regular check to see that it is still in place.

The mucothermic method
This is a more developed form of the rhythm method and it works by measuring both your temperature and your cervical mucus every day of the month on a special chart. At the time of ovulation a woman's temperature rises sharply and her cervical mucus changes quite considerably, becoming thinner, clearer and much more abundant. She may have a sensation of a wet vagina, whereas at other times of the month it may feel quite dry. As we said in the section on menstruation (pages 88-93), a few women always know when they are ovulating because they experience pain and possibly an increase of libido. Others notice no change at all, even in the cervical mucus, and for them the change in temperature is the only sure indication that they are ovulating.

In a woman with a regular pattern of menstrual cycles – and this method can only be used reliably by such a woman – ovulation occurs twelve to sixteen days before her next period. It is only after keeping a temperature chart for at least a year that you can be really sure that you know your cycle and its variations. As a very rough guide, the woman who does not want to conceive should

not have intercourse between the time that her vagina becomes noticeably wet and three full days after her temperature has risen. This is because the male sperm can live for as long as seventy-two hours inside her and her egg may survive for twenty-four hours. Obviously, the reverse applies for the woman who is trying to become pregnant. The chart above shows how a woman with a twenty-eight-day cycle might keep her mucothermic record.

RSC Rating. This method is only reliable for women with a high degree of motivation and the good fortune to have a regular menstrual pattern. For Safety it scores 100 per cent, because it produces no physical ill-effects. But as regards Convenience, which should include psychological well-being, this is a matter of individual temperament and lifestyle. Apart from those who are compelled to use it for religious reasons, only those women who can adapt easily to the limitation on intercourse and careful self-monitoring that this method involves should consider it. Of course, it is possible to use it in conjunction with another contraceptive such as a diaphragm or condom during the unsafe period, and this may appeal to women who are unhappy with the Pill or the IUD. However, it cannot be recommended to anyone who, for whatever reason, cannot

UTERUS

BLADDER

CERVIX

PUBIC BONE

VAGINA

URETHRA

FOLDED DIAPHRAGM

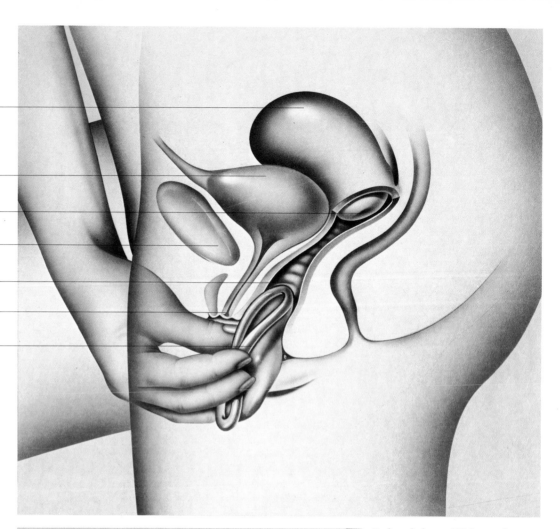

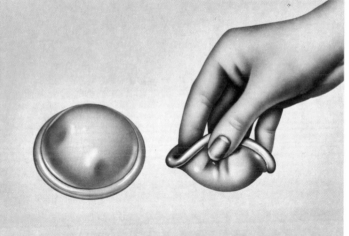

FOLDING DIAPHRAGM

risk pregnancy under any circumstances.

The diaphragm (Dutch Cap)
This is a dome-shaped, soft rubber cap mounted on a spring which holds it in place in the vagina over the cervix. Providing that it is combined with approximately one teaspoonful of spermicide jelly or cream, spread over both sides of the cap, it is an efficient contraceptive. Timing is also very important. It can be put in at any time before intercourse but it should be left for at least six hours afterwards. If you have intercourse again less than six hours after the first time, then you should add more spermicide without removing the diaphragm.

The diaphragm varies in size according to your internal measurements, so it must be fitted by a doctor, who will also show you how to insert it. It needs to be kept clean and dry and checked regularly for any signs of perforation or perishing. If you gain or lose more than 7 lb (3.2 kg), or have a child, you must check again with your doctor for size – or a different type of cap might fit you better. You should renew your cap once a year.

The cervical cap and the vault cap are smaller versions of the diaphragm which fit tightly over the cervix and are mainly

used by women whose vagina has become very stretched and whose muscles are not strong enough to hold the diaphragm. They are fitted, inserted and maintained in the same way.

RSC Rating. The diaphragm is very Reliable (a failure rate of between 2 and 8 per cent, depending on how carefully the woman uses it); it does extremely well on Safety, with no side-effects, unless you develop an allergy to the spermicide which is rare; and on Convenience it works well for

those who lead organized lives and can learn to look on it as a regular habit. What tends to put women off using it is the mess and bother of insertion, particularly if it is not always followed by intercourse. However, this is a method well worth considering, or perhaps trying again, if you have not been too happy with other methods of contraception.

The condom (sheath)
This is a thin rubber jacket about 7 in (17.5 cm) long which is rolled on to a man's erect penis just

Left and above: With practice, inserting a diaphragm is quick and easy. First, put spermicidal cream or jelly into dome, around rim and, if desired, on underside of diaphragm. Gently squeeze sides together and insert diaphragm into vagina in upward and backward direction, with folded edges facing forward wall of vagina. Ease into position with index finger. Once in position, spring rim of diaphragm returns it to original circular shape and it fits snugly across vagina covering cervix. When used to feeling cervix through the rubber, it is easy to check that diaphragm is in correct position. It can be inserted any time before intercourse, but must be left for at least six hours afterwards. If intercourse occurs again within that time, more

before intercourse. It may have a teat or a plain end; if the latter, then at least 1 in (2.5 cm) of space should be left at the tip as a precaution against bursting. The man must withdraw his penis immediately after ejaculation and before his erection subsides and remove the condom carefully, as there is a danger of the semen seeping out. One type to be avoided is the short one which just fits over the glans, the tip of the penis, because it slips off all too easily inside the vagina.

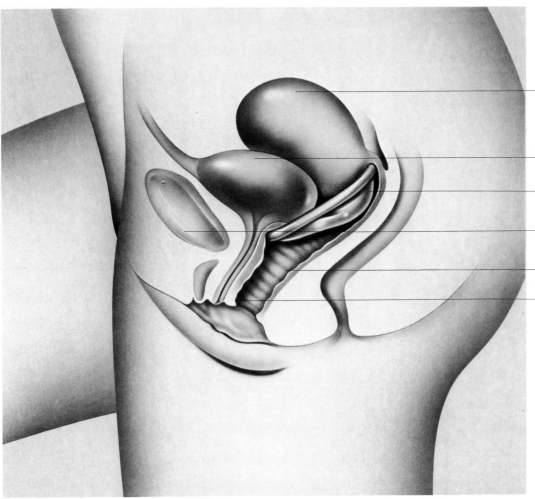

UTERUS

BLADDER

DIAPHRAGM IN POSITION

PUBIC BONE

VAGINA

URETHRA

spermicide must be added without disturbing diaphragm. To remove, hook index finger under spring rim. Take out and wash diaphragm carefully, dry, and check for any sign of perishing or perforation. Keep in clean, dry conditions.
Right: Cervical and vault caps are smaller versions of diaphragm. They fit tightly over cervix and are used if vagina has become stretched and muscles will not hold diaphragm in place. They are fitted, inserted and maintained in the same way.
Far right: Condoms are a safe and easy method of contraception if used with spermicide. However, since a condom must be fitted over a man's erect penis love-making is interrupted at a crucial point. Some couples also complain that condoms reduce sensitivity.

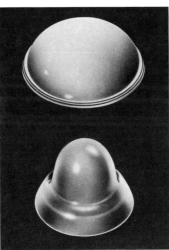

CERVICAL AND VAULT CAPS

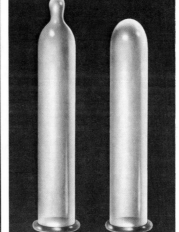

TEAT AND PLAIN CONDOMS

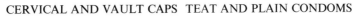

RSC Rating. The condom levels with the diaphragm for Reliability and Safety provided it is always used with a spermicide. Convenience is again a personal matter. It is relatively cheap and easy to buy – a major plus point. On the other hand, putting it on does interfere with love-making at a sensitive moment. However thin and lubricated the condom may be, it dulls sensation for the man, and his immediate withdrawal after orgasm tends to disturb post-coital enjoyment.

Sterilization
This is a permanent and final method of birth control. Only very occasionally is it either reversible or a failure, so if you decide on this method you must be absolutely certain that you do not wish to have any more children.

Female sterilization. This used to be a serious operation for a woman, involving a week or more in hospital and several weeks of convalescence, but today it usually involves no more than an overnight stay. Some doctors even

perform sterilization on an out-patient basis. It involves an operation on the Fallopian tubes so that the egg is prevented from passing through the tube to meet the sperm and become fertilized. Instead, it simply dissolves into the body.

Tying the tubes (tubal ligation) means an abdominal operation and a stay of several days in hospital. Nowadays this method is usually offered only when the woman has to be in hospital for another reason, say

giving birth to the child which she wishes to be her last. The advantage is that it affords the surgeon an excellent opportunity of examining other major organs in the woman's body.

However, if such an examination is not medically necessary and the doctor is confident of his skills, then the best and most convenient method is undoubtedly the laparoscopy. A laparoscope is a very thin, lighted telescope which is introduced through a minute abdominal incision. The Fallopian tubes are then cauterized by means of electrically heated forceps inserted through another tiny abdominal opening. The cuts are so small that they can be closed by a single stitch each, which is removed two or three days later. This is an excellent method of sterilization as long as it is done by skilled and experienced doctors. Make sure you have it done in a hospital or clinic where you know it is routine procedure.

Male sterilization or vasectomy. This is a much simpler operation. It can be done with a local anaesthetic in a doctor's surgery and involves cutting and tying, or clipping, the two ducts (vas deferens) which carry the sperm from the testes to the penis. A vasectomy is not immediately

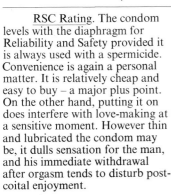

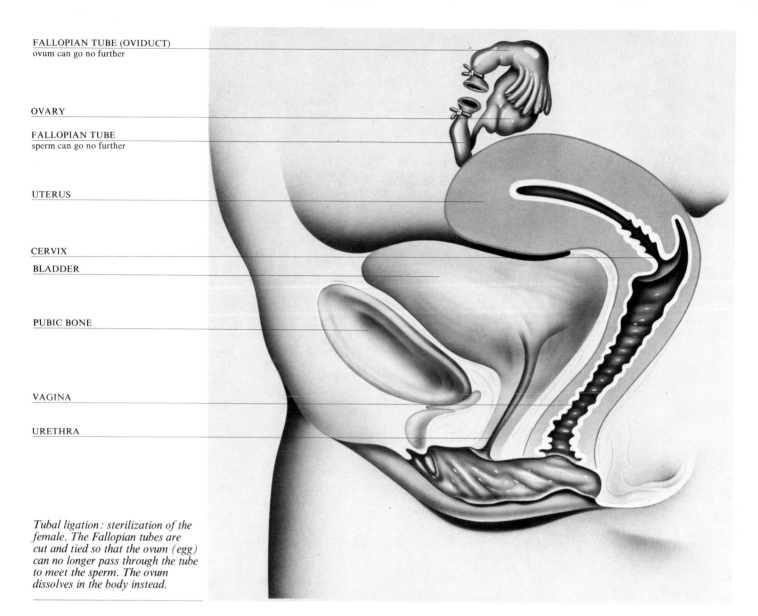

FALLOPIAN TUBE (OVIDUCT)
ovum can go no further

OVARY

FALLOPIAN TUBE
sperm can go no further

UTERUS

CERVIX

BLADDER

PUBIC BONE

VAGINA

URETHRA

Tubal ligation: sterilization of the female. The Fallopian tubes are cut and tied so that the ovum (egg) can no longer pass through the tube to meet the sperm. The ovum dissolves in the body instead.

effective because a man has to use up his stored sperm – usually about ten ejaculations – so, depending on the frequency of intercourse, this may mean that for up to six months the couple will need to use another contraceptive. A man cannot be cleared until two follow-up tests show that his semen has become completely sperm-free.

As for the woman, sterilization should be regarded as irreversible, although if a man does change his mind later on, perhaps because he has remarried or his children have died tragically, he has a better chance of having his fertility restored (30 per cent). However, this is not something to bear in mind when asking for the operation and most doctors doing it insist on careful counselling beforehand, as they do for women. Some insist on a signed agreement from the husband and wife, though this is not legally necessary. Women who ask for sterilization because they have decided that they never want

106

children will have difficulty in finding a doctor who will agree to do it, especially if they are under the age of thirty.

There are many reasons why it may be preferable for the man to be sterilized rather than his wife. Firstly, it is undoubtedly a safer and quicker procedure with no side-effects. (Female sterilization does sometimes produce menstrual problems.) Secondly, in no way does it affect sexual performance; indeed, many men who have had a vasectomy say that this is actually improved because the vasectomy has removed the fear of causing an unwanted pregnancy. However, the couple asking for a vasectomy must be certain that they want to remain monogamous because otherwise it could become a serious source of tension.

ABORTION
This is an emotive issue which continues to arouse strong feelings both for and against, despite a decade of liberal legislation in Britain and the United States. The

moral and other arguments which are employed in the debate are outside the scope of this book, but abortion is included in this section because it has a valid claim to be counted among the full range of birth-control measures available to a woman. Few people would say that it is the ideal form of contraception, but it is an essential back-up for the woman who has become pregnant accidentally and who cannot or does not wish to bear the child.

Abortion counselling should be an integral part of a responsible medical service, but unfortunately many doctors are ill-suited or disinclined to offer this to their patients. If you find yourself in this position and feel that you must have some unbiased advice before you make up your mind, then contact a Family Planning Clinic or one of the pregnancy advisory services, checking beforehand that it is a genuine charity and not serving as a cover-up for doctors who are more interested in your purse than your well-being.

Alternatively, try to contact a women's group* through your local newspaper; they will be able to put you in touch with an experienced counsellor.

The earlier you have an abortion the safer it is, so the first thing to do, if you suspect that you may be pregnant, is to go either to your doctor for a pregnancy test or to a pregnancy advisory centre or a Well-Woman Clinic. Depending on the stage of pregnancy, various types of abortion are available.

Interception (endometrial aspiration) can be done up to fourteen days after an overdue period. A plastic cannula (tube) is inserted through the cervix without dilating it and the uterine lining is gently pulled away by means of a syringe. Should the woman be pregnant – and at this stage it is impossible to establish definitely that she is – foetal material will also be extracted. This is not yet a common procedure, but many women and doctors are in favour of it because it is simple, relatively painless and quick. Since it

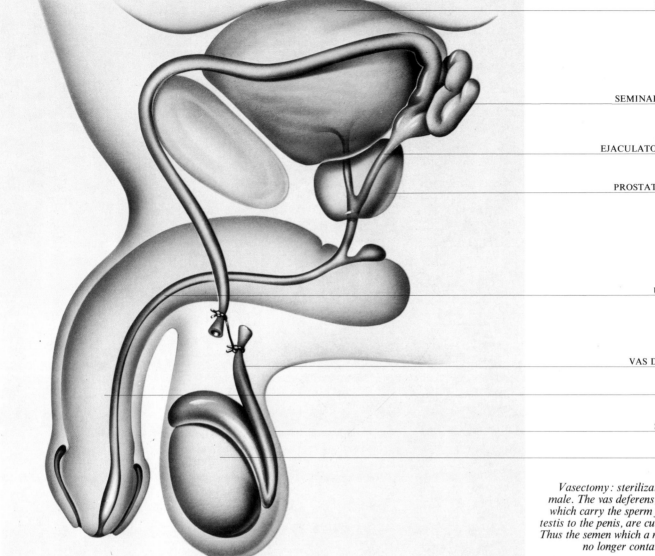

BLADDER

SEMINAL VESICLE

EJACULATORY DUCT

PROSTATE GLAND

URETHRA

VAS DEFERENS

PENIS

SCROTUM

TESTIS

Vasectomy: sterilization of the male. The vas deferens, the ducts which carry the sperm from each testis to the penis, are cut and tied. Thus the semen which a man ejects no longer contains sperm.

requires no anaesthetic it can be done in a doctor's surgery.

The advantages are obvious: emotional problems can be avoided as well as hospitalization. On the discount side, if the woman is not pregnant she has been put through an unnecessary procedure, and doctors also fear that sometimes not all the foetal material is removed, which may cause subsequent complications of bleeding and the need for an operation later.

Interception should not be confused with menstrual extraction, which is the process whereby the menses (menstrual blood and matter) are extracted on the first day of the period with a device called the Del'Em syringe. This is a growing practice in many women's self-help groups, but is not something you can do for yourself.

Vacuum aspiration is a recently-developed technique which is now the most favoured method for abortions done before the twelfth week. This is because it can

be done in an out-patient clinic under a local anaesthetic, and trauma is minimal. The doctor dilates the cervix with a plastic cannula as much as is necessary to remove all the foetal material, which is sucked out by means of an electric pump. The more advanced the pregnancy, the greater the amount of dilatation required and the wider the cannula.

Dilatation and curettage* is a similar procedure in that it involves clearing the uterus via the cervix and vagina. Again, depending on the stage of pregnancy, the cervix is dilated by a succession of metal rods gradually increasing in diameter until the cervix is open enough for the doctor to insert forceps to extract foetal material. The curetting part of the procedure involves scraping round the inside of the womb with a spoon-like instrument after this extraction, to make certain that nothing has been left behind.

This operation does involve a general anaesthetic and an

overnight stay in hospital. In the hands of very skilled doctors it can occasionally be extended to abortions over thirteen weeks, but usually a doctor prefers to wait until sixteen weeks when it is possible to induce an abortion by different means.

Amniocentesis and urea replacement is not the easiest way of having an abortion, as by this time – over sixteen weeks – the foetus will be far advanced and plainly recognizable. The abortion is induced by replacing the amniotic fluid* in which the foetus floats with a solution of urea, which has the effect of stimulating the uterus to expel its contents: a mini-labour, in short, which can be very painful and distressing.

Sometimes prostaglandins* are introduced into the amniotic fluid with the same effect. To speed up the process, which will anyway take several hours, the woman is usually put on to an oxytocin drip* (a synthetic hormone). Use of the drip also stimulates contractions of the uterus.

Hysterotomy is in effect a mini-Caesarian. It is a major abdominal operation which involves removing the foetus through the opened abdominal wall, and it leaves a scar. Hysterotomy used to be the traditional method of dealing with late abortions, but doctors now try to avoid it unless there is no alternative, as in the case of a young girl who may have concealed her pregnancy until a late date or an older menopausal woman who could not imagine that she might be pregnant.

Providing it is done in the first three months, the above-mentioned Mr Diggory and Dr McEwan say that 'the dangers from having an abortion are probably no greater than arise from being on the contraceptive Pill for a year. It carries less than one-tenth the risk of having a full-term delivery.' Here again, the practitioner is important. Patients are less likely to experience complications when treated by a skilled doctor.

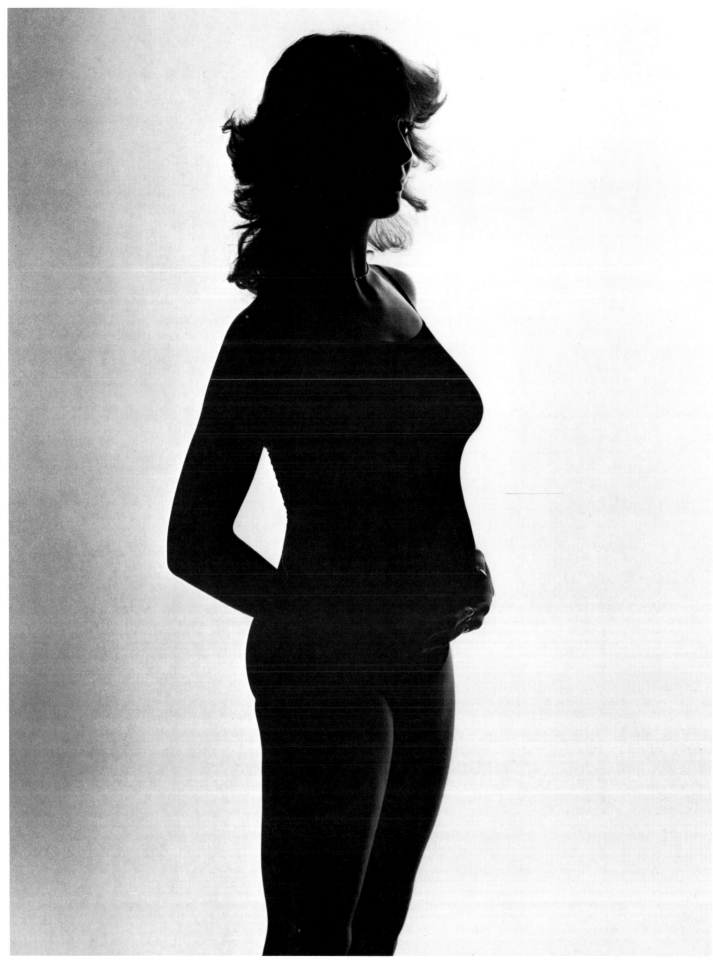

Pregnancy

If every woman waited for the perfect time to become pregnant the human race would die out. In place of the traditional woman's lot of endless childbirth and unmanageable families has come the potential freedom for every woman to conceive a child at the best possible time for her.

However, the decision can never be absolutely clear-cut. A late or a too-early marriage, a shortage of money, career development, a change of job or an illness can all interfere with trouble-free family planning. And underneath the rational decision-making runs the turbulent stream of biology. For all the options open to women to control their own destinies, there is an irrational strain that still leads us blindly into pregnancy. Pregnancy is one of the rare events in a human life which must be followed through to its natural conclusion. Abortion may be a possibility in the early stages and

accidents may bring it to an untimely end, but the average woman who conceives a child is on a through train to labour with no stops along the way. Mentally, emotionally and physically, pregnancy unrolls itself so slowly that the enormous responsibility it represents is realized only gradually. A professor of obstetrics once described a woman's change of attitude to herself during pregnancy as 'having missed a period, being pregnant and expecting a baby'.

The baby is almost the least real part of pregnancy. All the concentration on antenatal care, the preparations for labour, are aimed at seeing the pregnant woman through childbirth. Then she is on her own, like all those fictional heroines who fade into the sunset through marriage. Childbirth, like marriage, is not just a happy ending. It is the beginning of the most important commitment one human being can make to another.

CHANCES OF GETTING PREGNANT

Pregnancy is not an automatic result of sexual intercourse. The chances of pregnancy within one month for a woman in her early twenties who is having intercourse three or four times a week are only 30 per cent. Within two months they are 45 per cent and even within one year, only 80 per cent. The best time for having a baby biologically is around the age of twenty, but social factors may not be as favourable. The risks of child-bearing rise slightly over the age of thirty, but the thirty-year-old mother has an emotional stability and maturity, and usually an economic security, that the twenty-year-old may lack.

Age is one of the factors that affect fertility. The overall chances of a woman under twenty becoming pregnant some time are 95 per cent as compared with 83 per cent for a woman between thirty-one and thirty-five, but age is only one factor. General health is important. So is state of mind. Anxiety and tension are known to be inhibiting factors in conception and many are the women who, having written themselves off as infertile, become pregnant after deciding to adopt a child.

INFECTIOUS AND HEREDITARY DISEASES

Before you choose to become pregnant there is one precaution it is advisable to take: make sure you have been inoculated against, or have had, German measles (rubella). Once you are pregnant you cannot be inoculated and German measles contracted in the first three months of pregnancy is a major cause of abnormalities, such as deafness or blindness, in the unborn child.

If you think you have come into contact with anyone suffering

from German measles, report it straight away to your doctor. Blood tests will establish whether you have been infected; it is possible to have such a mild attack that you are not aware of it. On the other hand, you may have had it in the past without realizing and so be immune.

If tests prove that you have contracted German measles in the vital first three months of pregnancy, a therapeutic abortion is possible, and you should give the matter serious consideration.

Another precaution you may wish to take if you believe there could be a hereditary abnormality or condition in your family, such as serious mental illness or haemophilia,* is to ask your doctor to refer you to a genetic counsellor. He will not be able to make your decision for you, but he may be able to compute the risks to your unborn child and help you to make an informed choice.

Most other illnesses have no ill-effects on the unborn child, but a doctor might worry if you had a serious bout of influenza or a very high temperature in the first three months of pregnancy.

DETERMINING SEX

If you feel passionately about the sex of your child, there are techniques with some scientific respectability which may help you to determine it in advance, but none of them is 100 per cent certain. Of course it is wiser not to have a violent preference, since children whose parents really resent their sex usually suffer for it. However, if you want a girl, your chances might be improved by having intercourse until two or three days before ovulation,* then abstaining for a few days. This theoretically enables the acid environment of the vagina before ovulation to favour the sperm which are carrying the female

chromosome.* On the same theory, couples who want a boy should have intercourse as close as possible to the date of ovulation, when the alkaline environment of the vagina during ovulation favours the male sperm.

There is no guarantee that this procedure will produce a child of the sex you want, but it may tip the odds in your favour.

INFERTILITY

If you and your partner decide to go ahead and have a baby, if you both seem to be in good health and make love with reasonable frequency, say twice a week, then you have very good chances of conceiving, but it is quite possible that some months may go by without anything happening.

It is all too easy to become anxious and obsessive about conceiving a child once you have set your heart on it, and it is only natural that you would like the reasons for your apparent infertility investigated. Try not to be depressed by old wives' tales about fertility. It makes no difference if you have irregular or painful periods, nor does it matter if anyone else in your family has had fertility problems: high or low fertility is not hereditary.

If after about six months of trying to conceive nothing has happened, and it is worrying you, consulting a doctor will probably reassure you that nothing is wrong.

The doctor will first check your basic physical condition. He will want to give you an internal pelvic examination to make sure there is no abnormality or infection of the cervix. He will also want to check your husband's medical background for any previous illness, such as mumps, which may have affected his fertility. He will want to know the frequency of intercourse and whether, basic as it seems, you are actually having

full intercourse. Ignorance can be a very effective contraceptive.

If this initial consultation reveals no obvious problems, he will probably want to check that you are actually ovulating each month: bleeding once a month is no guarantee of this. The simplest way to check ovulation is to take your temperature regularly each morning. The temperature rises slightly when ovulation takes place, usually around the fourteenth day of the twenty-eight-day cycle. He will also arrange a post-coital test. This is done within twenty-four hours of intercourse to check the quantity and quality of sperm in the cervix. Finally, the doctor will X-ray the Fallopian tubes* to make sure that they are not blocked in any way. Further information may be obtained from hormone tests.

ARTIFICIAL INSEMINATION

There are two types of artificial insemination. The first, AIH (artificial insemination by the husband), consists of collecting the husband's seminal fluid* and introducing it with a special applicator into the wife's cervical canal. This is done if the husband is producing sperm but for some reason is unable to deposit it in the vagina. The second type, which is much more controversial, is AID (artificial insemination by donor) – in other words, using the seminal fluid of a carefully-chosen donor. This method can be used when the husband is unable to produce sufficiently fertile seminal fluid. There are obvious ethical, emotional and legal problems attached to this procedure. The so-called 'test-tube' baby method involves fertilizing the mother's egg with the husband's sperm outside the womb; the egg is then reintroduced for a 'normal' pregnancy. The method is still highly experimental.

PREGNANCY

Pregnancy tests

One day you will suspect that you are pregnant. The most obvious sign of pregnancy is the absence of your monthly period, if you are generally regular, but there are other signs. Women who are pregnant for the second time usually know without the help of a pregnancy test, but if this is the first time, there is something very cheering about the positive confirmation of a test. A simple chemical tester can be bought from the pharmacist so that you can do your test privately at home, or the pharmacist will do the test for you, but it is usually advisable to consult your doctor.

The basis of these pregnancy tests is to check on the presence of a hormone* called human chorionic gonadotrophin (HCG)* in your early morning urine. If the hormone is present you are certainly pregnant. If the test is negative, and you subsequently find you are pregnant, it simply means that you have had the test too soon; it should be done a minimum of thirteen days after the period was due, i.e. forty-one days from the first day of your last period.

The pregnancy test will confirm that yours is a genuine pregnancy and not just a period missed through illness, anxiety or fatigue. In any case, follow your own test by visiting the doctor to confirm pregnancy.

Another sign of pregnancy is a very obvious change in your breasts. They will be bigger, feel tender, and the blue veins will be noticeable. It is quite likely that you will feel sick or even be sick. This is the famous 'morning sickness', which may never actually manifest itself as sickness or confine itself only to the mornings. You may simply feel nauseous all the time, or you may feel sickened by certain foods or smells, by cigarettes or meat or alcohol.

You may feel an obsessive craving to eat certain foods – it could be anything from ice cream to oranges to lumps of coal – or nothing at all.

You may continue to feel exactly as normal, or you may feel emotionally unstable, unaccountably tearful and tired, sometimes to the point of exhaustion. At the same time, you will probably feel elated and excited. Congratulations. You are pregnant.

Feelings during pregnancy

Whether you feel happy or depressed or an uncontrollable mixture of both, you know that for the rest of your pregnancy your feelings are not entirely under your control. This is not because you are being particularly stupid or irritating but because the fast and sudden rise in hormone levels

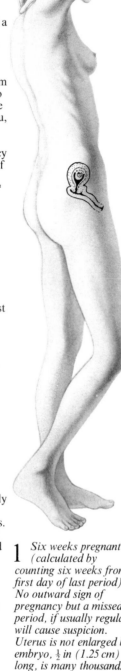

1 *Six weeks pregnant (calculated by counting six weeks from first day of last period): No outward sign of pregnancy but a missed period, if usually regular, will cause suspicion. Uterus is not enlarged but embryo, ½ in (1.25 cm) long, is many thousands of times larger than original ovum. It has a heart, just beginning to work, and nervous system. At this stage, placenta weighs more than embryo, which looks rather reptilian with an enormous head and small tail. The woman may notice her breasts swelling and becoming tender, often an early sign of pregnancy.*

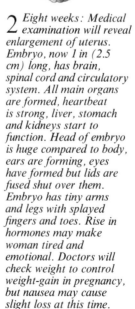

2 *Eight weeks: Medical examination will reveal enlargement of uterus. Embryo, now 1 in (2.5 cm) long, has brain, spinal cord and circulatory system. All main organs are formed, heartbeat is strong, liver, stomach and kidneys start to function. Head of embryo is huge compared to body, ears are forming, eyes have formed but lids are fused shut over them. Embryo has tiny arms and legs with splayed fingers and toes. Rise in hormones may make woman tired and emotional. Doctors will check weight to control weight-gain in pregnancy, but nausea may cause slight loss at this time.*

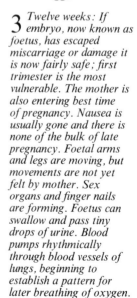

3 *Twelve weeks: If embryo, now known as foetus, has escaped miscarriage or damage it is now fairly safe; first trimester is the most vulnerable. The mother is also entering best time of pregnancy. Nausea is usually gone and there is none of the bulk of late pregnancy. Foetal arms and legs are moving, but movements are not yet felt by mother. Sex organs and finger nails are forming. Foetus can swallow and pass tiny drops of urine. Blood pumps rhythmically through blood vessels of lungs, beginning to establish a pattern for later breathing of oxygen.*

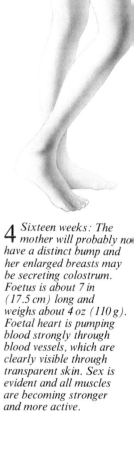

4 *Sixteen weeks: The mother will probably no have a distinct bump and her enlarged breasts may be secreting colostrum. Foetus is about 7 in (17.5 cm) long and weighs about 4 oz (110 g). Foetal heart is pumping blood strongly through blood vessels, which are clearly visible through transparent skin. Sex is evident and all muscles are becoming stronger and more active.*

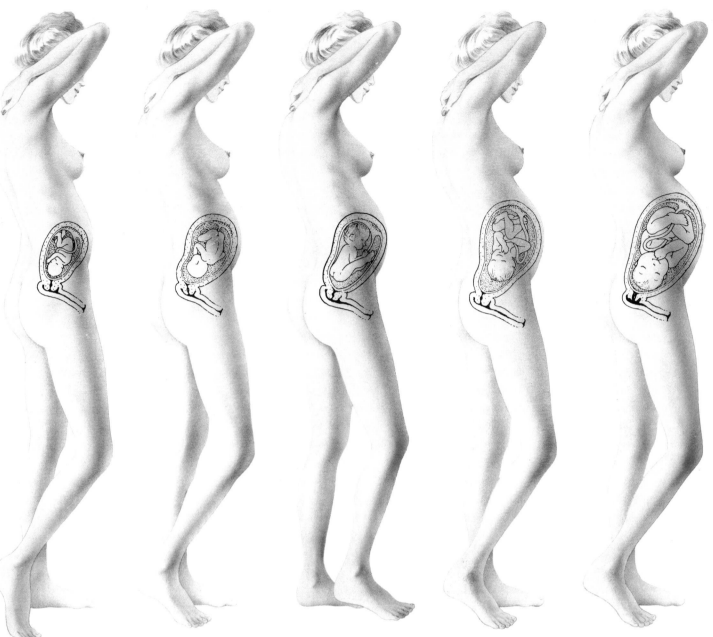

5 *Twenty weeks: Faint fluttering movement (quickening) can be felt by the mother as foetus swims around inside amniotic sac. It can already hiccup and suck its thumb and is becoming quite human in appearance, with a little hair on head, eyebrows and hair (lanugo) all over body. Lungs are strengthening but are still too immature to cope on their own outside uterus. Skin has become less transparent.*

6 *Twenty-four weeks: Foetus is gaining weight rapidly; it now weighs about 1½ lb (675 g) and is about 13 in (32.5 cm) long. The doctor can hear its heartbeat clearly with a stethoscope. Limb movements are strong enough to make mother's abdomen move. Eyelids can open but a fine membrane covers eyes. Head is still large in proportion to body, but fat is being deposited under skin to increase body size. The mother must watch her weight and rest as much as possible, as size of uterus is beginning to slow her down and cause fatigue.*

7 *Twenty-eight weeks: Baby is viable by law. If born, it can breathe and cry weakly; one in four will survive with intensive care in an incubator. It is still thin and wrinkled, with a red skin covered in protective waxy substance called vernix. Eyes are open and covering membrane gone. Increased pressure on the mother's stomach can cause heartburn and indigestion. Her joints stretch ready for labour, particularly in pelvis. She must watch her diet and eat small, nutritious meals. Her body heat rises and she may be short of breath and need to urinate frequently.*

8 *Thirty-two weeks: Baby is now growing at a tremendous rate and weighs about 4 lb (1.8 kg). Although still rather wrinkled, fat deposits are about sufficient to keep baby warm outside uterus. Lungs are well developed and baby now has a very good chance of survival if born prematurely. The mother's uterus may have grown up to twenty times its original size; life has become so crowded inside that her navel starts to protrude. Her heartbeat will have risen by up to ten beats a minute and small contractions will gradually become stronger and more frequent.*

9 *Thirty-six weeks: Baby weighs 5½ lb (2.5 kg) and although still termed premature has 90 per cent chance of survival if born. From now until full term, forty weeks, it will lose lanugo and bones will harden, although they must be soft enough to allow head through birth passage. Head should have settled down into birth position; if not, doctor may try to turn it. Uterus is now right up under rib cage. Leaning backwards to balance extra weight may cause backache. Rest is essential. Waiting may seem interminable, but birth date is near.*

during pregnancy – especially in the first three months – affects your emotions and makes you unstable. If you understand this, and if the people close to you are helped to understand it too, life will be a lot easier for you.

A woman who is pregnant can feel illogically happy, smug, excited, apprehensive, despairing and frightened in turn. Her perspective on life, however broad and far-ranging it may have been, does a somersault and turns inwards. Once she is sure that she is pregnant she is very much aware of another living being growing inside her.

The unborn baby, who can be forgotten most of the time by everyone else, who is just a foetus to her doctor and a lump to her family and friends, begins to be a real presence to her from the moment she knows of its existence. This is why miscarriage, even at an early stage, is such a deeply upsetting experience.

The real happiness and serenity of pregnancy can co-exist with moments of awful depression and panic. Women who have led a full working and social life wonder what they have let themselves in for. In the first three months, in particular, many women feel so low that they wonder rather bitterly when all the 'blooming' is going to begin.

Happily, by the end of the third month, life improves enormously. The middle three months – the second trimester – of pregnancy are the most stable emotionally and physically. The sickness and exhaustion of early pregnancy should magically disappear, you will begin to look better and you are a long way yet from the bulk of late pregnancy. You have enough energy to lead a normal life, so this is the time to make the most of work, travel and social life.

It is towards the end of pregnancy that you may begin to feel overwhelmed by it. Sheer size can make the simplest action an effort and you may not feel like going anywhere very much. For the first time in your life you may feel perfectly content to sit at home all day and stare into space. Interspersed with these periods of glorious lethargy will be terrific bursts of energy and nest-building when you may pack your hospital suitcase or spring-clean the house for the fifth time.

There is also a kind of pre-natal depression, when you might suddenly feel that you have been pregnant for ever and ever and that the pregnancy will never come to an end. Illogically, a kind of panic goes hand in hand with this as you realize for the first time that there is no way out of your condition but through the unknown gates of labour. You may look at your

112

enormous stomach and wonder how the baby is going to get out.

All these fluctuations of mood can be eased if the people near to you understand how closely they are related to your physical condition. Nothing is more infuriating to an already tearful and tired woman than being told to pull herself together or being asked brusquely what the matter is. Pregnancy is the matter and she just can't help it.

Bodily changes in pregnancy
A healthy non-pregnant woman leading a full and busy life can afford to take her body and its functions for granted. A pregnant woman is preoccupied by her body and its demands and changes. For the first time in her life it comes to dominate her with the extra-ordinary changes that are taking place within and without.

Apart from the feelings of nausea and fatigue, you may notice the need to urinate more frequently, especially towards the end of your pregnancy when there may be particularly startling moments when a sudden movement from the baby jams its head up against your bladder and you wonder how you are going to hold out. Never lose the opportunity to go to the lavatory, particularly in late pregnancy.

You may also find yourself constipated and consequently suffering from piles.* Piles are varicose veins* around the rectum which may be very uncomfortable. Varicose veins in the legs should disappear after pregnancy if you suffer from them, and may not occur with a first pregnancy at all. To avoid varicose veins in the legs, rest with your feet up as much as possible, and never cross your legs when sitting; to avoid piles, watch that you include plenty of fibre-rich foods such as bran cereals and wholemeal bread in your diet. If either of these conditions worries you, ask your doctor's advice.

You will not look noticeably pregnant until about the fourth month, when you will find that your belts need extra notches and your trousers fail to do up. By the end of the fourth month or the beginning of the fifth you may begin to notice the baby moving about inside you. It is very hard to detect for the first-time mother because the movements are slight, fluttery ones known as 'quickening', but they become stronger as time goes by.

It is commonplace to talk about the baby kicking, but an unborn baby does a great deal more than that. It heaves and turns and strange bumps appear outlined by the abdominal wall, which you will try to identify as elbow or knees or the head. Your whole abdomen can appear to shift from one side to the other, and

many a pregnant woman lies in her bath transfixed by the secret activity that is taking place inside her. Once the baby starts moving it becomes even more real to you and you can share it with your fascinated family.

By seven months you may be suffering from heartburn* or indigestion as your stomach is squeezed up, but your doctor can give you perfectly safe antacid tablets which will relieve the discomfort. Try sleeping propped up, too. This helps to prevent the acid stomach juices passing into the oesophagus, the passage for food from mouth to stomach.

By the eighth month your normally flat navel will protrude, pushed out by the full uterus.* You may find that your feet and ankles swell, especially towards the end of the day. Your joints, particularly the pelvic joints, will stretch, loosening themselves up for the business of labour.

You may also be aware of backache, particularly if you have to spend too long in one position, or if you have to carry things. Backache (see page 55) is partly a result of the extra weight you carry and the distorted balance of your body, and partly a result of the softened joints and ligaments, but it is mostly due to bad posture. You may find that lying on your side is better rest for you than lying on your back and eases the strain.

In late pregnancy you will also find that your body heat rises. You will notice this especially at night, when your husband needs the blankets on and you keep trying to push them back. You may also find that you get very short of breath, and not just with exercise, as the uterus occupies lung-expanding space.

You may find that you are sticking to one comfortable pair of shoes and that your stretched feet simply won't go into the rest, but they will return to normal after labour. Low-heeled, comfortable shoes will also help you keep your balance, which tends to be less sure in later pregnancy.

At eight months you might be advised to buy nursing bras for later: the front-fastening kind are best. Your breasts will grow still more between now and the milk coming in, but at this stage they are more or less the size they will be after pregnancy.

Throughout pregnancy, and indeed throughout a woman's reproductive life, the uterus contracts in little practice contractions. You will gradually notice these in pregnancy as the stomach hardens, stays hard for a few seconds and then relaxes. These are known as Braxton-Hicks contractions and they become more and more noticeable as pregnancy progresses. They are

occasionally mistaken for the much stronger, regular contractions of labour, but they are helping the uterus to get into training to push the baby out.

Apart from these outward physical signs, even more dramatic changes are taking place within the body. The blood supply, which is normally about 10 pt (5.7 litres), increases by between 25 and 40 per cent. Unless the red cells increase to match the extra supply anaemia* can result, which is the reason why most pregnant women are issued with iron pills at the antenatal visit. Many doctors feel that if the haemoglobin* level in the blood is regularly checked and found to be normal then there is no need for the automatic prescribing of iron.

As well as the increase in the blood supply, the uterus grows to twenty times its original size and the heartbeat rate goes up by ten beats a minute or about 14,000 beats a day. But despite all these dramatic changes, the heart and the uterus and the blood supply will all return to normal within a week or so of delivery.

Changes in the foetus
Of course, the most extraordinary developments of all are going on within the uterus. Even at six weeks old the embryonic heart is beginning to work, and by the seventh week, when the embryo* is only just over $\frac{1}{2}$ in (1.25 cm) long, it already has a circulatory system, an intestine, liver and kidneys, brain, spinal cord and the rudiments of ears and eyes. By the eighth week it is no longer called an embryo but a foetus.

By twelve weeks, all the major internal organs are formed, the sex of the foetus is clear, and from now on its life in the womb consists of maturing to the point where it can exist independently in the outside world. If it has escaped congenital abnormalities by three months, then it is fairly free from danger. The first trimester of pregnancy is the most vulnerable, both to abnormalities caused by drugs or disease and to the risk of miscarriage.

Ready for birth
After twenty weeks you will be able to feel the movements of the foetus for yourself; by that time it may even be sucking its thumb or hiccuping. At twenty-eight weeks the baby is viable by law. This means that if it is born prematurely, even stillborn, its birth must be registered. In fact its chances of survival, were it born at this age, are only 5 per cent.

After this stage the baby is coated with a greasy, cheesy substance called vernix, which protects it from the amniotic fluid* in which it floats. Vernix may well be present when the baby is born. By the thirty-sixth week the baby has a 90 per cent chance of

About three days after fertilization, the egg splits into two parts. The inner mass forms the embryo and the outer collection the placenta. This attaches itself to the mother by implantation in the endometrium,* the lining of the uterus, and to the embryo by the umbilical cord, through which the growing baby receives all its nourishment during pregnancy. The placenta, which resembles a sponge, also acts as the lung, liver, kidney and bowel of the foetus.

As the placenta needs a large supply of blood to pass the required nutrients to the baby, the volume of the mother's blood increases by up to 40 per cent. At no time does the blood of the mother and baby mix. The mother's blood provides oxygen and nourishment to the cells of the placenta, which in turn passes these to the foetus through the umbilical cord. This process also happens in reverse, with the placenta acting as a sieve to diffuse waste products from the baby's blood into the mother's circulation to be cleaned by her kidneys.

Although the placenta acts as a faithful guardian to the baby, some harmful substances do cross it. Certain diseases can be transferred, so that the baby can be born with chicken pox or show the dangerous effects of infection with German measles (rubella). Other diseases such as tuberculosis can also be transferred. Antibodies made by the mother in response to infection in the second half of her pregnancy will cross the placenta and help to protect the baby from infections after birth.

Certain drugs cross the placenta, as happened in the tragic thalidomide cases. Most doctors now recommend mothers to avoid all drugs unless they are specifically prescribed and essential. The most dangerous group of drugs for the foetus are narcotics, such as heroin and morphine. A baby born to a

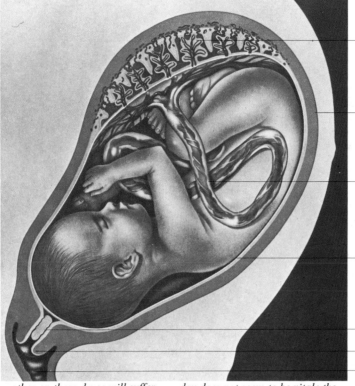

PLACENTA

UTERUS

UMBILICAL CORD

AMNIOTIC SAC

PLUG OF MUCUS

CERVIX

VAGINA

mother on these drugs will suffer from withdrawal symptoms from which it can die if it is not treated. The baby must be kept in hospital for several weeks to be 'weaned' from the drug. Alcohol also passes to the baby via the placenta, but this appears to do no harm provided the mother is not drinking heavily.

Doctors disagree on whether or not chemicals from cigarette smoking directly interfere with the foetus. But there are statistical associations that women who smoke have babies of a lower full-term birth weight and that some of these babies are slightly behind other children later in life, for example when learning in school. The number of cigarettes smoked per

day does not seem to be vital; the evidence is related to whether a mother smokes or not.

In some cases, the placenta fails to function efficiently during the pregnancy. This may be due to maternal illness such as kidney disease or high blood-pressure before pregnancy. Doctors will be on the lookout for this and for complications as a result of pregnancy, such as toxaemia, which affects the placenta causing bleeding. The placenta has a life of its own – youth, maturity and old age. If tests show that it is no longer working efficiently, thus endangering the baby, labour may be induced. If the placenta is wrongly placed in the uterus,

bleeding will result. An expectant mother with this complication may have to remain in hospital for as many weeks as possible in her term, to rest and allow the baby to grow 'in utero' rather than in the premature nursery. After this there is every chance of a completely healthy baby, but a high percentage are delivered by Caesarian section.

When the baby is born, the placenta becomes the 'afterbirth' and is expelled a short time after the baby. It will resemble a dinner plate and weigh about $1\frac{1}{2}$ lb (675 g). Blood goes on flowing from the placenta through the umbilical cord to the baby and an obstetrician or midwife will often not cut the cord until it stops pulsating.

---

survival, and it is now that it should have settled itself into the head-down position, ready for birth. A breech birth may take place when the baby has failed to turn itself head down and presents itself for delivery bottom first.

At forty weeks the pregnancy has officially arrived at term, but don't be disappointed if nothing happens on the appointed day. A lot of babies come earlier than expected and a lot come later. Nobody really knows why some babies are born earlier than expected, though certain conditions, such as multiple pregnancy, Rhesus incompatibility* and diabetes* carry a bigger risk of prematurity than normal. The chances of the baby's survival if it is born in the last four weeks of pregnancy are very good. The main threat to a premature baby

comes from breathing problems since its lungs are still immature.

If your baby is a day or two late, don't worry. It is obviously difficult to decide the exact day of conception and you should prepare yourself for a slight delay. To avoid feelings of anti-climax if the baby fails to arrive on the appointed day, it is a good idea to have activities planned so that you aren't sitting at home simply waiting for something to happen.

You may find that your doctor is unwilling to let you go too long over term, although you yourself might prefer to leave it to nature. He may have right on his side. Postmaturity has its dangers for babies, just as prematurity has. The greatest threat is that the placenta, which has been supplying the baby with oxygen, blood and nourishment, may begin

to falter so that the baby is starved. When this happens the baby is safest outside the womb, so listen carefully to your doctor if he wants to induce labour after term; there may be a sound medical reason for induction.

Antenatal care
Your best chances of a successful delivery and a healthy baby lie in the quality of your antenatal care. This is not simply a moral admonition, but a statistical fact. The maternity services are unique in their relationship with their patients. A pregnant woman is the one patient who walks into hospital as a healthy human being, and the co-operation which can be established between her and the people who take care of her, the help and education and clinical guidance which are available to her, have led to the safety of

modern childbirth.

Through antenatal clinics, either at the hospital where you will have your baby or with your doctor, through antenatal classes with other pregnant women and experienced teachers, you should be able to clear your mind of doubts and fears and prepare your body for labour. Conditions which might threaten your health and the health of your baby can be checked before they develop. In the past, the first contact a pregnant woman had with the medical services was when she went into labour – with sometimes catastrophic results – but nowadays she can be helped from confirmation of her pregnancy to a happy and healthy delivery.

The first check-up
Once your pregnancy is confirmed you will undergo a standard check-

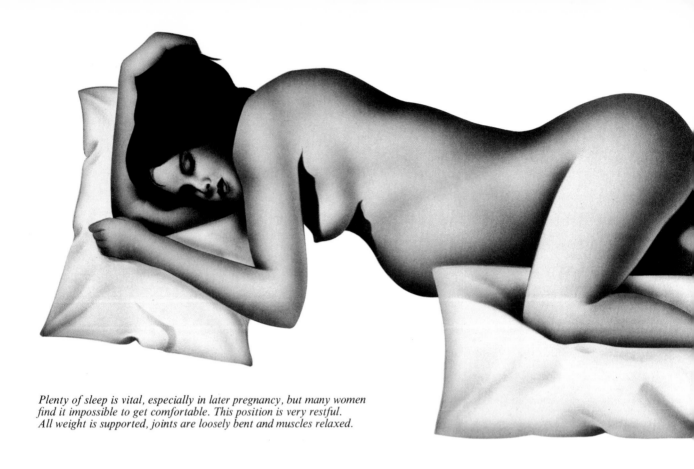

*Plenty of sleep is vital, especially in later pregnancy, but many women
find it impossible to get comfortable. This position is very restful.
All weight is supported, joints are loosely bent and muscles relaxed.*

up, either at the doctor's or at the
hospital's antenatal clinic. An
antenatal history will be recorded,
a physical examination will be
conducted and certain standard
tests will be carried out.

The maternity staff will want
to know as much about you as
possible, starting with your family
and social history – what work do
you and your husband do, are
there twins in the family, how long
have you been married? They will
want to know your obstetric and
menstrual history – do you have
regular periods, is this your first
pregnancy, is there a previous
history of miscarriage? They will
want to know if you have been in
hospital before and why, what
diseases or accidents you may
have had. They will want to check
your height and weight. Height
will help them to estimate the size
of your pelvis, and control of
weight is very important in
pregnancy (see page 115).

Your urine will be tested for
the presence of protein and sugar
and a blood sample will be taken.
The blood sample will enable them
to check the haemoglobin level,
which should not normally be
below 80 per cent, to know your
blood group and the Rhesus
factor,* and to do a routine test
called the Wassermann reaction
which indicates whether you have

ever had syphilis.* You may know
perfectly well that you haven't, but
syphilis can be transmitted to your
baby after the twentieth week of
pregnancy and cause abnormalities.
The Wassermann test is a routine
preventive measure applied to
everyone. Your blood-pressure
will also be taken.

The doctor will then check
the level of your uterus and
compare it with your estimated
dates. The EDD (estimated date of
delivery) is calculated from the
first day of your last period and is
done by working 280 days forward
from this. The doctor may also
perform an internal pelvic
examination to see that all is
normal within. Some women find
this unpleasant, but it is not painful
and it is a help to relax the internal
muscles as consciously as possible
– a technique which you will be
taught in your antenatal classes
and which will stand you in good
stead in labour. The first antenatal
visit is also the time to discuss the
likelihood of a home or hospital
delivery and to raise any doubts
and questions you may have.

Improvements in antenatal
·services will only come about as
pregnant women – the consumers
– make their wants and worries
known. This is easier said than
done. Antenatal clinics are often
rushed and busy places where

staff, though well-intentioned, can
be brusque. You may never see
the same person twice, and in a
teaching hospital you may be
confronted by a group of medical
students. You may have to wait
one or two hours before you are
seen. Your biggest problem is that
it takes a strong-minded woman
to get her questions answered and
her needs seen to under these
circumstances, and very few
pregnant women feel strong-
minded. On the contrary, they are
at their most vulnerable and
insecure and often the last place
they feel like a battle of wills is the
clinic or the labour ward. So sort
out problems while you feel fit
and healthy.

If you feel very strongly
about the way you have been
treated, then the right person to
complain to is the doctor in
charge of the unit. Ask who he is,
and if you don't feel strong
enough to fight alone, ask your
husband to see him with you.

Do attend antenatal classes.
These are much more relaxed and
responsive occasions than the
clinic and will give you self-
confidence and information that
will help you to deal sensibly with
medical and nursing staff.

Screening techniques
Once you have been to your first
antenatal check-up, you will be

asked to attend again at monthly
intervals until the twenty-eighth
week (i.e. twelve weeks before the
EDD), then every two weeks until
the last four weeks, when you will
be expected to attend each week.
During this period any
complications can be observed,
and you may come across screening
techniques that are unfamiliar to
you. The most common of these
is Ultrasound,* which is used to
check that the baby is the right
size for dates, to detect the position
of the placenta, to detect a
multiple pregnancy and to check
for the presence of certain
conditions and abnormalities.

Ultrasound has to a large
extent superseded X-rays, but
X-rays can still play an important
part, particularly where the shape
and size of your pelvis need special
assessment, for instance if it is a
breech birth. The need for X-ray
arises only in late pregnancy when
it can be used without danger to
the baby; X-rays are avoided in
early pregnancy when they can
damage the developing embryo.

There is no evidence to
suggest that Ultrasound is harmful
to you or the baby. It is also used
as part of a screening technique
called amniocentesis,* which can
detect certain abnormal conditions
such as mongolism (Down's
syndrome*) or spina bifida.*

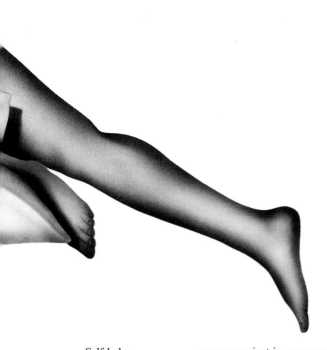

Self-help

The staff of the maternity unit, or your own doctor, will be keeping an eye out for any problems, but there is a great deal you can do to help yourself. You will be advised to lead as normal a life as possible during pregnancy, within the bounds of common sense and allowing for extra rest. Work, by all means. It is very foolish to throw up work at the first opportunity and then sink into depression through isolation and boredom. But if your work is physically demanding or dangerous, then think how it might be adapted to suit your condition. Now is the time to find out what benefits you may be able to claim, and what your rights are as regards maternity leave and your job being held open for you.

Travel, certainly, but avoid unpressurized aircraft which could limit the oxygen supply to your baby, and remember that airlines will not take a woman in the last four or five weeks of pregnancy and that after twenty-eight weeks you will need a doctor's certificate of fitness. Try to avoid too much travelling in the last months, though you may not feel like it anyway, and beware of lack of concentration when you drive. It is common sense not to go too far from home towards the end of pregnancy just in case you go into labour before time.

Exercise

You will be advised to take a 'normal' amount of exercise. If you are used to leading a very active life then carry on, unless you play a sport that is physically dangerous – use your common sense. Your body will tell you when it has had enough, so listen to it.

The extra weight you are carrying around, especially towards the end of pregnancy, will slow you down and make you tired. Allow for this and don't push yourself too hard. If you can get an hour or two's rest during the day, so much the better. If you have other children this would probably fit in well with their rest times; otherwise, make a time when you lie down with your feet up. It is important to get your feet higher than your pelvis. You can achieve this by lying on the floor with your feet on a stool or low chair, or by lying on the bed with pillows under your feet. Getting your feet at an angle of forty-five degrees gets a good transfusion of blood going, and reduces swelling in feet and ankles. It is a good tip for any time when your feet swell, not just in pregnancy.

There are specially adapted exercises for women to do in pregnancy (see page 59), and although they may seem rather gentle, they will help you to keep in condition if you do them regularly. They concentrate on the muscles that you will need during labour. Exercises for the pelvic floor* are vital before and after labour, both for a smooth delivery and for the quality of your sex-life afterwards.

Maternity clothes

The clothes that you wear during pregnancy should be comfortable above all, though they should also boost your morale if possible. High heels are not comfortable; nor are normal tights, which roll themselves below your bulge. You can buy special maternity tights or wear long socks, but no garters.

You must have properly designed bras as soon as your enlarged bosom needs them. The damage done to your breasts occurs with the extra weight of pregnancy and not through breast-feeding, so a supportive bra with the right cup size is essential, even if it means sacrificing an element of glamour.

Smocks and caftans that are not specifically designed for pregnant women are usually much prettier than things that are, but it is vital to try them on. Clothes that look loose on the hanger may not be cut generously enough around the bosom.

Weight-gain

As for your weight, there is the temptation – which should be ruthlessly resisted – to let yourself go in pregnancy. Not only is it risky to be over-weight, especially at the end of pregnancy, but you will find it difficult to lose extra weight afterwards. It is quite easy to calculate how much weight you should put on by the end of pregnancy by doing the following sum – the weight of the average baby is 7 lb (3.2 kg), the weight of the placenta will be $1\frac{1}{2}$ lb (675 g), the weight of the amniotic fluid is 2 lb (900 g), the weight of the uterus is 2 lb (900 g). Increased volume of the breasts accounts for $1\frac{1}{2}$ lb (675 g) and the increased blood volume is 4 lb (1.8 kg). This all adds up to 18 lb (8.1 kg). There may be extra fluid retention but it is unwise to let your extra weight creep above 28 lb (12.6 kg). However, if you are worried about your weight and wonder whether to diet, don't do so without consulting your doctor.

Early in pregnancy you may find there is no weight-gain, and there may even be a small weight-loss as nausea affects your normal appetite. This is nothing to worry about. On the other hand, your baby grows heavier at an increased rate during the last eight weeks of pregnancy: you will probably find that you gain as much as 1 lb (450 g) a week. This is why weight-loss or only tiny weight-gain at this stage may prompt your doctor to suggest Ultrasound scan to measure the size of the baby, or tests on your urine or a sample of blood in order to assess the efficiency of the placenta. But the baby may be growing perfectly well – and at *your* expense!

Diet, alcohol and smoking

A good diet in pregnancy is the same as a good diet at any other time, and that means plenty of fresh fruit, vegetables, meat, fish, eggs, cheese, milk. Make sure that your diet contains fibre to help you avoid constipation and don't eat anything that you know puts weight on you. The old saying 'eat enough for two' is sheer nonsense. The baby inside you will take enough for its needs whatever you eat. There is no reason why you shouldn't drink a moderate amount of alcohol, but remember that it crosses the placenta so don't give your baby a headache!

There is every reason why you shouldn't smoke cigarettes. There is statistical evidence that smoking affects the oxygen and blood supplies to the baby so that babies of smoking mothers can be smaller and less intelligent than they need be. Thirty cigarettes a day can reduce a baby's weight by as much as 10 per cent, so now you have a positive incentive to give up smoking.

Drugs

Since the thalidomide disaster most people are extremely cautious about taking drugs in pregnancy. If you are one of the very tiny percentage of women who have become pregnant while on the Pill – probably because you forgot one or two – don't worry: the pills you will have taken since you became pregnant will not harm the baby. But as a ground rule it is best not to take any, not even an aspirin or a travel sickness pill, without asking your doctor first. In fact, he will tell you that some drugs will do you and your baby no harm and he may, at different times, prescribe you anti-nausea pills, antacids for heartburn, aspirin for headaches and a mild sedative or a laxative.

The doctor will also prescribe iron tablets and maybe vitamin pills and calcium.

Teeth

The calcium is less to help your teeth than to build the baby's bones, but care of the teeth and gums is important during pregnancy, as they are particularly vulnerable then (see pages 200–203). Pregnant women in Britain are entitled to free dental care under the National Health Service; but all pregnant women should visit their dentist as soon as possible and take his advice.

The most common dental condition associated with pregnancy is gingivitis or bleeding gums, so you are likely to be

COMPLICATIONS IN LABOUR

A woman's labour and delivery are usually perfectly normal, but complications may arise where the birth needs extra care and emergency help must be at hand. About one pregnancy in ninety is a twin pregnancy. Although the combined weight of the twins will be greater than a single baby, usually both and certainly one will be under-weight and in need of special care. Twins are also frequently born prematurely. In Britain about 6 per cent of births, and in the United States 30 to 50 per cent, require delivery by forceps. These may be used to help the baby's head over the perineum, but more often they are required because the baby's head has not made sufficient progress during the second stage of labour. The mother will be given a local anaesthetic and usually an episiotomy* to ease the birth. About 4 per cent of babies present themselves for birth in the breech position. Labour is often normal, but if long, with maternal or foetal distress or danger of the cord being squeezed, thus depriving the baby of oxygen, a Caesarian section will be required.

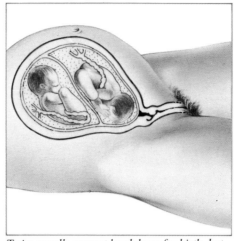
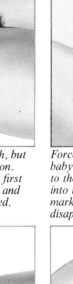

Twins usually present head down for birth, but sometimes one remains in a breech position. Labour should be quite normal; after the first delivery the second baby follows quickly, and labour is easier as cervix is already dilated.

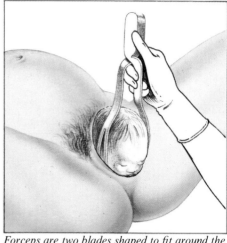

Forceps are two blades shaped to fit around the baby's head. After giving a local anaesthetic to the mother, they are inserted separately into the uterus and locked together. Any red marks left on the baby by the forceps soon disappear.

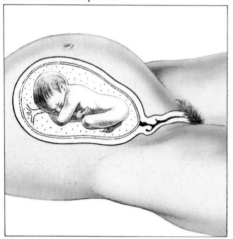

At thirty-six weeks most babies settle into a head down position. If not, the doctor will try to turn the baby. If this is not easily achieved he will leave it. Sometimes the baby turns back to its original, comfortable position.

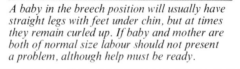

A baby in the breech position will usually have straight legs with feet under chin, but at times they remain curled up. If baby and mother are both of normal size labour should not present a problem, although help must be ready.

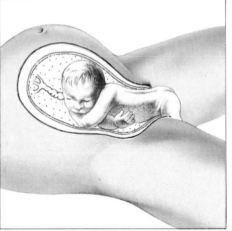

Usually the baby is born bottom first; legs, shoulders and head follow. If head is big and mother's pelvis small, cord may be squeezed depriving the baby of oxygen. If the baby is large, a Caesarian section may be necessary.

---

advised to keep your teeth and gums scrupulously clean. It seems to be the condition of the gums which leads to tooth decay rather than lack of calcium.

Love-making

You may get conflicting advice as to whether you can carry on a normal sexual relationship, but the general agreement is that as long as you feel like it there is no reason not to carry on as before. The only note of caution might be sounded if you have had a previous miscarriage, in which case you might be well advised to abstain at the times of greatest risk, which are at the missed periods of the fourth, eighth and twelfth week. Once the first three months are past the pregnancy should be well established.

If you find that your sexual drive is diminished, don't fret about it. Reassure yourself that it will return. However, you might be lucky enough to find that it is

even stronger. Many couples are turned on by the wife's pregnancy and feel closer together than before. Others feel more protective than lustful and you may find a new, gentler side to your husband. One reason for a woman's loss of sexual confidence may simply be that she feels lumpish and unattractive, in which case reassurance and flattery usually work wonders.

There are as many ways of reacting to pregnancy as there are people so don't be unduly disturbed – any changes in your normal feelings will usually put themselves right once pregnancy is over. You may find it rather uncomfortable to make love in the usual position with the man on top, even from the very first, because of your swollen and tender breasts, and certainly once your stomach starts to grow you will need to look for other positions.

It is easier for the woman to

lie on top at first, but in late pregnancy even this is uncomfortable and the man will find that he is unable to penetrate as deeply as before because of the shortage of space inside your crowded interior. Neither of you should worry that the man may penetrate into the womb and harm the baby or that he could break the waters. It is still easy to make love with the woman's back curved into the man's front and there are many other positions you can devise with imagination.

It can be rather depressing to feel yourself growing physically farther apart from your husband, but if pregnancy isn't always a time of wild passion, it can certainly be one of great tenderness and closeness.

True or false?

Above all in pregnancy, try to have confidence in yourself. Keep yourself as well-informed as you can. If you are going to be affected

by everything anyone tells you, then at least make sure that what you hear is correct by checking it out in the library or with your doctor. It is not true, for example, that raising your arms will twist the cord round the baby's neck or that some unhappy experience you have will transmit itself to the baby. Nor is it true that falling downstairs or having too hot a bath or taking a bumpy ride will cause a miscarriage – look at the many women who have tried all those things and failed.

Danger signs

However, there are certain danger signals in pregnancy which should be taken seriously and reported to your doctor at once, if only for your own peace of mind. The most common of these is vaginal bleeding. Any bleeding should be reported straight away, though it is quite possible to have slight bleeding during pregnancy without any further mishap. Nonetheless,

116

bleeding, particularly in early pregnancy, can be an indication of a threatened miscarriage. You will certainly be told to go straight to bed and rest until you can be seen.

Miscarriage, or loss of the pregnancy, is much more common than most people realize. This is because a large number – up to a third of all conceptions – abort themselves within the first month before they can be confirmed, and appear to be no more than a late, heavy period.

Most miscarriages occur within the first three months of pregnancy, and once a miscarriage is under way it is unmistakable. You will start with some bleeding and have stomach pains like period pains which will develop into regular contractions, accompanied by heavy loss of blood from the vagina.

There is absolutely nothing that can be done to stop a miscarriage once it's under way, but you must inform your doctor, who might wish to admit you to hospital for curettage or scraping of the womb under general anaesthetic, to make sure that all the products of conception are cleaned out and your womb is free of infection (D and C*).

Miscarriage is a miserable and a disappointing experience and it is of little comfort to tell yourself that there was very probably something wrong with the pregnancy. You will want to know when you can start trying to conceive again and you may be told to wait for six or, more normally, three months, but many women have disregarded this somewhat cautious advice with no ill-effects.

Bleeding in late pregnancy may mean that the placenta has positioned itself low down between the baby and the opening of the uterus. This can cause severe bleeding during labour and a Caesarian section* will have to be performed. Not strictly a miscarriage, an ectopic pregnancy* will mean that the pregnancy has to be terminated.

There are other danger signs during pregnancy which will be checked each time you attend your antenatal appointment. One of these is a rise in blood-pressure. Another is undue swelling of the legs, ankles and hands. Sometimes if you press the swollen skin with your finger the depression will remain for some seconds after you have taken your finger away – this condition is known as pitting oedema.*

When raised blood-pressure and oedema occur together with the presence of protein in the urine, the resulting condition is known as toxaemia, and it can also be associated with a sudden weight-gain. Unchecked, toxaemia can progress to pre-eclampsia, and

this can lead to the very dangerous condition, eclampsia. Nowadays it is extremely rare for it to go unchecked. If it occurs near or at term, the doctor may suggest induction. If it occurs earlier, the mother may well be admitted to hospital for bed-rest and observation.

These are only some of the conditions which can affect the pregnant woman, and it cannot be emphasized too strongly that if you have any doubts or fears whatsoever about the state of your pregnancy then you should confide them as soon as possible to your doctor. The sooner they are dismissed, cleared up or treated, the better it will be.

Hospital or home delivery?
The first decision which you will take, deliberately or not, is whether to have your baby at home or in hospital. For most women now there is no conscious choice, as statistics show that 96 per cent of women in Britain had their babies in a National Health Service maternity unit in 1976. And in the United States, of 3,326,632 live births in 1977, 98.5 per cent were attended by physicians and in hospital. The normal procedure is for your doctor to book you in once the pregnancy has been confirmed and from then on your care is either in the hands of the hospital or shared with the doctor.

Theoretically, mothers can have their babies at home, but they can sometimes be made to feel eccentric and dangerously self-willed if they insist. It is a decision which needs very careful thought.

Hospital delivery
The increasing dominance of hospital deliveries has undoubtedly coincided with the greater degree of safety for mother and baby in childbirth. In hospital there are the facilities to cope with every emergency: highly-skilled obstetric staff, twenty-four-hour nursing care, blood, surgical procedures, incubators* and paediatricians.

Some people find it more restful to cope with the first exhausting days of motherhood in hospital, where all other responsibilities are taken from them. Others find the routine and bustle of hospital and the added tumult of other people's babies far from restful. In a sympathetic maternity unit, those days of nursing care and enforced rest may be just what you need. On the other hand, many women resent the impersonality of hospitals. They fear the invasion of medical techniques into what they feel is their private experience.

To help you make your decision there are certain things you should know. Try to find out from the other women in your area what maternity care is like in the

hospital you will be going to, and whether it is sympathetic to its patients. Ask at the hospital whether husbands are allowed to be with their wives during labour. This is vital: more and more hospitals allow husbands to stay with their wives, but there are still pockets of resistance run by old-fashioned staff who prefer husbands to make themselves scarce. The presence of the person closest to you can give you all the courage you need to get through an overwhelming experience, and it is an extraordinary event for fathers, too. Many men who were initially unwilling to take part have come out of the delivery room feeling infinitely closer to their wife and to the baby they have just watched coming into the world.

Ask, too, if the hospital conducts its own antenatal classes. It is astonishing that some of the best obstetric units still fail to help their mothers in this way. Apart from the normal instruction, an advantage of hospital-run classes is that they introduce women to the labour ward itself, so that the machinery and the staff are familiar when the time comes to be admitted as a patient.

Ask what methods of pain relief the hospital staff advise and what they most frequently use, and ask if they are sympathetic to methods of natural childbirth* and if they will help you with your breathing exercises, if that is what you want.

Ask, above all, what their attitude is to mother and baby. You will find very few units who diverge so far from normal practice as to try the Leboyer method,* but you will want to know if you will at least be given your baby to hold as soon as she is born. Will she be allowed to stay with you in the ward? Will she be kept in a separate nursery and only brought to you at feeding times? The whole relationship between mother and baby can be deeply affected by their closeness at this early stage and the mother who is allowed to spend as much time as possible getting to know her newborn baby goes home with more confidence than the one who carries home a stranger.

There can be too much closeness, however. Mothers who have had their new babies by their beds day and night – and are roomed with other mothers and babies – often creep home exhausted. Perhaps the best arrangement is a ward with a nursery attached so that the baby can be left there, if need be, while you catch up on some sleep.

If the answers to all these questions satisfy you that the hospital is one which is sympathetic to its patients and doesn't automatically throw them beneath the wheels of the hospital

juggernaut, then you would do well to consider a hospital delivery.

Home delivery
Women who want a home delivery may be influenced by a previous unhappy hospital experience, or they may already have children and wish to keep the birth of a new baby as a family experience. They may worry that their home is inadequate for a successful delivery, but the basic requirements for a home labour are few – some midwives narrow it down to a telephone in working order in case of emergencies. Heating must be to 70°F·(19°C), but so it should be to welcome home a new baby. If the option is open to you, the midwife or doctor will advise on any equipment or alterations that might be needed.

The time to discuss a home delivery is when your pregnancy is confirmed by your doctor, but do not be surprised if he tries to dissuade you. The medical profession have been trained to look for problems and they are essentially conservative and risk-conscious. There is a rule of thumb by which they will assess your suitability for home delivery, and the risk of complications goes up slightly if you are 5 ft (1.5 m) or under and therefore likely to have a small pelvis, if you have a previous history of complications, if it is your first baby or your fourth, if you are over thirty-five or under seventeen, if you have Rhesus antibodies in your blood or if it is a multiple pregnancy. Later complications, such as toxaemia, could also change your plans.

However, if the doctor is satisfied that you don't present undue problems he can arrange for the community midwife to deliver your baby, and will either continue your antenatal care himself or share it with the hospital.

For women in Britain, there is a third alternative to home or hospital delivery, and that is delivery in a GP-run maternity unit situated in a normal hospital. This combines the advantages of hospital services in case of emergency with the care of your own GP. However, this alternative is not open to everybody. There are only 3,849 beds in GP maternity units compared with 17,512 in consultant units.

Whatever you decide, try to take all the factors into account and make a rational, not a purely emotional, decision. There is a strong and justifiable reaction against too much intervention in childbirth by the medical profession, but it has never been safer to be pregnant or to deliver a child than it is now and it may be literally throwing the baby out with the bath water to reject modern obstetrics from some exaggerated earth-mother point of view.

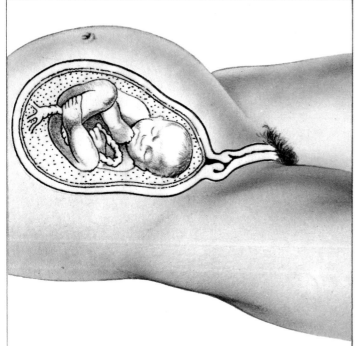

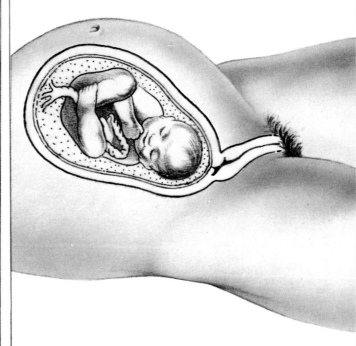

Around the fortieth week of pregnancy, contractions of past few months begin to build up, coming at regular intervals of thirteen to fifteen minutes. The regularity of contractions marks the onset of labour. At this stage, baby should be lying head down, facing one of mother's hips. The cervix has softened but still forms a sleeve at entrance of uterus. Muscles of uterus now start to pull cervix up, a process called cervical effacement. As contractions increase to ten-minute intervals and cervix shortens, plug of mucus which blocked neck of cervix comes away.

By full effacement, when muscles of uterus have pulled cervix up round baby's head, contractions will be coming every three to five minutes and lasting up to ninety seconds. The cervix is now flush with uterus and forms beginning of birth canal. The baby will have its chin well tucked in and crown of head forwards. The waters of the amniotic sac may still be intact. Full effacement may take eight to nine hours in a first pregnancy, about four in subsequent pregnancies. Contractions are easy to handle – the mother can talk to her husband, read, rest or watch television.

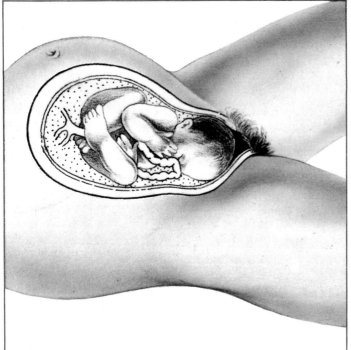

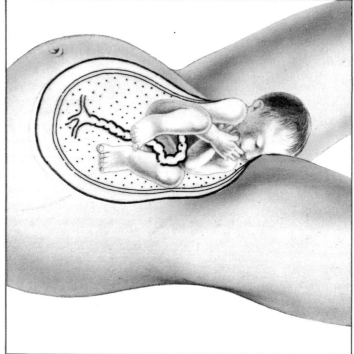

The baby's head has now completely turned to face its mother's back, to enable it to squeeze through pelvic arch. With each contraction, baby's head presses harder on perineum, until attendants can see top of head. The perineum is very stretched and it is vital to control pushing in case it tears. The doctor may make an incision, called an episiotomy, after a local anaesthetic in vulval tissue. This stage of labour can take up to two hours for a first pregnancy. If it is difficult, too long, or involves maternal or foetal distress, the doctor may intervene.

A few really hard pushes under guidance from the doctor and finally baby's head clears perineum. First the back of head, then eyes, nose, mouth and chin are visible. As baby's head emerges, it turns back to its original position to face its mother's hip, its shoulders turn to fit under bones of pelvis, and the worst is over. The rest of the birth follows quickly. The shoulders emerge and delivery is almost complete. One or two more pushes by the mother are all that is needed for baby finally to clear birth passage.

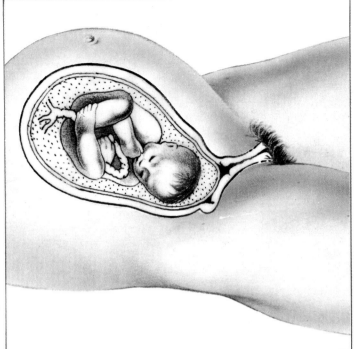

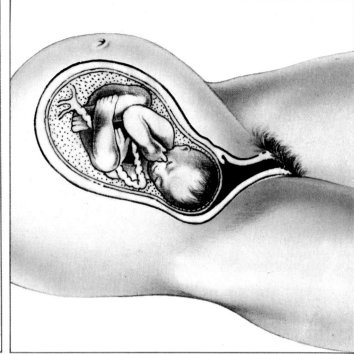

The cervix now starts to dilate a little wider with each contraction. The amniotic sac bulges forwards. When half-way dilatation is reached, contractions get stronger and more frequent, every three to five minutes. The mother may need a painkilling injection or gas and oxygen as baby pushes into birth canal. Breathing and relaxation exercises are invaluable now. As full dilatation approaches, she may feel nausea and cramp and need help and encouragement. Complete dilatation takes about three to five hours for a first baby, and then the first stage of labour is over.

The second stage of labour begins with powerful contractions every two to five minutes. The uterus and vagina have now formed a continuous birth passage for baby to pass through. Its head begins to turn to face mother's back, amniotic sac breaks expelling waters, and delivery begins. The mother will have an overwhelming desire to bear down to push baby out. In antenatal classes she learned to control pushing to help attendants guide baby safely through delivery. There will be pressure on bladder and rectum, so she is given nothing to eat or drink during labour.

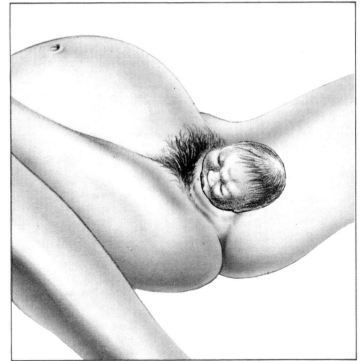

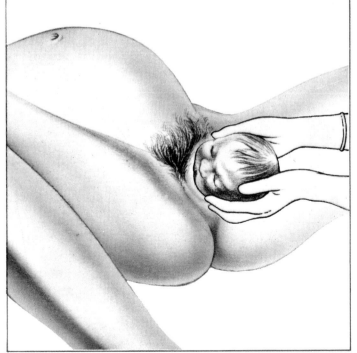

Often the baby is crying as it leaves the mother's body. If it is not, the doctor may hold it upside down so that mucus will drain from lungs. All passages will be cleared so that baby can breathe easily. The umbilical cord will be clamped and severed. The baby will be wet and possibly smeared with blood or covered with waxy substance, vernix, which protected it in the womb. The baby will be dried and wrapped warmly and given to the mother. She may wish to put her baby to the breast, though there is no milk yet, only colostrum.

Now the mother enters the final stage of labour. As baby's head or shoulders emerged, she was given an injection of ergometrine. This speeds up expulsion of 'afterbirth' or placenta, now separated from wall of uterus, and causes uterus to contract strongly to prevent blood loss. The doctor may apply pressure to abdomen just above pubic bone to help uterus expel placenta. The process takes twenty to thirty minutes. If there was an episiotomy, it will now be stitched up under local anaesthetic. Then the mother can have a well-deserved rest.

PREPARING FOR LABOUR

Antenatal classes

Once your pregnancy is confirmed, you will be curious about everything to do with your condition, and the best starting point for gathering further information and learning how to cope with your own pregnancy is the antenatal class. It is very likely that your hospital runs classes, but if it doesn't there are other classes run by childbirth organizations such as the National Childbirth Trust* in Britain and the International Childbirth Education Association of America,* which also offer help in the form of literature and counselling.

Antenatal classes are invaluable, not simply for information, which you can find in books, but for the self-confidence they give you in dispelling ignorance, and the moral support you get from other women in the same situation as yourself.

Apart from the basic physiology of pregnancy and labour, the aim of antenatal classes is to familiarize you with the experience and the trappings of labour. You should be told about the different methods of pain relief and the growing technology that surrounds childbirth, and you will be taught methods of relaxation to help you through labour itself. Most antenatal courses include husbands or have fathers' nights, when the men will be helped to understand what you have been taught and shown positive ways in which they can help you. By repeated 'labour rehearsals' the teacher will try to instil into you the different kinds of contractions you will experience and the way to ride them.

Only the most enthusiastic natural-childbirth supporter will claim that labour can be absolutely painless, and there are very few women, however well-prepared, who aren't taken by surprise when it comes to real contractions. But many women have been helped enormously by remembering their instruction and by having something to do to help themselves stay in control.

No woman should feel herself a 'failure' if she finds that in spite of relaxation classes she needs the help of painkilling drugs when it comes to the real thing. There is no shame in making the most of the advances of modern medicine: it makes better sense than being a martyr and too worn out after the event to respond to and enjoy your baby.

Most antenatal teachers teach a mixture of methods and ideas, and only the most rigid purists would try to dissuade mothers from taking advantage of everything that modern obstetrics has to offer. In order to help them make sensible choices when the time comes, classes are told about the different forms of pain relief such as the inhalation of a gas and oxygen mixture,* the injection of pethidine* (demeral) and the use of epidural* anaesthesia. They are also told in advance about the monitoring devices they may find in the delivery room.

Monitoring devices

The monitoring of the foetal heart during labour means that the doctors and midwives will be able to keep a close check on the effect that labour is having on the baby. If the monitor shows them that the heart rate is slowing down more than is safe because the baby is under severe stress, then they can take steps to deliver the baby quickly. In order to monitor the baby's heart, the mother will either have the monitoring devices slipped under a belt which will be eased over her stomach or a small electrode may be fitted directly on to the baby's head inside the birth canal.

Should the baby prove to be in distress in the second stage of labour, this is one indication for a forceps* delivery, which may sound alarming but is performed to protect the baby from undue pressure as it passes through the pelvis. For a forceps delivery on a mother who has not had an epidural, the doctor will administer a local anaesthetic called a pudendal block* to deaden pain in the pelvic region.

Episiotomy

The doctor delivering your baby may think it is necessary to perform an episiotomy.* During labour the perineum, the region between vagina and rectum, may tear. The episiotomy is a clean surgical cut performed to pre-empt the tear, both in order to make more space for the baby to come out and also to be easily and cleanly repairable.

There has recently been a great deal of discussion about episiotomies, and there is no doubt that they can give trouble if they are performed by inexpert hands. If this really worries you, then ask about it at an antenatal visit and make it clear that you want your stitches to be put in by someone experienced. A neatly sewn episiotomy can return a woman's vagina to normal much more efficiently than a tear or irreparable stretching of the muscle. The stitches are undeniably sore, and the postnatal ward is full of women who sit down extremely carefully, but the worst is over within a few days. You will find it extremely uncomfortable to make love while the stitches are still there, but everything should be back to normal in six weeks or so.

Caesarian section

Although antenatal classes are there to prepare you for a normal, self-starting vaginal delivery, they should also tell you about possible interventions in labour such as Caesarian section, which is relatively common, and induction, which is very common.

In some instances, for example if the pelvis is small, Caesarian section is necessary. This is the final intervention, undertaken when all efforts to help the baby to be born normally have failed, and it is undertaken for the safety of both mother and child. It involves bypassing vaginal delivery and extracting the baby from the uterus surgically through an incision in the abdominal wall.

One of the disadvantages of Caesarian section from the mother's point of view is that it deprives her of the satisfaction of seeing her own child born, and of that first essential contact. If you feel very deeply about this, ask the obstetrician if he will perform the operation under a local anaesthetic. This means that you remain fully conscious during the operation, although you will feel no pain and a screen will be placed across your stomach so that you don't see it taking place. But you will be conscious as your child is brought into the world.

Induction

Induction means the starting of labour by artificial means, either by breaking the bag of amniotic fluid which surrounds the baby and setting the uterus into action that way, or by the administration of a drug through an intravenous drip, and sometimes by a combination of the two. Both methods stimulate contraction of the uterus.

An induced labour is a speeded-up labour, and so a less controllable one from the woman's point of view. Women also suspect that in many cases labour has been induced for the social convenience of the doctor, though women themselves are not guiltless of this. Doctors will say that there are usually sound medical reasons for induction, and there are even cases where a socio-medical argument has some weight! It would be tragic if a baby died or suffered unnecessarily because the paediatrician was off duty or the ward was understaffed.

However, despite the doctors' protests, the drop in the rate of induction shows that it is not being used quite as freely as it was. The rule, as in every aspect of pregnancy, is to ask firmly for the reasons and to be prepared to accept a reasonable case.

LABOUR

Every woman having her first baby is beset by the fear that the onset of labour will pass her by. She may have been having practice contractions for weeks – will she really know when the time comes to rush to hospital or to call the midwife? In fact, when the time comes there is no mistaking it.

There are three basic signs that labour is on its way. They may come to you in any order and at any time, but when any one of them comes to you will know that, at last, the show is on the road. Definite contractions, much stronger than the contractions you have been having intermittently for weeks, will start occurring *regularly*. It is the regularity that is probably the clearest indication of labour. If they come at clear intervals and keep on coming, then you know you are on your way. This is the most common sign of the onset of labour.

The breaking of the waters is the sign that alarms first-time mothers most. When the membranes holding the amniotic fluid round the baby break and 2 pt (1.2 litres) or so of water leaks or gushes out, will you be in bed? Will you be in the supermarket or out to dinner? Some people advise wearing a sanitary pad during the very end of pregnancy and it might be wise to put a plastic sheet over the mattress, but despite the potential embarrassment, most women find that they are not caught unawares in public and often the waters will be broken for you when you reach hospital.

The third sign is the 'show', the plug of blood-streaked mucus that comes away from the cervix.

Your hospital or midwife will probably tell you when you should present yourself – usually when contractions are coming every ten or fifteen minutes, but the time of day should also play some part in your calculations. If you live half an hour from the hospital and it is rush hour, allow yourself extra time to get there. In Britain you are entitled to use the ambulance service: just dial 999 and tell them that you are in labour and which hospital you need to go to. In the United States, you may use the emergency services, though there may be a small charge. If you are being taken by car, make sure it has enough petrol in the tank, and don't drive yourself. Don't use public transport and don't be surprised if an unhappy taxi-driver refuses to take you.

You should have had a case packed and ready in advance with at least three front-opening nightdresses – you will be surprised at how milk spreads, even if you have had an injection to 'dry it up' if you are not breast-feeding – toilet things and reading or writing materials, although you may never get round to reading or writing after all. You won't need anything for the baby while you are in hospital, though you will need warm clothes and shawls to take her home in.

120

What happens to you once you are really in labour is something so highly personal that no two experiences of childbirth are exactly the same. The fact that most women advise each other from their own personal experience only makes a clear account of labour more difficult.

The basic physiological stages are the same for everyone, but the way in which you feel them and cope with them, the time it all takes, the help you are given, your physical sensations and emotions are unique to you. A first baby can appear after thirty-six hours, or it can arrive in three; usually it appears after about twelve. Sympathetic attendants can make the whole experience the most memorably rewarding of your life, or unsympathetic ones can turn it into a nightmare. If you yourself have prepared, both mentally and physically, for the work you have to do now, you will have given yourself the best possible chance of making it a positive experience. But on no account feel a failure if it is all much more overwhelming and painful than you expected, or if you need help. Shout if you feel like it, take the pain relief that is offered and thank God for modern obstetrics.

Stages of labour
Antenatal classes will have taught you to be aware of the three stages of labour. The average length of labour is between six and twelve hours and the first stage is by far the longest part. This is when the uterus contracts regularly and strongly in order to open or dilate the cervix so that the baby may pass through. When the cervix is fully dilated at 4 in (10 cm), the first stage is over.

The second stage brings the strongest, most overwhelming sensation. It is quite common for women to vomit, for the most well-bred to swear like troopers and even for some women to try to get up and go home. The strength of the muscle contractions can bring on all or any of these reactions. If any of this happens to you, remind yourself that it is a sign that the worst is nearly over.

What happens next can really take you by surprise – you will find that your whole body can become doubled up by an overwhelming, irresistible urge to push downwards with tremendous force, just as if you were opening your bowels. The pushing is to get the baby out, but it feels as if every part of your body that can open is opening out.

There is nothing refined and romantic about childbirth. It is an extraordinarily earthy, physical process in which inhibitions simply vanish. If they don't, then you could be making the whole business much more difficult for yourself. You need to control this extraordinary urge to push with the help of your doctor or midwife, who will make quite sure that the cervix is fully dilated. Your antenatal classes will have taught you the technique for this.

However overwhelming the second stage is, it is also exciting because you know you are nearly there. The attendants can see the baby's head and will be encouraging you all the way. It is quite likely that excitement and exhaustion will be fighting a fierce battle within you and any training you have had will be very useful to you in keeping control.

The second stage is comparatively short: up to two hours for a first baby and less for subsequent babies. When the head is out you know that one last real effort will push the body out too, and then your baby has left your body and is being helped to take her first breath. The attendants may be sucking any mucus from her airways through a fine tube and they may wish to wrap her warmly, but once everything is seen to be all right she should be given to you – you have worked very hard for her.

You may or may not have noticed that, as the baby was born, you were given an injection of ergometrine.* This is routinely given to encourage the uterus to continue contracting in order to expel the placenta. The delivery of the placenta is the third stage of labour and may last an hour.

Reactions to the baby
So much has been written about how you will or should feel at the sight of your baby that it is best to disregard it all and accept the experience as it comes to you. You may feel very elated. You may feel full of renewed energy. You may feel deeply moved. You may feel so physically exhausted and battered that you couldn't care less if it's a baby or a litter of kittens. You may feel shocked at the sight of your new-born baby if you were expecting something pink and rounded and sweetly clean. New-born babies are a peculiar-looking lot: they can be funny, distorted shapes from the stress of birth and strange, unlovely colours for the same reason. They are usually smeared with blood and vernix and they may be covered with hair, have bloodshot eyes and birthmarks. Most of these features will have disappeared within a few weeks.

Don't feel guilty or abnormal if you aren't immediately emotional about the small, wet creature you should be holding in your arms. At the moment of delivery you will have been through such a violent physical, mental and emotional experience that it is quite normal for you to feel simply drained, peaceful and ready for sleep.

The postnatal period
Once your stitches have been inserted and your baby is sleeping after her exhausting experience, the nurses will wash you down and dress you in a clean nightdress and bring you refreshment if you want it. They may also make you pass water, which seems like a cruel refinement after everything you've been through, but the bladder needs encouragement to start working again right away.

When you are finally left alone do not be surprised if the sleep you have been longing for refuses to come. You are very keyed-up emotionally and you may be too excited to get to sleep, even though you are extremely tired. When you surface from this first rest you have a great many adjustments to make, new things to learn and a new person to care for. You may feel as though you deserve a long holiday, but there is no time for that now. You are into the time-consuming business of being a mother.

Regaining your figure
The first thing you may be interested in is your own body. Your stomach, if you are lucky, will have flattened a great deal, but the average postnatal ward is full of women who still look four or five months pregnant. The uterus will take up to six weeks to return to its normal pre-pregnant size, and the abdominal muscles seem enormously stretched, but you will be surprised how effective postnatal exercises are if you force yourself to do them immediately (see page 59). The general slackness of your body can only be pulled together by exercise.

You will have lost around 20 lb (9 kg) in weight. Anything over that you must diet to lose, but if you are breast-feeding, don't diet without consulting the doctor.

Postnatal depression
The majority of women feel unreasonably emotional and weepy a few days after labour and this irrational depression may last a week or so. It comes partly from the anti-climax after birth, partly from changes in hormone levels and partly from sheer exhaustion. There is nothing you can do about it except to make sure that your husband understands its physical basis and doesn't take it personally.

In fewer cases, postnatal depression can last for weeks rather than days and an understanding husband and doctor are essential. In very rare cases it can go hand in hand with delusions, hallucinations and suicidal feelings – this is called puerperal psychosis and must have the serious attention of a doctor. But it is important to recognize that most postnatal depression is normal, that it has a physical cause and that there is no need at all to feel guilty or ashamed of it.

For mothers whose experience of childbirth has been unhappy, the depression is more severe. Where a baby is stillborn the shock and misery of the mother are all too often compounded by the attitude of hospital staff who, maybe through embarrassment, find it very difficult to help the parents through their grief. There is an increasing willingness to look at the situation now and it is being realized that the last thing mothers of stillborn babies need is a conspiracy of silence from everyone round them.

Mothers of children who encounter problems at birth, or who need incubation in special-care units, also need extra time and sympathy from hard-worked staff, and a sympathetic unit will do their best to draw the mother into the care and the progress of her new child. The feelings of a mother for her child can be deeply affected by a difficult delivery or separation after birth: recent research has shown that early separation of mother and child is a likely cause of child-battering. In an attempt to strengthen the bond between mothers and babies separated by the glass of the incubator, one Scottish hospital takes a photograph of the baby which the mother keeps beside her at all times. A duplicate is supplied to the proud father, too.

Going home
Happily, most mothers only have to face the routine problems of adjusting to a new baby.

Going home is a very big moment. When you and your brand-new baby find yourselves alone without the help of nursing staff and with the additional problems of housework and cooking, you may feel happy to be home, but apprehensive, frightened and exhausted as well. Extra help is vital. Understanding husbands can transform your life by shouldering a lot of the housework, and if a relative or friend – best of all, a granny – can be persuaded to stay or call regularly, your life will be much easier. You will be surprised at how weak and easily tired you can become and how exhausting a tiny baby can be when it is with you twenty-four hours a day. It is essential that at some point in the twenty-four hours you are able to hand the baby over to somebody else and recuperate alone.

New babies are a source of mystery and bewilderment to new mothers. When she cries you won't know why, though 90 per cent of the time it seems to be hunger, and there will be times when you feel you would do anything to stop her crying, including throwing her down or hitting her. If you find these feelings overwhelming, physically distance yourself from the baby until you have recovered a little equilibrium. If the problem is persistent, seek help urgently from your Health Visitor or doctor. You may be really unlucky and have a baby who suffers from three months colic.* This is a condition for which there is no magic cure. The baby simply screams inconsolably every evening for hours on end and your only consolation may be the knowledge that it almost always stops at three months old. Handing the baby over sometimes to a third person while you have an evening off, preferably out of the house, may help your sanity, together with the knowledge that there is light at the end of the tunnel.

However, luckily for the future of the human race, most babies sleep quite a lot and can be so funny and captivating when they are awake that they store up enough goodwill to see you through the bad times. You may also find that a good baby book can be very reassuring in these first muddled, exhausting weeks (see Suggested Reading, page 223).

Above all, don't make your husband feel that he has been ousted from your timetable and affections. A new baby can be very threatening to a husband and other children as well as being a nice new toy, so be aware of their reactions and don't concentrate on the baby to the exclusion of the rest of your family.

Breast-feeding or bottle? Your most urgent practical problem when you arrive home is feeding. You will probably be asked at your antenatal clinic whether you wish to breast- or bottle-feed. Breast milk is the ideal food for babies, no matter how close the imitations. It provides the baby with natural protection against a number of ailments and infections; it is exactly suited to a baby's digestion; it is impossible to over-feed a breast-fed baby; and it helps you to regain your figure, too, because breast-feeding actually causes the womb to contract, making your abdomen flatter, and because the baby takes excess calories from you. It is free and it is marvellously convenient because it bypasses the business of mixing feeds and sterilizing bottles. The breast-feeding mother's response to her baby's hunger is spontaneous and immediate and the physical closeness of breast-feeding builds a warm and sensuous bond between a mother and her child.

It may be this very sensuousness, the sheer sexuality of breast-feeding, that puts some mothers off. Certainly, nothing can quite prepare a new mother for the extraordinary power and strength of a baby's suck. It is one of the

great natural forces, and unless you are very careful to begin with, it can make your nipples very sore.

Some people like to put the baby to the breast immediately after birth – not that there is any milk yet, but in order to stimulate the sucking reflex. Some babies are born with a very strong, instinctive suck and others take time to get going. Although there is no milk, there is a substance called colostrum which you may have noticed during pregnancy. It contains nourishment for the baby until the milk is produced, about the third day. For the first couple of days after birth the baby exists off her own fat and the little colostrum she gets from you.

at first you put the baby to the breast for only a couple of minutes each side, and work up slowly to the average time of ten minutes a side. This is for your own protection, since cracked nipples can be extremely painful. Massaging them with breast cream helps to keep them supple, and they will return to normal in time.

Once a baby has established her own routine she will generally want to be fed every three to four hours, but there are good reasons for 'demand' rather than routine feeding to begin with. One is that a hungry baby is a crying, miserable baby. The other is the way in which the breast milk supply establishes itself. The

making up any deficiency as they otherwise would by stimulation from your baby's sucking.

It takes a few weeks to establish a satisfactory breast-feeding routine, but the emotional rewards and the great simplicity of the whole system make it all worth while. There is also some evidence that breast-feeding offers a defence against cancer of the breast, and that it acts as a kind of natural contraceptive, though it would be extremely unwise to rely on breast-feeding alone.

If despite all this you find the idea of breast-feeding distasteful, painful or simply difficult, then choose to enjoy the advantages of bottle-feeding, which undeniably gives you more freedom. Working mothers may have no option unless they choose to express milk during the day, but remember that even a few weeks' breast-feeding is better than none.

Getting back to normal
In the meantime, your body is slowly returning to normal. After delivery you will have a vaginal discharge called the lochia, which is similar to a normal period, although it can continue for up to six weeks. You will also find that you tire very easily and you should pick up the threads of normal life gradually. The tiredness following labour and pregnancy is compounded by broken sleep and it is a time for raw nerves and heightened emotion as well as great happiness. Don't push yourself – undue tiredness will also affect your milk supply, so rest when you can.

Most of all, you will probably be looking forward to resuming a normal married life. It seems years since you weren't separated from your husband by a great lump or were able to hold each other really close. You can resume sexual relations as soon as it is comfortable, which may be some weeks if you have had stitches. Don't force yourself if you feel tight and sore – just take things gently, and if you don't feel like sex to begin with don't worry, because that's quite common, too.

Six weeks after delivery, the doctor will want to check your stitches and make sure that everything has returned to normal internally. A specimen of your urine will be tested for protein and sugar as before. This is the time to discuss what contraception you want to use in future, and to have an IUD or diaphragm fitted. If you are breast-feeding and want to take the Pill, you will be recommended one which does not inhibit the flow of milk.

Raise any questions or problems you may have now, because the postnatal check-up is the last contact you will have with the maternity services . . . until the next time.

TEN GOLDEN RULES FOR SURVIVING A NEW BABY

1 Rest at every possible opportunity. Don't stand when you can sit, don't sit when you can lie down, and don't just lie down if you can sleep: an exhausted mother is no use to her baby.

2 Cut the housework to the tolerable minimum.

3 Cut cooking to the tolerable minimum – if possible get meals from the freezer and the nearest take-away. At a time such as this a freezer, well stocked by you while you feel fit, is a life-saver. If you don't have one, see whether a neighbour will 'lend' you space – people rarely keep them full.

4 Never turn down an offer of real help.

5 Beware of visitors: they can be time-consuming and tiring.

6 Get a good, comprehensive book on baby-care (see page 223), but use it as it suits you.

Don't feel that there is a standard set of rules applicable to every baby. Go by the baby, not by the book.

7 Hand the baby into someone else's arms at least once a day, and walk away, closing the door behind you.

8 If in doubt, ring your doctor, home midwifery service, Health Visitor or local childbirth organization counsellor for reassurance. That is what they are there for. Whatever problem you have has been experienced by thousands of people before you.

9 Use disposable nappies or nappy liners to start with, unless you can find a nappy laundering service.

10 Economize on expensive and unnecessary equipment for the baby; spend the money instead on a washing machine, tumble-dryer or freezer. The baby will benefit more from a calm mother than a gold-plated rattle.

When the milk does come in you will notice an astonishing change in your breasts. They will be as full and hard and round as if they were made of marble. The extreme fullness can also be painful, and can be relieved by expressing a little milk – the hospital will show you how – or by taking a hot bath so that some of the milk leaks out. One of the penalties of breast-feeding is leaking milk and specially-made breast pads can save both your clothes and the social embarrassment of stains suddenly appearing down your front.

It is usually suggested that

system is one of beautiful simplicity – if you put your baby to the breast whenever she is hungry, the baby herself will be letting your breasts know how much milk she needs. Breast milk works on a supply and demand system: if the baby feeds often you will produce more milk to satisfy her. If you make the baby wait, then your breasts get the message that they should produce less milk, so the baby goes doubly hungry. For this reason it is not a good idea to supplement what may seem like an inadequate breast-milk supply with bottle feeds. You will simply prevent your breasts from

Menopause, a fresh start

The menopause arrives at a time in many women's lives when other circumstances are causing them concern. If they are married, for example, and have devoted their lives to caring for a husband and growing family, they now find that they are no longer needed in the same way. Unmarried, divorced, widowed or childless, no woman in her menopausal years can entirely escape feelings of loss, questioning and regret. They are natural to this time of life and we should not forget that men are also affected by the mid-life crisis and may become equally depressed, but at least they seem to be spared the sneaky tricks that hormones play on women.

Not only is the menopause a highly individual phenomenon, it is also a relatively new one. A hundred years ago the average woman could expect to live forty-two years and, often as not, would then die, worn out by child-bearing. Today her average lifespan has increased to seventy-five years, almost half a lifetime again. It is not surprising, therefore, if we are still learning how to have time on our side rather than on our hands, but the improved medical understanding of menopause and treatment of the symptoms it may produce will help women to make the most of this gift of extra years.

Physically, the end of the menopause marks the end of a woman's reproductive life. Her ovaries cease to respond to her pituitary hormones* so that she produces less oestrogen* and progesterone.* As her oestrogen level declines so does her egg production and quality, hence the greatly increased risk of producing a deformed baby when a woman is in her forties.

Oestrogen is not linked to sex-drive, however, so there is no reason why this should diminish. In the same way that the average age for puberty is coming down, the average age for menopause is going up, so that today British and American women can expect it round the age of fifty or more. However, it is not abnormal for a woman to have a natural, healthy menopause in her mid-thirties, while another, equally healthy, may be nearly sixty before it happens. If a woman's ovaries are surgically removed because of disease or other abnormalities, she will have an artificial menopause (see uterine disorders, page 220).

Approximately 15 per cent of women sail through menopause without any problems. The rest will know that they are having it, but only 10 per cent of these will suffer any serious problems.

Menopause can last as long as five years or can happen abruptly. The safe rule for contraception is that a woman under fifty should continue using a preventive for two years after her last period, a woman over fifty for one year. In this way a late pregnancy will not be misinterpreted as a sign of menopause.

MENOPAUSAL SYMPTOMS

If you notice any of these menstrual changes in yourself, you will know that you are entering the menopause:
1 Periods become irregular.
2 Menstrual flow becomes lighter.
3 Gap between periods is longer.

The following symptoms may appear during the menopause, but they are not common to all women, nor is it likely that one woman will be unlucky enough to experience them all:
1 Hot flushes. A sudden sensation of feeling very hot and flushed, creeping up from chest to neck, shoulders and face, which happens without warning at any time and causes great embarrassment to women.
2 Itching in the genitals and other parts of the body.
3 Weight-gain.
4 Sagging breasts, tired-looking skin, wrinkles, lank hair.
5 Dizziness, palpitations, headaches.
6 Nausea, flatulence, constipation.
7 Anxiety, nervousness, irritability, depression, lack of energy, lack of concentration.
8 Vaginal atrophy can occur two or three years after the menopause. The lining of the vagina becomes thin and dry and may shrink, making intercourse very painful.

LONG-TERM EFFECTS OF MENOPAUSE

1 Osteoporosis* where the bones become increasingly brittle due to loss of calcium.
2 Greater tendency to arthritis, arteriosclerosis and coronary disease.

HORMONE REPLACEMENT THERAPY

Apart from the weight-gain, which can be kept under control by sensible dieting and exercise, all these symptoms are largely caused by the dramatic fall-off in oestrogen which occurs when the ovaries cease production. Some women appear to compensate for this oestrogen deficiency through their adrenal glands* which also produce oestrogen, but for those who do not, hormone replacement therapy (HRT) is an alternative and effective solution. However, although it undoubtedly benefits the skin, oestrogen treatment is not the magic elixir of youth. It neither delays the process of ageing nor does it eliminate it, *but properly prescribed and monitored* it can certainly relieve some of these distressing symptoms.

The oestrogen used is a natural one, unlike the synthetic variety contained in the Pill. It is usually administered on the basis of three weeks on, one week off to prevent over-stimulation of the uterine lining which would cause bleeding. Doctors who are cautious about the prolonged use of HRT give this as one of their reasons, because any post-menopausal bleeding requires clinical investigation. The role of oestrogen in cancer is still uncertain, but to exclude this risk progestogen is now routinely included in the third week. HRT may not cause the actual cancer, but it may heighten a predisposition towards it, and it undoubtedly makes an existing breast or uterine cancer grow faster. Most doctors, therefore, now tend to the view that it is better to treat menopausal symptoms as they occur in an individual woman according to her needs, rather than to prescribe HRT as an automatic and long-term palliative. Hot flushes, for instance, can be kept under control by oestrogen tablets; vaginal atrophy can be halted by the local application of oestrogen pastes or ointments; and painful intercourse, because of dryness, can be eased by using a lubricant cream or jelly. HRT undoubtedly helps with many of the psychological symptoms, and women who have experienced the transformation from a state of misery to a renewed state of well-being describe it as little short of amazing.

However, medical opinion is sharply divided about the benefits of continuous therapy into old age, particularly when it is done with an oestrogen implant, where it is not so easy to control the dosage. The increase of endometrial cancer* in older women in the United States, where HRT has been widely used for many years, does give cause for concern. The best advice we can give to women is to seek out a doctor or clinic specializing in menopausal problems, where oestrogen levels can be estimated and replacement therapy instituted if it is indicated.

AFTER THE MENOPAUSE

So far modern medicine has succeeded in enabling more people to become old people, but there is no point in living longer if all it means is that you suffer for longer the disabilities of old age. What we must hope for now is that scientists will find a way to control the rate of ageing so as to enable us to carry the vigour, interests and pleasures of our middle years into old age.

We have deliberately avoided mentioning any of the miracle cures that are claimed to rejuvenate people – cellular therapy, royal jelly, blood replacement and the like – because to date the only proven miracle about them is the way they line a few doctors' pockets. However, if spending money makes you feel good, there is no harm in trying them. But there is a sounder way of feeling good: eat sensibly, exercise carefully and if you want to drink and smoke, do so in moderation.

As women, we count ourselves lucky that the menopause comes at an age when we are physically and mentally still in our prime. Nature kindly discharges us of our reproductive responsibilities, leaving us free to start a new life with renewed energy and optimism. Society, however, still needs to be convinced that older women can make a useful contribution. Better and more opportunities should be provided for anyone wanting to make a career change or start a completely new life. In the last decade women have waged a successful campaign against sexism. Now they have a new battle to fight, on behalf of men as well as themselves, against the cruelly wasteful doctrine of ageism which relegates anyone past their first youth to the rubbish heap. The declining birth rate combined with increased longevity gives the advantage of numbers to the generation now in its forties, so why not make 'Life begins at fifty' a triumphant slogan for the last quarter of this century?

Meanwhile, there are things that we can do for ourselves now. For a start, live each day as it comes. Never give up anything because you have persuaded yourself, or allowed others to persuade you, that you are too old – sex, for instance. If you have a job which you enjoy, keep at it and if, finally, it becomes too much physically, find another. Never turn your back on new interests, new friends or new ideas. We may not be able to stop the clock, but we *must* stop watching it.

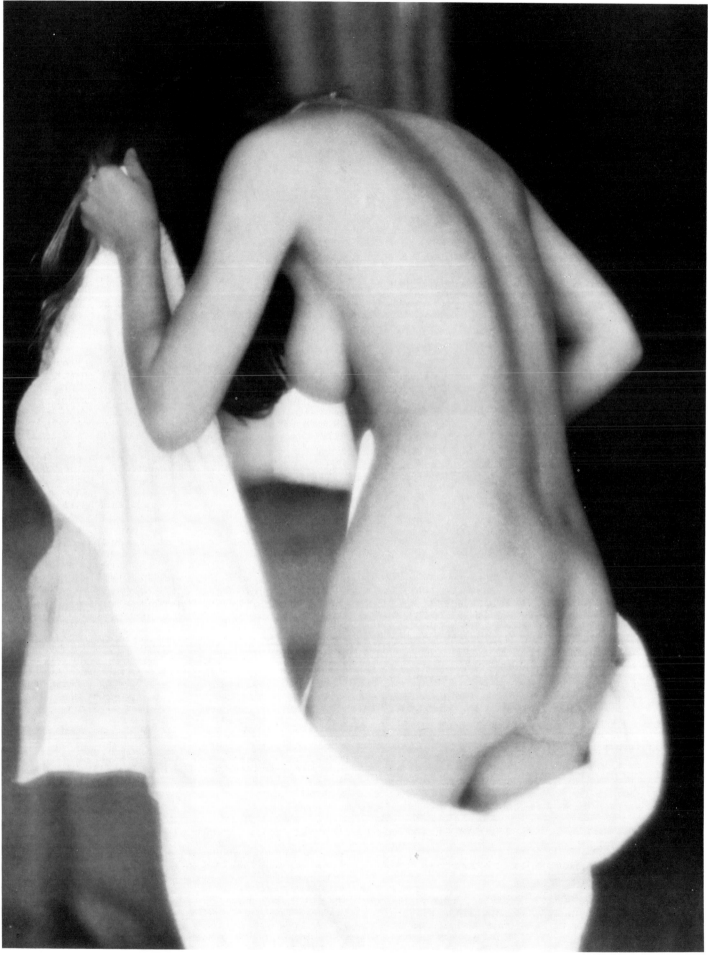

Clean Outside and In

The average woman in the sixteenth century took a bath once a year and carried a pomander for the sake of her nose, and other people's. The average woman today takes a bath once a day, and consigns the quaint pomander to her wardrobe to perfume her clothes. Our ancestors would think we were fanatical, while we take a dim view of their standards of hygiene, believing that the daily wash is essential to clean the pores of the skin and to remove unpleasant body smells.

Washing frees the pores of sweat and oily sebum, which are continually being secreted by glands in the skin. These glands perform the vital task of lubricating the *skin, but the mixture of sweat and sebum traps dead skin cells and dirt, which can clog the pores and stop the skin breathing, besides making it look grey and dingy and causing spots and blackheads.*

Neither sweat nor sebum smells unpleasant in itself – indeed, the faintly salty smell of sweat on the skin can be healthy and attractive. The body smells we object to arise when air cannot circulate freely over the surface of the skin because of clothes, and so moisture cannot evaporate. When this happens bacteria attack the trapped moisture and, as it breaks down, it gives off the smell that turns people into social outcasts.

Unless you play an active sport which obviously calls for a shower-off afterwards, one bath, shower or all-over wash per day is enough for anyone. If you love the bath so much that you are tempted to plunge in morning and evening, remember that the body's natural oils are destroyed by soap and water, and it takes a few hours for the natural balance to be restored.

If you find you feel panicky about having got your hands dirty, or about not having washed for a couple of hours, it is probably a sign that something deeper and more radical is wrong in your life and you should seek the advice of your doctor.

SHOWERS

The quickest and most effective way to get your whole body clean is to have a shower. Other benefits are that it uses far less water than a bath; that a really hard shower (hail storm water-pressure rather than English drizzle) is invigorating, making the skin tingle and glow and speeding up your circulation, providing it isn't too hot; that you can wash your hair in it at the same time; and that the water being hurled at you is clean, as opposed to the scummy stuff you wallow in in the bath.

If you can bear to have the water progressively cooler as you shower, this will close the pores as effectively as any skin tonic.

Whatever kind of shower you opt for, whether it is in the bathroom, over the bath, or tucked into a cupboard, it is worth investing in a curtain or reinforced glass panel to keep the water in: you can't enjoy a good vigorous splash if you are worried about spilling water.

BATHS

If a shower wakes you up, and is thus ideal in the morning, a bath is the way to relax. You can lessen the soporific effect by having a tepid or cool bath, but a warm bath is most people's favourite way of unwinding.

The ideal temperature is body heat, around 98–100°F (36–37°C). It is worth testing with a thermometer just to see how much too hot you have been having it. A hot bath makes your heart thump, and heightens your susceptibility to the cold outside the tropical atmosphere you have created in the bathroom. It dilates the blood vessels, turning you lobster-red and increasing the chance that tiny blood capillaries may burst, leaving you with permanent broken veins.* As if that were not enough, it speeds up the wrinkling, ageing process of the skin. And, incidentally, too hot a bath makes you sweat, which defeats the object of the exercise.

THE BEST OF BOTH WORLDS

For health, hygiene, and a bit of wallowing thrown in, you can combine bath and shower in Japanese fashion. Soap and wash off under the shower first, then get into a deep, warm bath for a soak in clean water.

For a more invigorating effect, wash in the bath, before or after your soak, then shower off to rinse away soap and scum. If you don't possess a shower, you can follow this second method just as well using a few jugfuls of clean rinsing water.

BATH ADDITIVES

Unlike perfume (see page 217), body and bath products have always been considered a bit of a wicked luxury – the kind of thing you might be given as a treat at Christmas, but which you would feel a little furtive about buying yourself. However, if you live in a hard-water area the addition of bath salts is not just a luxury but a practical way of protecting your skin from drying out, while making the water smell nicer. Bath salts, however, do not make aches and pains disappear; any soothing effect is due to the warmth of the water, and to its depth. Foam and bubble baths serve the same purpose, with the bubbles an 'extra' to make you feel like a film star. But whereas bath salts consist of sodium carbonate (washing soda), foam baths and bubble baths are mild detergents – not as devastating as a squeeze of washing-up liquid, but nonetheless related. They do not float out the dirt so that you can lie back and get clean without lifting a finger. There is no substitute for rubbing the dirt off with soap or some other cleanser and your hands or flannel. Look on bath salts and foam baths as pleasant extras; don't spurn the psychological effect, but don't expect wonders. On the negative side, if you should suffer from vaginitis* your bath salts or additive may be causing the irritation.

You can expect rather more of bath oils, a boon to anyone with dry skin because they protect you from the drying effects of water. They are most effective added to the bath, or in some cases rubbed into your body before you get into it, though more usually when you have dried off. They can be too oily for anyone with greasy or delicate skin. Many perfume houses include a bath oil in their range of products, so you can complement your favourite perfume. But body oils do not have to be expensive. If you are using the oil for the sake of your skin, and not for the fragrance, any vegetable oil such as olive, maize or peanut will do for a bath oil, but avoid the mineral oils such as baby oil as these are not so easily absorbed.

If you want a really effective reviver to add to the bath, go for products which contain the pure essences known for their soothing properties, such as pine, horse-chestnut and mint.

SPECIAL BATHS

Once in a while, if you can find the time, give yourself a relaxing special bath to soothe and smooth your skin. You could time this to coincide with your home facial (see page 139) – in which case apply your face mask just before you hop into the bath and let it dry while you soak.

Depending on what you put in the water, a bath can be nourishing, stimulating, toning, soothing or simply relaxing. Easy additions to the bath water are: 1 cup of vinegar to soften water and soothe dry and itching skin *or* 1 tablespoon of ground oatmeal to soothe and soften *or* 1 cup of powdered milk to nourish skin and combat dryness *or* 1 large spoon of honey to relieve tiredness or sleeplessness *or* orange or lemon peel for a lovely smell *or* three tablespoons of laundry starch to tighten and smooth skin *or* two handfuls of Epsom salts to combat tiredness.

Herb baths are a traditional beauty treatment. You will need to make a couple of small muslin pouches with drawstring necks, to prevent the plumbing getting clogged up with bits of leaf and stalk. Into a pouch put whatever herb or herbs you have chosen for your bath, and allow it to soak in the hot water like a tea bag.

Popular herbs for the bath are: camomile flowers, elder-flowers or thyme for soothing and softening the skin; mint or rosemary for stimulating the circulation; blackberry leaves for clearing the skin; comfrey for chapped, sore or spotty skin; lavender for a beautiful smell. These are available from herbalists and healthfood shops.

Body scrubs help to combat gooseflesh, blackheads or skin that is feeling a bit wintry and sallow. The simplest way is to scrub with soap and water and your bath mitt, loofah or brush, but sea salt rubbed all over as you stand in the bath makes a good stimulating scrub, as does sugar rubbed in with your soap lather. Or you can fill your muslin bag with ground oatmeal or bran, from healthfood shops, and scrub with that.

BATH EQUIPMENT

Washing. Flannels and sponges for washing are useful, but not necessary; washing is best done with the hands. Doctors say that hand-washing keeps you literally in touch with the condition of your skin, aware of any lumps, bumps and changes in texture, and it is obviously more hygienic.

If you prefer a flannel, keep it well-rinsed and squeezed out and, weather permitting, give it an airing on the washing line or window sill. Each week give your flannel a whirl in the washing-machine, or boil it up the good old-fashioned way with a table-spoon of vinegar or lemon juice to remove all the slime-generating soap. Don't hang on to a flannel for years: it doesn't cost much to buy a new and hygienic one.

Sponges are expensive, but with the right care they last for years, so it is an investment to get a good one. Biggest is not best, more of it to rot; a 5-in (12-cm) diameter is plenty. Look for a small root at the back of the sponge – this is the point at which it was cut off the rock on which it was growing. The smaller the root, the less likely the sponge is to tear.

A sponge is made of protein and as such is prone to attack from the alkali in soaps and bath additives. Always squeeze it out gently after use in clear, warm water and leave to dry on a rack where the moisture can get away, not on the edge of the bath where moisture will collect and rot the base. Don't cram a sponge into a plastic bag – it needs room to breathe.

Scrubbing. Loofahs are actually vegetables, and their biggest enemy is acid. Treat them to careful rinsing and draining, as with sponges, to stop them going black and mouldy. Never add vinegar or lemon juice to rinsing water for loofahs or sponges as that treatment is much too harsh for once-living things. Whereas sponges are soft and luxurious and not strictly necessary, the loofah, or alternatively a hemp glove, is an abrasive and valuable tool to get rid of the layer of dead skin cells which soap and water glide over. A loofah provides the friction to nudge off sluggish, grimy, dead cells and the most effective time to use it is before you get into the bath or shower. If this seems too spartan, you can soften the blow by wielding it in the bath.

The use of a loofah, hemp glove or natural-bristle, long-handled back brush is good at all times, but is especially important when you are on a strict diet or fast. Under these circumstances the body is throwing off poisons rapidly and these need to be scrubbed off the skin.

Pumice stone is very porous volcanic rock and works best if you work up a good lather with soap then rub gently at hardened skin in a circular movement.

Soap. Even dermatologists* can't agree on whether soap is positively good or bad for the skin.

The theory that it is bad is based on the fact that skin is naturally a little acid, while most soap is alkaline. Hence the soap temporarily destroys the skin's protective acid mantle. However, as the balance is restored in one to three hours, the damage is not permanent. The anti-soap lobby claim that the drying effect of soap is cumulative; years of washing will take their toll in the form of skin prematurely dry and wrinkled. Certainly, you can feel the drying effect of soap on the skin; it is this very feeling that makes some people say they 'feel clean', but often this means that soap has been left on skin which has not been adequately and thoroughly rinsed. Nowadays most soaps contain moisturizers such as cold cream to mitigate the drying effect, though this does not alter their alkalinity.

Most people can do their skin no harm by using soap; it is only those with particularly dry or sensitive skin who should use the special acid-balanced soaps, which are not strictly soap at all, and cleansers.

BATHTIME TREATMENTS

Bulge-reducing. One treatment that combines friction with a weight-losing treatment is to use a friction glove. Even if weight-loss is not your worry, the glove is an excellent way of putting paid to gooseflesh and achieving a healthy, pink glow.

Gooseflesh. This usually crops up on thighs, buttocks or upper arms. Stimulate the circulation by scrubbing regularly with bath mitt or loofah in the bath. Scrub with sea salt once in a while, or with sugar or a bag filled with oatmeal or bran. Massage thoroughly with hand cream or body lotion.

Horny and discoloured elbows and knees. Regular attention is important but you could start on these neglected areas with a blitz treatment. First massage elbows and knees with cleansing cream and tissue off. Pumice the areas with soap and water while in your bath and rub with water and sea salt or oatmeal or bran bag, or with sugar mixed with a little vegetable oil. Rinse. After your bath rub a cut lemon over the elbows and knees and allow juice to dry, then massage in body lotion or hand cream. You may re-do the blitz treatment once a week or once a month, but in between times be sure to pumice and massage with hand cream or body lotion.

Spotty chest and back. This is common among greasy-skinned women and adolescents. Keep the areas clean by washing regularly and scrubbing, if not too blemished and tender, with a bath brush, loofah, special abrasive sponge

or bath mitt and medicated soap. Stimulate circulation by splashing with cool or cold water or slapping the areas with a cold flannel. Make sure towels, bras, petticoats and so on are always clean, as well as your hair. Dust with baby powder or pat with astringent to absorb excess grease. Consider some ultra-violet sun-lamp treatments, and try to get your body into the sun and sea as these will help to dry out excess grease.

BATHTIME BONUSES

Make use of the bath to do other beauty treatments. It is the ideal relaxing place for a face mask to work well, or just a simple steam treatment, preparation for which involves no more than thoroughly cleansing your face of all make-up – don't apply any toner or moisturizer – before getting into the bath. The steam from the bath will do the rest. Having a quick bath *after* making-up sets your make-up in the same way that spraying your face and neck sparingly with a mineral-water spray keeps make-up fresh.

The bath is a good place to give yourself a manicure. Rub softening cuticle cream into nails on hands and feet before getting in, and it will work even better with warmth and water to help. Massage cream into cuticles with a very soft nail-brush.

Speedy pick-up bath. When time is at a premium and you have an hour or less in which to transform yourself for an evening date after a long, hard day, snap into a quick routine.

Run a warm bath and add bath oil, foam or salts.
Put your going-out clothes to hang in the bathroom.
Take off make-up.
Depending on hairstyle and current condition, tuck hair under a cap, put it in rollers and steam set, or if it is short and easy, shampoo it in the shower-off after your bath.
Apply a mask (see page 139), have eye pads and a cool drink to hand on the side of the bath.
Get in and soak for ten minutes before you soap.
Shower off and remove face pack.
Dry off (hair too if need be), moisturize skin, etc.
Dress, apply make-up, do hair, check nails.

AFTER-BATH EQUIPMENT

After your bath or shower a large, rough, cotton towel is the most effective rub down. Talcum powder makes you smell nice, helps you slide into clothes, and is soothing and absorbent, but it is no substitute for a thorough job with the towel, especially in between the toes.

Body lotion or oil replaces lost moisture, though go easy on grease-prone areas. You can be

generous on feet, elbows and knees, and it is a good chance to massage podgy areas such as thighs and buttocks. Finish with a splash of cologne, by which time your body will have cooled down and be ready for deodorant and/or anti-perspirant. Leaving this till last means the deodorant doesn't have to work overtime. Do not use an anti-perspirant before you go to bed; it is not a good idea to inhibit natural perspiration twenty-four hours a day.

SWEAT AND BODY ODOUR

Everyone sweats, but there is no need to smell unless you are careless. Sweat only becomes smelly in the parts of the body where fresh air does not easily circulate – i.e. the feet, crotch and armpits. In these places the sweat does not evaporate quickly and so lingers around to be decomposed by bacteria.

What makes you sweat? The body is equipped with eccrine sweat glands,* which cover the whole skin surface, and apocrine sweat glands,* which are concentrated only in the armpits, groin, around the nipples and navel. A change in body temperature brought about by a hot day, a stuffy office, an energetic game of tennis, a spicy curry or a high fever activates the eccrine glands. The evaporation of the sweat they produce (which is 99 per cent water, 1 per cent waste salts) cools the body down again, and acts as an efficient temperature control.

The apocrine (scent) glands respond to emotional and nervous change. The sweat they produce has a slightly 'earthy' smell which used to be thought sexy, as it was intended to be, but is now considered primitive and embarrassing. Our natural sexy smell is shunned in favour of the more civilized Chanel No 5.

On average you lose about 1 pt (600 ml) of sweat a day, but this doesn't allow for the fact that some people just do sweat more than others. If you really can't keep pace with your sweat production, there could be an underlying medical problem. Your sweating might have a nervous origin, in which case your doctor may be able to prescribe a mild sedative.

Armpits can be protected by either anti-perspirants or deodorants. Anti-perspirants are formulated to prevent some of the sweat getting through to the surface of the skin, so they curb both wetness and smell and are essential for anyone who sweats a great deal. Some brands come in different strengths – for those who sweat a lot and those who sweat less. Deodorants only prevent smell, they cannot reduce wetness.

You can use both products –

one in the morning and one in the evening – or either, but you must be sure to wash regularly as well. Also see that your clothes are clean – the smell of sweat seems to cling doggedly to sweaters and dresses. There are special dress shields available from haberdashers and stores to protect your clothes if you sweat excessively.

Shaving the armpits helps to combat smelliness because the sweat cannot then cling to the underarm hair. But do not use a deodorant or anti-perspirant immediately after shaving unless it says you may on the bottle; it can sting like mad and cause a rash. Best to shave before going to bed and then apply deodorant or anti-perspirant the next morning.

Feet. Nowadays there are all sorts of foot sprays and powders to help control smelly feet – but washing is the first essential.

Vaginal hygiene. If women can get worried about underarm odour, they can get obsessive about vaginal odour. It is quite normal to have vaginal secretions, and these have a characteristic but inoffensive smell. Only when there is some vaginal infection* present (see page 221) do they smell unpleasant. If you are at all worried consult your doctor. However, for women who prefer to be totally aseptic and odourless, just as effective and far safer than vaginal deodorants* is soap and water, especially when applied with hand rather than flannel. The easiest and most pleasant way to ensure vaginal cleanliness is to wash in that marvellous French invention, the bidet. Vaginal deodorants in the form of impregnated tissues do come in useful though, if you are travelling long distances and do not have access to soap, water and privacy. Obviously, extra cleanliness is advisable during menstruation, when the smell from discharge can be unpleasant. However, the use of tampons, changed at regular intervals during the day, will reduce the problem to a minimum.

Douching. External cleansing is one thing, but should you cleanse internally? It is a matter of personal preference. The healthy vagina maintains its own cleanliness through the action of normal bacteria and the secretion of mucus. Douching temporarily destroys these bacteria, even if it is done with plain tap water, but too frequent douching with a strong proprietary solution can cause irritation. Hence, if you must douche, don't do it more than twice a week, unless it is specifically advised by your doctor.

Never douche during pregnancy, or for at least a month after the baby is born. During late pregnancy and until the internal organs have returned to normal, the cervical os (opening) and canal

may be slightly open and fluid could get into the uterus* and cause infection.

If you use spermicides for contraception, remember that douching after intercouse will destroy your protection.

ALTERNATIVE BATHS

Turkish baths. The ancient custom of Turkish bathing is based on a progression from hot to warm to cold chambers, finishing with a body shampoo and warm shower graduating to cold. The steam heat in the hot room, which is endured as long as is comfortable and safe, encourages the flow of perspiration, so cleansing the pores of the skin.

As the heat can, literally, go to your head, many beauty salons have devised units which encase the body in steam while keeping the head out of it.

Saunas. Saunas have taken over from the Turkish bath as the

Although anyone with any respiratory or heart trouble should never take a sauna bath, for the generally healthy it is very enjoyable. Any weight-loss is temporary, the water-loss it represents should be replaced, but it is an encouraging way to start a diet. You should not take a sauna bath while actually on a strict diet or fast, however, when you may be in a weakened state. Nor should you sauna for at least two hours after a meal. Alcohol should be avoided for two hours afterwards.

CLEAN INSIDE

No matter how clean you keep the outside of your body, it is the inside that finally matters. If your internal system is functioning properly this will be reflected in a healthy appearance; if it is not, this will also manifest itself, and in a variety of disagreeable ways. Constipation, a sluggish digestion and over-indulgence in food,

bran, which help to pump waste matter through the digestive system so that bowels are opened regularly and effectively. Constipation is usually caused by a diet which is too high in fat and too low in roughage, but it can also be the result of insufficient exercise or simply not allowing enough time in your morning routine to go to the lavatory. Constipation can be temporarily remedied by drinking plenty of water and eating dried fruit, or by taking one of the patent laxative products, but it is far better to take steps to prevent it occurring in the first place.

There are a number of products on the market containing sodium bicarbonate and citric acid, which can be taken in powder or tablet form after over-indulgence in food or alcohol. They are useful aids against indigestion or hangovers but should not become part of your way of life, since this would imply a regular over-indulgence and the way to inner cleanliness and health is through sensible eating, drinking and living habits.

The after-effects of alcohol, food – particularly rich, garlicky or spicy food – and nicotine are often immediately recognizable in bad breath. Short-term disguise, for that is all it is, can be obtained by thoroughly brushing your teeth, chewing a coffee bean, bay leaf, parsley or some form of spearmint, or using a patent 'breath deodorizer'. But these so-called remedies are only superficial – using them is rather like spraying a room which is basically dirty with an air-freshener. In order to remove the smell completely one has to clean the room out, and so it is with our digestive system. However, if you suffer from persistent bad breath, and you know that over-indulgence or bad teeth aren't the cause, you should see your doctor in case there is some malfunction in your digestive system.

Deep breathing, fresh air and exercise also contribute to keeping you clean inside. If your circulation and muscles are in good running order you are far better equipped to digest your food. Exercise also makes you sweat and this provides an important way of ridding the body of waste. This is one reason why saunas have become increasingly popular in the West as the sweating and subsequent bathing or rinsing helps to clean our bodies both inside and out.

In striving to achieve a healthier and more beautiful you, remember that what goes on inside your body is vital. Treat it with respect, feed it sparingly, exercise it regularly, keep it clean, and the results will be obvious for you and others to see.

EXCESSIVE SWEATING

Many factors contribute to the excessive production of sweat, the liquid discharge of the eccrine and apocrine glands. Among these are heat, nervous tension, sexual stimulation, mild infections, certain drugs and the menopause. The problem can be controlled to some extent by anti-perspirants. These differ in strength, so experiment until you find one that suits you. Wearing loose-fitting clothes, especially under arms or around crotch, will allow sweat to evaporate more quickly. A bland diet may also help: highly-spiced foods, alcohol and caffeine-based drinks can contribute to excessive sweating. Odour is caused when lingering sweat is decomposed by bacteria. Regular washing and use

of a deodorant will minimize this.

Hyperhidrosis is the term used for excessive sweating in localized areas, usually palms of the hands, forehead and soles of the feet. Emotional stress plays a large part in sweating of the hands. Anti-perspirants or cooling applications can help, and in more severe cases sedatives can be useful, but it is far better to tackle the problem by learning to relax (see page 59). Where hyperhidrosis of the palms persists to a stage where the sufferer is permanently troubled, surgery can be an answer. This involves cutting out the nerves in the neck which are responsible for the sweating of palms, and the operation generally offers a permanent cure.

---

favourite way of cleansing the skin by steam heat.

The traditional sauna is a log cabin lined with pine boards, heated by an electric or gas stove to a temperature of 176°–230°F (80°–110°C). Lying on top of the stove are several hard rocks, made of peridotite, a granite which can withstand extreme temperatures.

By ladling water on to the rocks periodically, the hot, dry air in the sauna is made suddenly humid, and though by this action the air is cooled, it feels hotter to the bather. Some people like to sweat in the dry heat, others prefer to keep ladling as they get used to the 'steam shock'. Experts claim that the sudden ionization of the air by the water produces maximum benefit.

Unlike other forms of bathing, you don't stay in the sauna for a long soak, but alternate short spells with a cool shower in a warm adjacent room.

alcohol or cigarettes can result in a feeling of heaviness, indigestion, wind (flatulence), blotchy complexion, spots, broken veins, discoloured teeth and bad breath.

One of the first rules for keeping clean inside is to drink plenty of water, a minimum of 2 pt (1.2 litres) a day. Except in rare cases of excessive fluid retention, we cannot drink too much. Water literally flushes out our system, our kidneys in particular, and helps rid the body of toxic waste material through urine and perspiration.

A citric acid, such as lemon juice, with water is a well-known aid to cleansing the digestive tract and many women start the day with a glass of water with a little lemon juice added, preferably freshly squeezed.

A second rule is to see that your diet contains plenty of roughage, such as raw vegetables, fruit, wholemeal products and

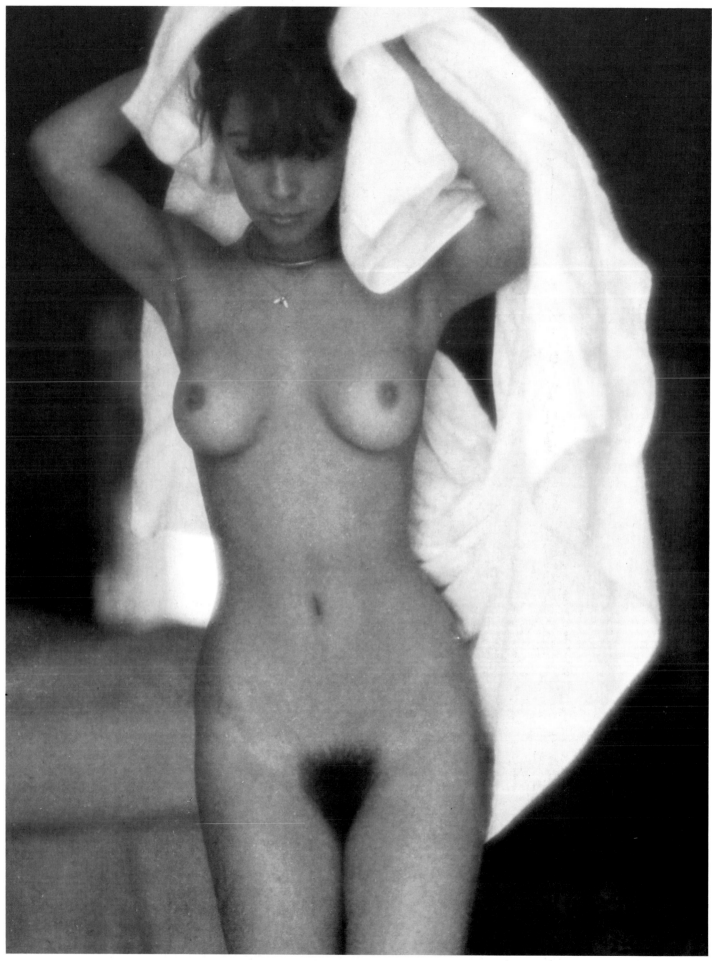

Body Hair

In the Western world, society's rules about what is and what is not 'nice' to look at in the way of a woman's body hair have changed a great deal in the past twenty years. There was a time when around the age of sixteen schoolgirls automatically acquired miniature pink plastic ladies' razors with which they ruthlessly scraped the blonde fluff from their legs each week. Whether the fluff would have turned into something thicker and uglier, no one knows, because they never waited to find out. At that time Frenchwomen with their unshaven armpits seemed shockingly wanton, flaunting all this dark and private growth on the beach.

Nowadays social attitudes are far freer – in fact there is a certain amount of pressure from feminists for women not to de-hair themselves at all – or at least, for them to start thinking about the question and not simply conform to convention. Increasing numbers of women do not remove the hair from their legs, though many who have bravely taken this stand happen to have fair hair and the merest hint of pretty blonde down on their legs. Certainly no one would stare at an unshaven armpit now, and young women no longer wear swimsuits with built-in skirts across the front for fear that a stray pubic hair might expose itself.

In the Sixties – when no one even talked about such matters – Mary Quant bravely predicted that pubic hair would become a fashion *emphasis*, and although this hasn't yet come true we have certainly lost a great many of our inhibitions. What is known as full frontal nudity (which really means the exposure of pubic hair) has now become perfectly acceptable on the stage and screen, and nude bathing and sunbathing are no longer thought of as something only indulged in by a few fanatics in nudist colonies.

This means that we are less likely to grow up in total ignorance of what other women's naked bodies look like, and that in itself may save a lot of misery. But body hair can still cause great distress – a thick moustache or hairy chest is not fun for a woman, however liberated she is, and women still worry about what is 'normal' – are they the only ones with hairs around the nipples, on the tummy, on the thighs?

It is in fact hard to define what is 'normal', because this varies so much from race to race. Chinese, Japanese, American Indians and Eskimos (in other words, the Mongolian races) have very little body or facial hair. Negroes have a little more, and the white races have the most. But even within the white races are huge differences – fair-haired women have less, or at any rate less *obvious* body and facial hair than dark-haired women. In other words, the body hair you have is, like your colouring, determined by heredity, and 'normal' can mean anything from a sparse downy growth of body hair to a thick thatch on legs, arms, pubic area and under arms, with none, a few or a lot of hairs on the face, around the nipples or on the tummy or upper thighs.

There are two types of body hair. The first is the kind we have from babyhood onwards – the hair on our scalps, eyebrows, eyelashes (which, incidentally, like the tiny hairs in the nose and

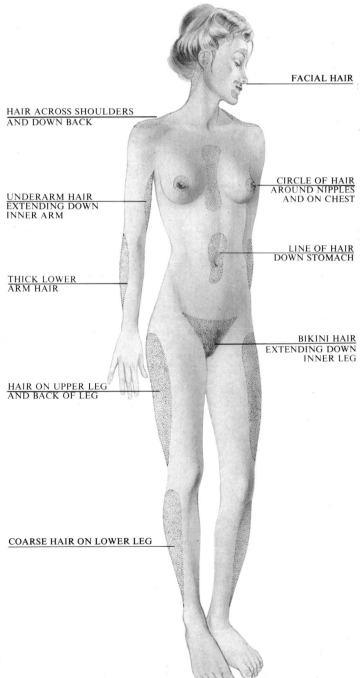

HAIR ACROSS SHOULDERS AND DOWN BACK

UNDERARM HAIR EXTENDING DOWN INNER ARM

THICK LOWER ARM HAIR

HAIR ON UPPER LEG AND BACK OF LEG

COARSE HAIR ON LOWER LEG

FACIAL HAIR

CIRCLE OF HAIR AROUND NIPPLES AND ON CHEST

LINE OF HAIR DOWN STOMACH

BIKINI HAIR EXTENDING DOWN INNER LEG

We are covered in hair, but 'superfluous' hair often comes with puberty. The illustration shows areas where body hair can cause distress.

ears act as filters against dust), and the fine down we have all over our bodies. This hair is distributed in exactly the same way on both sexes. Then there is the hair that develops at puberty. Where this grows differs between the sexes. Boys develop hair on the beard area of the face, in the armpits, in the pubic area and on the abdomen. Some also have thick hair on the chest, arms, legs and thighs. On girls the pubertal hair grows in the armpits and in the pubic area, where it forms a definite triangle with a straight line where the hair ends on the abdominal wall. There may also be the occasional dark hair around the breasts, and thick hair on the legs and arms and possibly the lip. Pubertal hair is of a different texture from that on the scalp. It is coarse and usually curly, so that a man may have hair on his head that is straight and fine whereas the hair of his beard and sideboards will be coarse, perhaps curly, and possibly even of a different colour.

This growth of hair at puberty is triggered off by hormones.* We all have hormones of the opposite sex, but it is only when women have an *excess* of the male hormone testosterone* that they also have excess body hair. Unfortunately at present there is no convenient, simple tablet that will reduce the amount of testosterone in women who have too much, so it is necessary to deal with the problem of excess hair in some other way. Methods of hair removal are talked about in detail later in this chapter.

A sudden growth of body or facial hair after puberty may be caused by going on the Pill, or changing from one kind to another, or a course of hormone treatment. Unfortunately, the hair doesn't disappear even if you stop the Pill or treatment.

Many myths and theories surround the subject of body hair – none of them proven. There is, for instance, a lingering idea that women with a lot of body hair are more highly sexed than women with less. Perhaps this is linked to the feeling that body hair is primitive and 'animal', leading one to imagine that the woman with a lot might be uninhibited and aggressively sexual.

It may also have something to do with the idea that women with a higher level of the male hormone testosterone might show certain male qualities, such as an active, rather than passive, sexuality.

Different societies have often held conflicting views on body hair. In ancient Egypt, neither men nor women allowed *any* body hair to remain – it was thought ugly and unhygienic – and in ancient Greece, too, the women made themselves hairless. This is still the custom in some parts of the world; a Turkish woman, for instance, may have to endure the agony of having every single hair removed from her body before her wedding. By contrast, pubic hair wigs (called merkins) were popular in England in the seventeenth century.

Within Western society, habits are very varied. There are some who do not bother at all with their body hair, though most women probably attempt to do something about the hair in their armpits and on their legs and upper lips. A few go the whole hog and even de-hair their arms or remove their pubic hair, usually to please a sexual partner who prefers them that way. For many women, abnormally positioned or unusually thick facial or body hair is a real problem, causing endless anguish and unhappiness. Unfortunately, there is still no simple, painless, permanent and quick method of hair removal for any of us. How unfair that nature should have given humans balding heads instead of balding legs! Perhaps, some day, someone will invent the perfect depilatory, but in the meantime here is a summary of the methods available to us today – all of them boring, some of them painful and only one of them permanent.

BLEACHING

Bleaching will not take away unwanted hair, but it strips all colour out of the hair, transforming an ugly dark growth into a prettier blonde one. More and more women are finding it an *excellent* way of coping with facial hair – particularly a moustache – for it leaves no shiny bald patches and there is no stubbly regrowth. Unless the hair is very coarse and thick, bleaching a moustache simply leaves a natural-looking blonde down on the upper lip which becomes more sparse as you repeat the process. This is because bleaching is so damaging to the hair shaft that, over time, it

weakens and thins the growth.

Bleaching legs and arms is more time-consuming and messy, and requires a good deal more patience – and bleach, of course. It is really only worth doing if the growth is dark but meagre, often the case on arms. If you have already shaved or used a depilatory on your legs, it is probably too late to consider bleaching as the hair will be coarse and bristly and bleaching will not cure that, it will only change the colour. But young girls who have never shaved their legs, and are a little worried about the darkening growth on them, should try bleaching before becoming trapped by any other method.

Bleaching can be done in a beauty salon, but it is so easy to achieve at home by yourself that it would be silly not to try – though by all means have one treatment at a beauty salon first and learn some of the tricks of the trade by watching the beauty therapist at work.

Bleaches for facial and body hair are available from chemists or stores. Some of them have to be mixed with hydrogen peroxide before being applied to the hair, others have their own 'activator' packed with them. Always follow the instructions on commercial bleaches. The first time you bleach it is absolutely vital to do a patch test on a small area of skin the day before, just to make sure you are not too sensitive for the mixture (see page 178).

The bleach is plastered over the hair, either with a spatula supplied with the product or with the tips of your fingers (wash them afterwards). Be sure that all the hairs are well covered. Most bleaches have to be left on for fifteen minutes or more. You may test how things are proceeding by scraping off a little bleach after that time and inspecting the colour of the hairs beneath. If they are bleached pale yellow or white, rinse off the bleach thoroughly with warm water; if not, re-cover the hairs with bleach and leave on a little longer before rinsing. The bleach often tingles on the skin while it is working. Do not be alarmed, this is normal – but if it should tingle to the point of being painful, rinse off. After bleaching you may notice that the skin itself looks bleached, or that there are little bleached white spots on the skin – peroxide burns. But don't worry, all reverts to normal more or less straight away, and you may, of course, soothe with a little cream. Remember, the purpose of bleaching is to strip all colour from the hair, leaving it white rather than gingery. The first time you bleach you may need to repeat the application in order to achieve this – but the second bleaching should be at least

twenty-four hours after the first. After this, bleach regularly, say every week or two, and you will only need to use one application.

DEPILATORY PRODUCTS

There is a wide choice of these in the shops, designed for use on the face, legs, underarms and pubic area. Whether to use a cream, lotion or aerosol is entirely a matter of preference, for they are all more or less the same when it comes to efficiency. Most women seem to prefer the easy-to-control cream for facial hair and the more economical lotions for leg hair removal.

Depilatories literally melt the hair down to where it emerges from the skin, and their main advantage is that they leave the skin feeling smooth and soft and of course nick-free. Disadvantages are that they work out quite expensive when used regularly, that the melting process 'chops' the hairs, leaving them with blunt ends which develop into stubble, and that they are messy and time-consuming to apply. Many women use depilatories on smaller areas such as their underarms or to tidy the pubic hair on their thighs, while still using a razor on their legs and bleach on their faces. If your skin is sensitive, you might be wise to do a patch test first (see page 178).

Never use a deodorant or anti-perspirant immediately after using a depilatory.

SHAVING

This is probably the most popular way to remove leg and underarm hair as it is quick, easy, and not too messy. Shaving must *never* be done on the arms, face, nipples or tummy, as it cuts the hairs off bluntly, leaving them looking and feeling coarse and bristly – and twice the problem they were before you started. And shaving the pubic hair that grows on the tops of the thighs often makes the skin there very spotty – beware.

Shaving does not change the fundamental texture or thickness of the hair, but it does chop off the fine, tapered – perhaps blonde – ends of the hairs so that they definitely look darker and feel more bristly. For this reason it is best not to shave if you have only a fine growth of hair on the legs: either leave it alone altogether or try bleaching first.

There are dozens of both ordinary safety-razors and electric razors around, some of them specifically designed for ladies. But on the whole men's razors, of either sort, are more efficient than the ladies' versions. And the safety-razor is best, for though it does have to be used with some care to prevent it nicking the skin and it must have a slippery base to work on, soap and water is the

most usual, it gives a closer shave than the electric ones.

Shaving has to be done fairly frequently because the stubble of new growth is quickly felt. Keep your razor ready to use with your bath things so that you remember to whizz up your legs and down the armpits once every few days after your bath. Shaving is extremely drying so be sure to rub hand or body lotion into your legs to keep them looking smooth and glossy instead of parched and flaky. Incidentally, baby oil or vegetable cooking oil smoothed on to wet legs is as efficient for shaving as soap and water, and less drying. Do not use a deodorant or an anti-perspirant in your armpits immediately after shaving unless it specifically says you may on the bottle. It is best to shave at night and apply the deodorant the next morning.

ABRASION

There are hair-removing mitts in the shops designed to *rub* away hair on the legs and arms – but they are not suitable for use anywhere else. These mitts are coated with the very finest sandpaper and they should be used on the legs only when the hair has been shaved off fairly recently – rubbing away whole legfuls of long hair would make the skin underneath very sore indeed, and could even produce friction burns. Once the hair has been shaved you should use the gloves every day or so, going over your legs with gently circular movements to rub away any stubble that has grown in the meantime.

On the arms you *can* use the mitts simply to thin down a too-thick growth. But do not *ever* be tempted to shave your arms in order to use the hair-removing glove more effectively; you will regret it forever. In fact it is far, far better to leave the hairs on your arms just as they are – any attempt to get rid of them is likely to make the problem worse. Bleaching arm hair is the only way.

PLUCKING

This is perfect for eyebrows, or for the odd few hairs that sprout round the chin, the nipples or the stomach. Hairs sprouting from a mole* should not be plucked without asking a doctor first, but you may *cut* them down to skin level as a temporary measure.

Plucking eyebrows
Plucking the eyebrows is a little painful at first, but it is worth doing if your brows are ragged and straggly – somehow neat brows help to make one's skin look better. One warning though: once you have plucked a lot away, the stubble does look fairly awful as it regrows, so always err on the cautious side.

Basic rules

1 Choose good tweezers with either square or slanted ends, not pointed, and always check when you buy them that the prongs meet firmly with no gaps.

2 Dab astringent on brows just before you begin: it gives you a better grip with the tweezers.

3 Always pluck brows in a good light to save your nerves and patience. Best of all, simply take a chair, hand-mirror and tweezers to a window.

4 Plucking should be done in stages – remove a few hairs from both brows and see how they look, rather than working away on one brow and then having to make the other match at the end, even if it's a disaster.

5 Never pluck hairs from above the brow, only from *underneath*, and from *in between* the brows where straggly hairs very often make not just the brows but the whole appearance untidy.

6 Pluck one hair at a time and pull it out quickly in the direction it is growing. Immediately put a finger on the same place for a second to stop the pain.

7 Plucking becomes much less painful the more you do it, and what is more, it weakens the hair growth so that eventually you may only be plucking a couple of really persistent hairs.

Ideal eyebrow

The object of plucking the brows is not to reduce them to a Jean Harlow pencil line – or indeed to do anything drastic at all – it is simply to bring out their *natural* arch. Before embarking on an eyebrow-plucking session it is important to study your whole face. The ideal eyebrow is a gentle curve that starts above the inner corner of the eye and finishes where a pencil slanted from the side of your nostril, past the outer corner of your eye, meets the brow (see illustration). See how your brows match up to the ideal by brushing them upwards – a toothbrush makes a good eyebrow brush – and then across in the direction they grow. You are

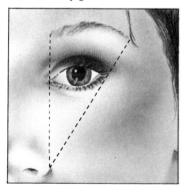

The inner corner of a perfect brow should align with a pencil held vertically alongside nose. Slanting pencil across outer corner of eye gives correct brow length.

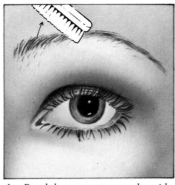

1 Brush brows up to reveal untidy stragglers which need removing. An old toothbrush will do for this.

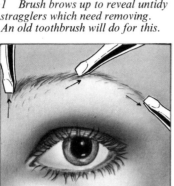

3 Pluck away stray hairs by pulling firmly in direction of growth. Only pluck one hair at a time.

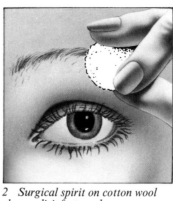

2 Surgical spirit on cotton wool cleans, disinfects and removes excess oil to give good tweezer grip.

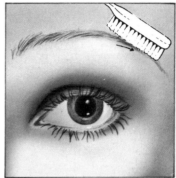

4 Never pluck hairs above brow. Brush brows into shape and allow skin to settle before using make-up.

better off without hairs that straggle across the bridge of your nose, so be fairly ruthless with any growth between your brows, so long as you do not pluck them back to beyond the inner corner of the eye.

As for what to pluck from underneath, this depends on you. Some brows are curved, some are almost straight. Tidy the brows but don't force a curve into a straight brow unless you are pretty sure of what you are doing – you might be taking away an unusual but charming feature of your face. Pluck too little rather than too much. Finish with a good splash of cold water or dab with a mild skin-freshener and apply a little moisturizer or cream. Brush the brows to show off their new shape. In a beauty salon they often remove the hairs between the brow with a strip of wax, but this is a little fiddly to bother with at home, unless you are waxing another area at the same time.

WAXING

This is the age-old traditional way of removing body hair. It is popular because the hairs are tugged out by their roots and therefore regrowth takes much longer than with any other method, apart from electrolysis. Waxing over a long period of time will also weaken the growth of the hair, until eventually you might only have hair left on small

patches of your legs.

It should be said that electrologists are very much against either tweezing or waxing, for these can distort the hair follicle. This means that if you ever decide to try electrolysis after waxing the operator may have to treat the same hairs over and over again, for the distorted hair follicle could prevent the electric probe reaching the root of the hair. This is something to consider if you have a heavy growth of hair on the lip, chest, or around the nipples which could be permanently removed by electrolysis, but it will probably not worry many women when it comes to the problem of removing leg hair: to have these removed by electrolysis would be a costly job taking a great deal of time.

Waxing can be done anywhere on the body, though it is more painful in some parts than others. It can also be done quite easily at home once you have developed the knack, and this is well worth learning as regular salon waxing adds up to a great deal of expense.

There are several kinds of wax, but the principle is the same. The most popular is a mixture of beeswax and resin, which is warmed enough to make it runny but not enough to burn the skin. Thin strips are applied to the area with the back of a spoon or spatula going against the direction

in which the hair grows. The strip is allowed to cool a little, is patted briskly to make sure it is gripping the hairs underneath, and is then ripped off quickly – bringing the hairs with it. Although painful at first – the first strip is always the worst – one does get used to it, and so many women do it or have it done that it can't be intolerable. A spray that numbs the skin, available at large chemists or drugstores, can be used first to prevent pain on limbs but not on the face.

Waxing is excellent for legs and for tidying the pubic area, i.e. if your pubic hair grows on to thighs or tummy – this is known in beauty salons as a bikini wax. It is also good for moustaches, though some women complain that they develop a rash of tiny red spots after moustache waxing. Underarm waxing is less popular since it can be very painful. One of the secrets of keeping waxing as painfree as possible is to do it *often* – once every three or four weeks. In this way you are coping with fewer hairs at a time, and the whole process is much more comfortable.

Waxing should not be done too often as the hairs must be allowed to grow at least $\frac{1}{4}$ in (6 mm) in between treatments so that the wax has something to grip. There is no pain after waxing, though sometimes the pores look red for a few hours. Frequently, new hairs, weakened by the waxing treatment, grow just *under* the skin. Usually, rubbing the waxed areas regularly with a loofah or bath mitt will keep the skin soft enough to allow the hair through, but just occasionally an under-skin hair will turn into a spot and it must be helped out with a sterilized pin or needle. Dab with antiseptic or surgical spirit afterwards.

After waxing, the new growth will feel a little less stubbly than it does with shaving or depilatory cream. After some time, possibly even a couple of years, you will notice that the hair growth is thinning out in patches.

Home waxing

The best way to learn how to wax at home is to have a couple of treatments done at a good salon. Watch the beauty therapist like a hawk to see exactly what she does, so that you can copy her technique at home, and don't be afraid to ask questions. In particular, watch how she uses her finger nails to flick up the end of a strip of wax to use as her 'hold' for ripping it off. Notice how she immediately rubs a stripped area with her hand to take the pain away. Watch the direction in which she applies the wax to the hairs on your legs – this is done *against* the way the hair grows and, curiously, though it is usually from ankle to knee in

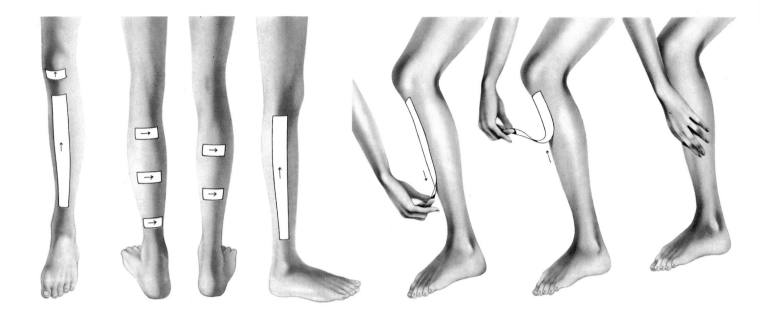

Apply wax in strips as shown in illustrations above, using first pattern of strips in each case and then fitting second pattern between. Wax should be applied against the growth of the hairs, usually up from ankle to knee at front and sides but across width on back of legs. When fitting second pattern of strips, try to cover exactly area not waxed before to avoid leaving straggling hairs. If you go over an area which has already been waxed you will find it very tender. At first you may need to wax one strip at a time, but as you become more proficient you will be able to manage two or three which makes the process quicker.

Apply a strip of wax and wait a few seconds until strip has set but not hardened. Press briskly with fingers to make sure it adheres to hairs underneath, then quickly, before it sets hard, flick up a corner of wax to give a firm hold from the end of the strip which enables you to pull against the hair growth in the direction the wax was originally applied. Seize the flap and pull the strip off sharply. Wax left adhering to the leg can be picked up by pressing a still-soft piece of wax on top of it. Rub a cool hand over the stripped area to take away sting and then start on the next strip.

the front of the leg, it will probably be across the calves and back of the thighs. When you feel confident have a go yourself.

To wax at home you need:
old newspapers
1 old saucepan (you will not be able to cook in it again)
1 old teaspoon
wax.

Depilatory wax can be bought in chemists or drugstores or department stores or, if you can find out where they are, from wholesale suppliers to the beauty trade. It can also be made at home by heating together equal quantities of white beeswax and block resin (order from chemists or drugstores) in your saucepan. Stir together thoroughly when melted and allow to cool in the pan so that you can store it until you need it. If you are buying a commercial wax for your legs, you will probably need more than one or even two packets since many of these are sold in very tight-fisted quantities. Leg waxing can be done much more quickly if you have at least half a 6-in (15-cm) diameter panful of melted wax. You will need far less for a moustache!

Leg wax can be used over and over again, though it will get more and more disgusting-looking as it clogs up with old hairs. Moustache wax is best used fresh each time to avoid any risk of infection. Most women will not want to buy a special wax heater

with thermostatic control as used in salons, but a pan on a low heat does just as well – though it takes much longer as the wax must be melted completely, and then allowed to cool to a workable temperature.

Melt the wax over a very, very low heat, and while it is cooling afterwards, stir it with the teaspoon from time to time until it is the consistency of thickish runny honey. It is wise to combine leg waxing with some other activity in the kitchen so that the long time spent waiting for the wax first to melt and then to cool is not totally wasted. Test a little wax on a finger or wrist: it should feel hot, but not un-bearably so.

Leg wax. Lay out some sheets of newspaper and, wearing only underpants on your lower half, sit yourself on the paper with legs in front of you and pan of wax and spoon close at hand. Do one leg at a time. Gather up a spoonful of wax, winding it round and round the spoon to prevent it dripping, and apply a strip of wax with the back of the spoon, working upwards from ankle to knee. Add more wax as you go – the strip should be about 1½–2 in (4–5 cm) wide and not spread too thinly or it will break when you try to pull it off. Put the spoon back in the pan, wait a few seconds until the strip has set a little but not hardened, press it briskly with your fingers

to make sure it is adhering to the hairs underneath, and then quickly, *before it has set hard*, pick a little flap of wax away from the skin near the ankle with your finger nails to give you a 'hold' on the strip. Seize this flap firmly and pull the strip off your leg sharply. Wax that gets left behind or breaks can be 'picked up' later by pressing a still-soft strip of wax on it, or it can be waxed again over the top. You will notice the beauty therapist doing either of these in a salon treatment. Rub your hand over the stripped section of your leg to ease the sting and then proceed to wax another strip until the whole leg is done. Before completing both legs you will probably need to melt down your wax at least once more.

It is important to work fast and efficiently, for you must never allow the wax to set hard or it will become brittle and break off too easily. You might despair the first time, but it gets easier and easier. Soon you will probably have the confidence to apply two or even three strips at a time, making the whole operation much quicker.

At first do not attempt more than a simple half-leg wax, i.e. from knee to ankle, but as you become more efficient at it you can move on to the backs of the thighs. You may never need to do the finer hair on the fronts. Before attempting to tidy any pubic hair on the thighs it is best, once again,

to book yourself a professional treatment so that you can see exactly how to proceed.

Moustache wax. Clean the area thoroughly of all grease and make-up and dab with witch hazel or surgical spirit. Apply a thin strip of wax from the outer corner of the lip, going against the growth of the hair, to the middle of the lip. Allow to cool slightly, and pat

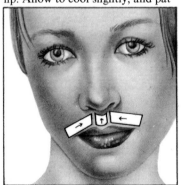

Lip waxing can be achieved with two strips of wax from corner of mouth to centre, or two side strips and one upward in centre of lip.

down firmly with finger tips to make sure the wax is adhering to the hairs. Now, pulling from the outside edge, rip off the wax and immediately press finger tips, or even an ice cube which you have at hand in a bowl, on the waxed area to relieve the sting. Repeat on the other side of the lip. You may need to apply a tiny third patch in an upward direction in the centre of your lip. Apply a soothing lotion such as calamine, or a gentle antiseptic, to the waxed area. Be sure not to wax any more of the face than the narrow hairy part of the lip – you do not want shiny bald patches on your cheeks.

Chin wax. Follow the same basic method. Apply the wax in small strips to make it easier to cope with the curved surface you are now working on. Apply soothing lotion or gentle antiseptic lotion afterwards.

Do not use make-up immediately after either lip or chin waxing, unless it is medicated; it is important to allow the areas a few hours to settle down. Do not wax the lip or chin if there are any spots or pimples, cuts or cold sores in the areas to be waxed.

After any waxing treatment, check to see that the wax has not missed any stray hairs. If it has, simply pluck them out with tweezers, or, if there are many, re-wax the area, but make sure the wax is not too hot, as an area that has already been waxed is ultra-sensitive.

Types of wax
In addition to the usual depilatory wax, made of beeswax and resin, several other types are available. Cold wax comes in a tube or pot ready to use. It is applied with a spatula and removed by pressing strips of cloth on to it which are then ripped off taking the wax, and hairs, with them. Also available are strips of cloth or paper with a coating of sticky wax already applied – these are stuck on the legs like giant strips of elastoplast and ripped off. Or there is a type of 'wax' popular in the Middle East made of 1 lb (450 gm) granulated sugar, 10 fl oz (300 ml) water and 1 fl oz (30 ml) lemon juice. This mixture is boiled for ten to twenty minutes until it is a medium honey colour and a small piece is soft and malleable when allowed to cool on a plate. When judged ready, take off the flame and allow to cool. Knead the toffee mixture for about five minutes while still warm. Then take small pieces of the toffee off the main lump and spread them on the unwanted hair, going against the direction of growth. Press each strip firmly down with the fingers and then rip off with a firm upward movement. Store toffee 'wax' in a jar, and when next needed, warm it up by placing the jar in a pan of water which you bring to the boil.

The standard beeswax and resin depilatory wax which we have talked about is the most reliable version of all the waxes, and is used in most beauty salons.

There is also a new waxing *treatment* available which claims to stop the hair growth altogether.

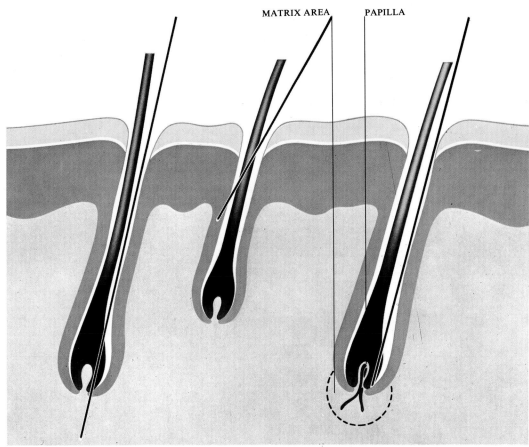

For electrolysis to be effective with minimum regrowth, angle and depth must be correct for each hair follicle. Left: Probe is too deep, ineffective for removing hair as papilla has been missed. Centre: Probe is too shallow to reach papilla and angle could cause surface burns. Right: Probe is at correct angle and depth to remove hair permanently.

The waxing session involved is like any other except that a chemical is rubbed or electrically massaged into the skin immediately after the hairs have been waxed away. This lotion is supposed to weaken the hair so much that after between five and fifteen treatments it does not regrow. The treatment has been available for a couple of years and is vastly expensive, but so far not proven to be effective. Certainly the treatment offers no overnight cure for unwanted hair.

ELECTROLYSIS
This is the *only* permanent method of removing hair. Because it is slow, sometimes painful, and expensive, it is really only suitable for smallish areas such as moustaches, chins, chests, upper arms, shoulders and hairs around the nipples. For any woman with a heavy and disfiguring hair growth in these areas, electrolysis is the only real answer.

The very first kind of electrolysis ever used for hair removal was called the galvanic method. This involved the use of a direct current and the patient had to be earthed; it was also slow. There are a few electrologists still using this method, but by far the more popular type nowadays

is electrolysis by short wave diathermy. This involves the operator inserting an electrode into the hair follicle until it reaches the hair root (or papilla). An indirect electric current is then sent down the electrode which cauterizes the papilla and kills it. If done accurately, nothing should ever grow there again. Often, because of distortions in the papilla, or because more than one hair is growing in the follicle, several sessions of diathermy will be necessary.

Electrolysis is a very skilled and tricky business: if the electrode is put in too deeply, or too shallowly, it will miss the papilla and not kill the hair. If the probe is not precisely in the centre of a hair follicle it might cause a small burn on the skin. For these reasons it is important to go to a really good electrologist. Make sure yours has the necessary qualifications and belongs to a recognized professional institute. There are many people performing electrolysis, but not all of them do a good job. Once in the hands of a competent operator, however, results are impressive.

The speed of electrolysis depends on where the hair is and whether or not the client has previously waxed or tweezed the

area – in which case the follicle may be distorted, making it harder to find the papilla with the electrode. Speed is less important in the long term than accuracy, but a skilled operator can tackle 100-700 hairs in one hour.

Some women find electrolysis more painful than others, and some areas are more sensitive than others – but this varies from person to person. It is possible to invest in a painkilling spray for the skin, available at large chemists or drugstores, but this is supposed to be used only on the body, not on the face. Electrolysis sometimes leaves tiny burns or leads to small spots forming in the area, but neither is serious and both will disappear in a few days. The operator will explain what, if anything, the area should be treated with, and whether or not you may wear make-up on it while it is recovering.

A new type of electrolysis was launched some years ago which involves holding each offending hair in special tweezers through which an electric current is sent down the hair itself to the root. It is completely painless. Unfortunately, independent tests appear to have shown that this method of electrolysis does not prevent the hair growing again.

133

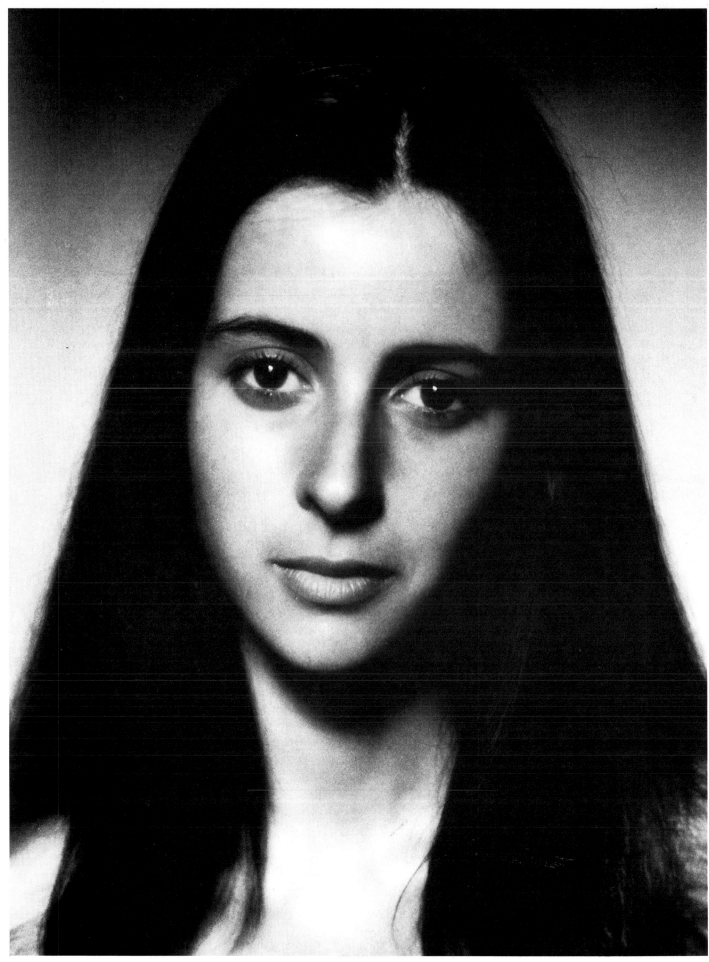

Skin

Whatever you may read in advertisements and in the beauty columns of newspapers and magazines, the first step to being sensible about your skin is to realize that there are no miracles in the business of caring for it. Your skin is like friends or children, it behaves well or badly depending on its character and the amount of time and attention that you are prepared to give it. So you will not read here of any wonder cream that will whisk away the years or give you beauty overnight. Dreadfully dull it may sound, the best advice often does, but skin-care is a lifetime's work. This does not mean that you must dedicate hours a day to it or, indeed, spend a lot of money on it; what is important is to develop good habits and a simple daily skin-care routine that you do night and morning as automatically as cleaning your teeth. This is the soundest beauty tip that anyone can give you. Act on it now – you'll regret it if you don't! Because the skin is constantly renewing itself – old cells wearing away to be replaced by new ones all the time – long-term care and good habits are the only ones that work. It is one of the unfair facts of life that the destructive things you do to yourself – too much alcohol, too many cigarettes, not enough sleep, poor diet – all show more quickly on your face than the positive ones.

WHAT IS SKIN?

Very simply, the skin is made up of two main layers. The outer one, called the epidermis, consists of a top layer of dead cells (this is the part we touch and see) which are constantly being sloughed off and replaced by new ones from the lower, living part of the epidermis. The dermis is a thicker layer beneath the epidermis. It contains the elastic tissue which accounts for the resiliency of the skin, the blood vessels, sweat glands,* sebaceous glands* and hair follicles. Under the dermis lie layers of fat which separate the skin from the muscle and bone of the body, and cushion and support it. This is why, if you crash-diet too cruelly, your skin may sag a little. Skin is the largest overall constituent of the body, weighing around 6 lb (2.7 kg) and covering an area of approximately 17 sq ft (1.6 sq m). It has been estimated that a piece of skin the size of a 5p piece or a nickel contains a dozen blood vessels, twenty-five nerve endings, a hundred sweat glands and an almost unbelievable three million cells.

The skin looks after itself to a certain extent, producing its own oils and moisture for lubrication. But the sebaceous glands which do this don't always act perfectly – they may produce too much sebum (oil) or too little – and the way in which we live does not always help. Central heating, sunbathing and pollution all take moisture from the skin, leaving it dehydrated; if you have experienced the way central heating can crack and warp furniture by drying it out, you will understand what it is doing to your skin. Moisture is as important to skin as oil, for it plumps out, smooths and softens the layer of dead cells on top of the skin. After all, any soldier can tell you that the best way to keep leather looking good is by combining spit and polish, and what is that if it isn't moisture and lubricant?

The point of a regular skin-care routine is that it will keep the outer layer of skin evenly lubricated and moisturized and protected from the environment all the time; it will stimulate the circulation (the blood is a 'messenger' rushing around the body supplying the cells with their needs); and it will speed up the sloughing-off process of the dead cells which in turn will keep the skin fresh and young-looking.

Fresh air and exercise also stimulate the circulation. Countess Csaky, a well-known London beauty expert, tries to walk 8 miles (12.8 km) every weekend – and she is in her seventies. Good diet provides the vitamins and minerals that the body and skin need. Enough sleep, you know instinctively what is right for you, rests and regenerates. Research has shown that both alcohol and cigarette-smoking are ageing – you have only to look at your face after a heavy night out to take the point.

Diet is dealt with fully in another chapter in this book (see page 34), but certain vitamins are particularly important to the skin: Vitamin A, found in eggs, butter, milk, cheese, carrots, spinach, broccoli, kidneys, lamb's liver and fish oils; Vitamin B, found in yeast, wholemeal bread, cereal, wheatgerm, green leafy vegetables, liver and kidneys; Vitamin C, found in citrus fruits, cabbage, potatoes, blackcurrants, broccoli, sprouts, watercress. You do not need to follow any special diet for a good-looking skin, just eat sensibly, which means meat, including offal, fish, eggs, cheese, milk, fruit, wholemeal or rye bread, potatoes and all vegetables, particularly the green ones.

Housewives and office workers often fall into the trap of skipping lunch or relying on snacks or 'processed' sandwiches. Much healthier and just as easy to organize would be a hard-boiled egg and a tomato, a piece of cheese and an apple, or a mug of milk and a piece of fruit.

A balanced diet should not need supplementing with vitamins, but if you have doubts or are on a slimming diet you can buy multi-vitamin tablets from any pharmacist without a prescription.

Don't forget to drink plenty of water – it is not fattening and helps to flush out and clear the system (see page 127). Many people like to start the day with a glass of water sharpened with a little freshly squeezed, or bottled but unsweetened, lemon juice. One beauty therapist suggests adding a dessertspoon of honey to this mixture if you are spotty; another drinks no less than eight glasses of water a day between meals. As an alternative to wine try pepping up fizzy mineral water at lunch or dinner with ice and a slice of lemon.

WHAT IS YOUR SKIN TYPE?

Though the daily routine you will follow is basically the same for all types of skin – the essential steps are cleaning, toning, also called stimulating or freshening, and nourishing – the products you use will depend on whether your skin is oily, dry, a combination of both, or balanced. You inherit your skin type and cannot change it, though you can control excess oil or combat dryness. Below are general guidelines for caring for different skin types. There can be no absolute rules as all skins have their own peculiarities. Your own regular skin-care routine will evolve through trial and error.

Dry skin is most often associated with women who are fair-haired and light-skinned. This is a fine-textured skin (i.e. no enlarged pores) which often feels 'tight', particularly if it has been in water or wind or cold weather. It chaps easily, can look flaky, and though it is envied in youth when it may escape going through a greasy or spotty phase, it does not wear well and needs care from an early age.

Some dry-skinned women have a tendency to broken veins,* known technically as split or dilated capillaries. These may affect quite large areas of the face, giving it the appearance of having patchy red cheeks. This type of skin – indeed any skin which suffers from broken veins – should not be steamed, roughly handled, or subjected to extremes of temperature (i.e. splashing with hot and cold water). Any drastic treatments can worsen the condition, so only the mildest of products and the gentlest of routines should be used (see Skin Problems, page 143).

Greasy skin is more common among dark-haired women and black women. This is often a sallow skin which, after washing, soon develops a film of grease, particularly round the cheeks and nose. Your skin, if it is this type, will always be greasy in the morning when you wake up. The pores of a greasy skin are often enlarged and it is sometimes called 'orange peel' skin. It is prone to blackheads and is sometimes spotty. The great consolation is that this skin ages well; it gets better as it gets older.

A combination skin is one that is oily down the central part of the face – the middle of the forehead, the nose and the chin – but it is dry and feels 'tight' everywhere else.

A balanced skin is neither greasy nor dry but just right. It is sometimes called a normal skin, but it is not normal at all – quite rare, in fact. If you are lucky enough to have this kind of skin you should maintain it sensibly: do not use any harsh products that may over-stimulate the oil glands and be sure it is kept moisturized so that it does not dry out either.

Both greasy and dry skins can be sensitive – to sun, wind, emotions, food and drink, as well as to what you put on them and how you handle them. Both greasy and dry skins can develop allergies* to the cosmetics or skin-care products that you use. And any kind of skin can go through a bad patch in adolescence when the hormones* of the body are changing

SKIN

The body's protective covering and largest organ, skin weighs around 6 lb (2.7 kg), with an area of about 17 sq ft (1.6 sq m). It is thickest on palms of hands and soles of feet, where it may be $\frac{1}{8}$ in (3 mm) thick. On eyelids it may be as thin as $\frac{1}{25}$ in (about 1 mm).

SWEAT PORE
Sweat composition varies, but consists mainly of water with some salts dissolved in it, plus small quantities of urea and lactic acid. Sweat emerges from sweat pore on skin surface and regulates body temperature by cooling skin as it evaporates.

PAPILLA
This is supplied with many small blood vessels providing essential nourishment for hair growth. New hair cells, forming the root, grow from papilla and push up older cells, which change into keratin, die, and become part of hair shaft. Degeneration of the papilla, caused by illness or chemicals applied to scalp, leads to loss of hair.

SWEAT DUCT
Tube through which sweat passes to skin surface.

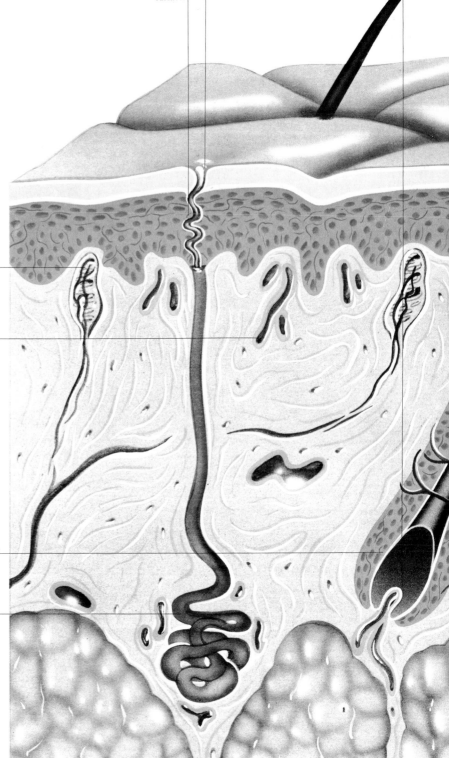

NERVE ENDING
These are embedded in skin and, especially those in finger tips, provide brain with information on relative degrees of temperature, touch and pain.

BLOOD CAPILLARY
These supply skin with food and oxygen and remove waste products; sweat glands and hair follicles have a network of capillaries supplying them. Capillaries beneath skin surface (epidermis) play an important part in temperature control. Blood vessels dilate at high temperature and carry more blood to surface to be cooled by air. Reddening of skin, known as flushing or blushing, is caused by increased volume of blood dilating vessels beneath skin surface.

HAIR FOLLICLE
Pocket in skin formed by downgrowth of epidermis from which hair grows and emerges.

SWEAT GLAND
Coiled tube of secretory cells absorbing fluid from surrounding cells and capillaries. Fluid passes through sweat duct to reach skin surface. Sweat is composed of free-flowing liquid of eccrine glands and milky secretion of apocrine glands. Eccrine glands, widely distributed over body and stimulated by heat or nervous tension, are not usually an odour problem. At times of stress, apocrine and eccrine sweat is secreted. Apocrine sweat glands are closely associated with hair follicles, particularly with hair in armpits and pubic area. They are stimulated by the same hormones which cause hair growth in puberty. Bacteria breaking down this sweat produces body odour.

ERECTOR MUSCLE

Attached to wall of hair follicle and lower layer of epidermis. Muscle contraction pulls hair upright, causing whole follicle to be raised to a higher level than surrounding skin. This is triggered off by shock, fear or cold. When hairs are erect, air is trapped next to skin to help keep body warm.

NERVE

Different types register touch, pain or pressure. Pacinian corpuscle relates to pressure; hair plexus transmits messages of touch or pain in relation to hair.

EPIDERMIS

The skin's outer layer is itself made up of three distinct layers:

CORNIFIED (KERATINOUS) LAYER

Constituted entirely of flat, dead cells, this makes a tough barrier both waterproof and bacteria resistant. Cells are continuously worn away and replaced by other dead cells from beneath. Keratin is the protein of which hair and nails are also formed.

GRANULAR LAYER

This consists of living cells newly produced from germinative layer. The cells are gradually pushed to outside, cornified layer by accumulation of new cells beneath. As cells move towards surface they produce keratin within themselves until filled with fibrous matter, and then they die.

GERMINATIVE LAYER

Continuous layer of cells, dividing actively and constantly producing new epidermis. In this layer cells are called melanocytes and produce melanin, the pigment which determines skin colouring and protects by absorbing sun's ultra-violet rays.
Melanocyte cells are equally distributed in light or dark skin, the difference between them being the productive capacity of each melanocyte rather than their number.

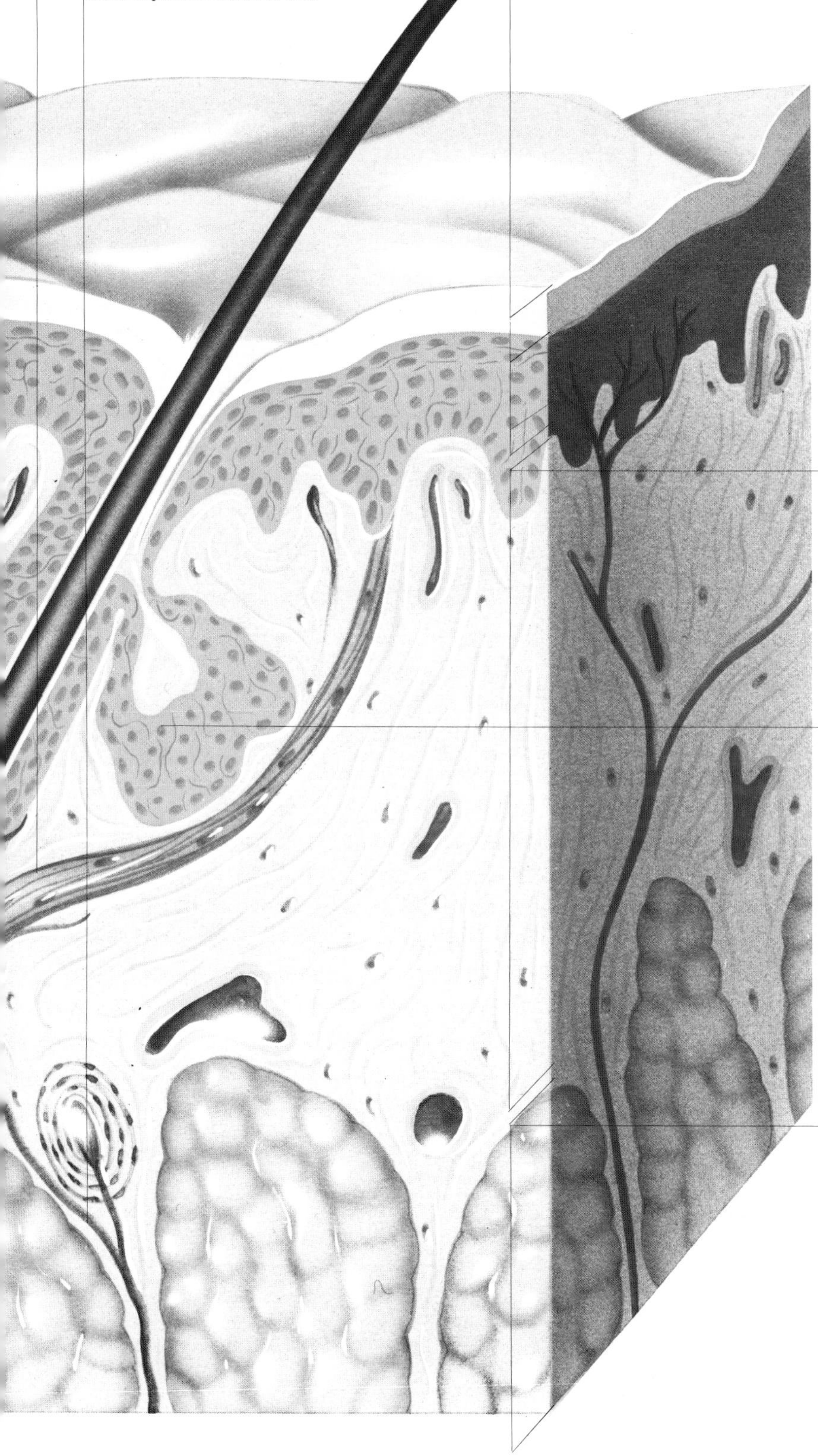

DERMIS

Inner, thicker layer beneath epidermis. Elastic tissue which accounts for skin resilience, containing blood vessels, sweat glands, sebaceous glands, hair follicles and nerve endings. The dermis has relatively few cells and consists largely of collagen fibres produced by fibroblast cells, which also play an important part in wound healing.

SEBACEOUS GLAND

Opening directly into hair follicle, these glands produce an oily secretion known as sebum. Each follicle contains up to three glands. Sebum gives hair water-repellent qualities and is valuable as a skin lubricant, keeping epidermis supple and preventing dryness through evaporation. Fatty acids in sebum are thought to help prevent harmful build-up of bacteria and fungi. Secretion of sebum is continuous along follicle to skin and hair; amount produced is greatly influenced by diet and hormones. Peak production is at puberty, often causing skin eruptions.

SUBCUTANEOUS FAT

Fatty (adipose) tissue in numerous cells beneath dermis. Vital functions: food reserves, laid down if more calories are consumed than are required immediately, and layer of insulation to keep body warm. Layers of fat also separate skin from muscle and bone to cushion and support.

and sometimes cause excess greasiness and acne.

Most women will know their own skin type, but if you have doubts, you can consult a store beautician – pick one working behind the counter for any of the well-known cosmetic companies – who will look at your skin and suggest suitable products. Don't be dazzled by sales talk into spending your week's salary on a carrier bag full of goodies; you do not really need more than a cleanser, a toner or freshener (you may not even need this if your skin is fairly dry), a moisturizer, perhaps a face mask and, if your skin is dry or you are aged thirty or over, a night cream or skin food. All make-up needs are dealt with in the following chapter. Choose the smallest size of each product the first time around, in case you or your skin do not like it.

Better still, if you have the money and the time, book a facial with a good local beauty therapist. She will massage and clean your face thoroughly, diagnose your skin type and suggest suitable treatment. She may gently squeeze any blackheads and she will probably apply a face mask. It is up to you whether you choose to be made up afterwards. It can be flattering or you can emerge looking like a Red Indian chief in war paint, but it does seem a waste of the facial to slap make-up on to the newly-cleansed skin. Make-up lessons are a different matter, dealt with in the next chapter.

WHAT PRODUCTS?

Sadly, there are too few shops that offer independent advice on make-up and skin-care. If you are lucky enough to have one in your area, consult the expert there before buying anything. Otherwise, you are probably left having to shop around in department stores and you will obviously not find the Revlon sales lady advising you that an Estée Lauder product would be better for you than hers. For this reason, selecting products that please you is largely a matter of trial and error: you will only know after you have bought something whether or not you like it and if it suits your skin.

Any of the brand names available in large stores and pharmacists are safe to use, though if you have a sensitive skin or have suffered from allergies it is probably wisest to go for the ranges of hypo-allergenic* products. These have as many as possible of the potentially irritating ingredients, such as perfume, screened out of them.

Most manufacturers' ranges are pretty much the same; they watch each other like hawks and are quick to reproduce a rival's good ideas. Remember that the most expensive products are not

necessarily the best – a large percentage of the price of today's cosmetics goes not on the ingredients at all, but on covering the costs of advertising and packaging.

You may like to try concocting your own skin-care products. It takes a little time but is not difficult and can be great fun, particularly if you persuade a friend to join in. On pages 218-19 you will find recipes for cleansers, toners, nourishing creams, moisturizers, face masks and bath aids, devised by Clare Maxwell-Hudson, well-known for her research into natural do-it-yourself beauty treatments.

Many women find the vast array of bottles and jars on sale too confusing to cope with. The following are the basic categories.

Cleansers

Cleansers divide into four broad groups:
1 The greasy kind (oils, creams, cold creams, lotions) that melt on the skin and float off make-up and dirt and must be removed with tissues.
2 The kind you use with water. Do not be afraid of a daily soap and water wash, which can often be the simple answer to skin problems. Soap will not hurt or dry the skin, provided you *rinse and rinse again* to remove all traces. You also have a choice between special facial 'soaps' that are used with water and lotions and creams that you massage on to the face but rinse off with water. These are called 'rinsable cleansers'. Many women use a greasy cleanser and follow this up with a good wash with facial soap or rinsable cleanser because they do not feel clean unless they have used soap and water.
3 Alcohol-based lotions that are applied on cotton wool and astonish by the quantity of dirt they seem to remove. These are only for greasy and spotty skins, and are better for morning and daytime cleansing than a full-scale evening clean-up.
4 Cleansing pads – pieces of lint impregnated with eye make-up remover or cleanser. These are useful for a quick clean-up during the day and for removing eye make-up at night, but for the rest of the face, a more thorough cleanse at night is advisable.

Dry skins can choose a greasy cleanser, followed up if you wish with a cool splash, or a wash with facial soap or rinsable cleanser.

Greasy skins may also use greasy cleansers, but they *must* follow up with a wash with facial soap and water.

Greasy skins benefit from using a complexion brush, or at least a well-textured flannel, during the wash. The brush may be made of soft bristle or rubber

(it can even be a man's shaving brush) and you should scrub gently all over the face, avoiding the tender eye area, using small circular movements. The use of a brush stimulates the circulation, removes dead cells and helps to unclog pores. It should *not* be used with ordinary toilet soap as that would be far too drying, but in conjunction with a special facial soap or a rinsable cleanser.

Greasy skins may find an alcohol-based cleanser a good idea for a quick clean-up during the day or before going out in the evening. These lotions should not be used on dry parts of the face such as around the eyes, so at night it is probably better to stick to the routine for greasy skins outlined above.

Combination skins should follow the routine for greasy skins.

Balanced skins may use the routine for either dry or greasy skins, depending on what seems to suit their skin best.

Toners, fresheners and astringents

These lotions basically serve the same function – to close the pores and stimulate the circulation – but they vary in strength, astringent being the strongest. Some women do not use a toner or freshener at all, they simply splash the face with cool or cold water, which also closes the pores and stimulates the circulation.

Dry skins should choose the mildest of skin fresheners, or use cool or cold water instead, and must never use an astringent.

Greasy skins should use a toner or an astringent, as the alcohol in these stronger products will also remove surface grease.

Combination skins should only use a toner or astringent on the central greasy panel of the face and a mild freshener on the rest.

Balanced skins should choose a mild skin toner or freshener, not an astringent.

Moisturizers

Moisturizers are essential for all skins. Their purpose is to prevent the skin losing its moisture and to add more, helping to plump out the dead cells on the surface of the skin.

Moisturizer should be used before making up in the morning, for it will protect your skin from the rigours of the day. Many girls prefer not to wear any heavy make-up on their skins, but they should still smooth on a light film of moisturizer. In a poll taken among a dozen or so beauties to find out what products they considered indispensable, moisturizer was the first on every list. So make moisturizer a habit.

At night, women over thirty or with dry skin should use a nourishing cream or a skin food instead of a moisturizer, but greasy skins should stick to a light grease-

free moisturizer which will not encourage spots, except around the eye area where a richer cream may be used.

Dry skins should use the richer moisturizers that contain both grease and water.

Greasy skins must avoid the rich moisturizers and choose instead one of the grease-free versions.

Combination skins should use a grease-free moisturizer with perhaps an occasional 'treat' of skin food for the dry areas.

Balanced skins may choose either kind of moisturizer.

Skin foods, night creams, nourishing creams

These are richer, greasier creams intended for dry skins or for older skins. Anyone over the age of twenty-five or thirty should consider using one, remembering that prevention is better than cure and that wrinkles do not simply appear overnight at a certain age. These creams vary in texture from light, for younger women, to heavy, for those in their forties, though the skin itself is a better gauge than age in years. They should be massaged in at night instead of a moisturizer, and any surplus should be dabbed off with a tissue.

Many of these creams contain special ingredients that claim to slow the advancing years. Some of these may suit your skin very well, but *none* of them performs miracles. These are some of the most common:
1 Hormones are added to some creams designed for older women whose own hormone levels are changing. There are legal limits as to how much hormone can be added, but never be tempted to buy 'quack' products – settle for a reputable brand which will at least be perfectly safe. Their value is very debatable; some hormone specialists insist that hormones cannot be absorbed through the skin, and therefore the hormone element in these creams would seem to be valueless, only the simple lubricating ingredients in them could do some good.
2 Enzymes are contained in some creams and these purport to work away at the dead layer of cells on the face, making it softer.
3 Acid-balanced or pH products. The skin has a protective acid mantle. The extent of acidity or alkalinity is measured on a scale of 1 to 14 and the pH (per hydrogen) factor or measurement of the skin's acidity is between 4.5 and 5.5. Soap is usually alkaline or has a pH factor of above 7, so it temporarily destroys the skin's acid mantle. For this reason, some products nowadays are acid-balanced to match the skin and so maintain the natural acid coating. The pH figure 7 is neutral, less than 7 is acid, and more than 7 is alkaline.

4   Firming creams. These are of no long-lasting benefit to the skin, since they simply act on the surface, temporarily tightening it so that small lines are smoothed out. They come in mask form – to be washed off after a few minutes – or as lotions which should be worn under make-up.

5   Soluble collagen is added to certain creams in an attempt to replace the natural loss of collagen that comes with age. Collagen fibres are a constituent of the skin which maintain its elasticity and its capacity to absorb water.

6   Vitamins. A couple of years ago there was a positive craze for Vitamin E, and it was claimed to be a miraculous healer for spotty or sore skins and even burns and cuts. Though there seems to be no medical proof of this, there are still women who are addicts and Vitamin E creams and oils are still on the market. Vitamin A is also to be found in some skin-care creams; it is said to counteract dry, scaly skin.

Eye creams, throat creams and wrinkle creams

These are designed for the most sensitive skin area, round the eyes, and the most neglected skin area, the throat. Since they are only applied in these areas, they may be used on both greasy and dry skins. Some eye and wrinkle creams are quickly absorbed by the skin and may be worn under make-up during the day, but the greasier ones are best used at night in small quantities. Surplus cream should be tissued off before you go to sleep as some of these creams can leave the eyes looking a bit puffy in the morning.

Masks

Masks are an occasional treatment designed to tighten the pores of a greasy skin or to nourish a dry skin. Be sure to pick one suitable for your type of skin. Greasy skins may use a face mask every few days, dry or sensitive skins not more than once a week. Masks wash off or peel off. Go carefully with the type that peels off as some people do experience difficulties, such as masks refusing to set or come off evenly, or pulling the tiny hairs of the face.

Skin peeling or exfoliating treatments

These are designed to remove dead cells from the surface of the skin, leaving it softer and more tender. Some of these products can leave your face feeling sore because they have tiny abrasive bits in them; it's rather like rubbing your face with a pot scourer.

Pore grains to be rubbed only on the open-pored, 'orange peel' areas of the face are a good compromise.

If you cleanse your face correctly, massaging in your cleansing cream, scrubbing with a complexion brush or face flannel,

and so on, you should not find it necessary to buy skin-peelers or exfoliators at all.

A mild and easy do-it-yourself exfoliating treatment is simply to scrub your face once a week or so with fine ground oatmeal from a healthfood shop. Keep the oatmeal by the wash-basin in a jar. Mix a little into a paste with some water in the palm of your hand and then rub on to the face with small circular movements. Rinse off.

Alternatively, you may add a little sugar to the soapy lather when you wash your face. Massage the sugar gently into your face with the lather and rinse off.

YOUR SKIN-CARE ROUTINE

Having chosen your products to suit your skin type, you must now allow yourself an extra few minutes, night and morning, to complete your routine. It must become as automatic as cleaning your teeth. Your skin is changing – sloughing-off dead cells and growing new ones – all the time. There is no point in wasting money on skin-care products unless you are going to use them regularly. Any beautician will tell you how different a cared-for skin looks from one that gets hit-and-miss treatment.

The secret of beauty care is not to aim too high. No matter how good your intentions, you are far more likely to spend five minutes a day on a simple routine than hours a week fiddling round with a host of exotic products.

At night

1   Cleansing. Pour a little cleansing milk or lotion or oil into the palm of one hand, rub the hands together and massage into the face using the expert's movements in the illustration on page 140. Or put a couple of blobs of cream on to your face and massage in using the same movements.

Tissue off the cream, and dirt, with gentle upward movements. Repeat, but this time spend a little longer on the massage. Now simply splash your face with cool water, or wash with special facial soap or rinsable cleanser. Dry, and you are ready for the next step.

If you do *not* use cleansing cream, but prefer to wash with water, massage the facial soap lather or rinsable cleanser lather into your face with the fingers – or a complexion brush – following the movements in the illustration. In this way you will not miss out on a nightly massage.

2   Toning. If you do not use a skin toner or freshener or astringent, be sure to splash your face after cleansing with cold or cool water to close the pores and stimulate the circulation. If you do use skin toner, now pat it on to the greasier areas of your face with

cotton wool.

3   Feeding. Pour a little moisturizer or put a little skin food into the palm of one hand, rub the hands together and then massage the moisturizer or skin food gently on to the face with the same sort of movements as shown on pages 140 and 141. In the course of this massage, lightly circle the eyes with the finger tips very gently twenty times; be sure there is enough cream to keep your fingers slipping on the skin. If you use an eye or wrinkle cream at night, circle this in round the eyes instead of moisturizer or skin food. Leave creams on for as long as you can, up to twenty minutes, but always tissue off any surplus before going to bed.

The whole routine can be accomplished in five minutes once it becomes a habit, and you are not only cleansing, toning and feeding your skin, but stimulating the circulation, removing dead cells and generally giving yourself a nightly beauty treatment.

In the morning

All skins may simply be washed with facial soap or rinsable cleanser if you feel it wakes you up in the morning, or greasy and combination skins may be cleansed with an alcohol-based cleanser applied on cotton wool, or dry and normal skins may be cleansed with a greasy cleansing cream or milk. After cleansing, tone the skin as at night with cool water or skin toner, astringent or freshener. After this, all skins *must* use moisturizer. Some women prefer to massage the moisturizer on to their *wet* faces, which helps to retain as much moisture as possible on the skin.

Moisturizer can go under a powder base, it can act as a base – just pat your powder on top – and it is an essential protector for those who prefer to wear no make-up on the skin. There are some tinted moisturizers on the market which are excellent for a natural-looking make-up, or for those who feel they need a little colour but hate to wear a thick, opaque base.

Taking stock

Once in a while – it could be every week or every month – try to take an hour off to give yourself a facial and take stock of your face. Do your eyebrows need plucking (see page 130)? Does your moustache need bleaching or waxing (see pages 130, 131)? Is your skin changing – getting drier for instance? In which case, you must switch to richer products or start using a night cream.

FACIALS

A facial can be quite a morale-booster, especially on those days when you feel down in the dumps over your looks. If you have the time and money you can be pampered by a professional, but

you can give yourself an effective facial quite easily at home.

Home facials

Start by collecting together all the things you will need:
scarf or bath cap to protect your hair
a greasy cleanser
a facial sauna, available from large stores, or a bowl of boiling water
tissues
skin toner or freshener
face mask, chosen to suit your skin type.

Step 1

Put your hair in bath cap or wrap with scarf. Take a blob of cleansing cream and massage it into your face using the movements shown overleaf. Spend as long as you can on this, but don't be rough and don't drag the skin. Tissue off and repeat.

Step 2

Put your face into your facial sauna or lean over your pan of boiling water with the towel over your head, exactly as though you were inhaling for a cold. Do not get too close to the water or the heat might cause broken veins. You may add some herbs to the water – elderflowers or camomile are traditional favourites, but you could just use some thyme or rosemary from the kitchen cupboard. Steam your face for as long as you can bear it – it is a very tedious business – up to fifteen or twenty minutes.

Step 3

With a clean tissue, very, very gently press out minor black-heads. Don't tackle any more serious offenders as this will just cause spots (see page 145).

Step 4

Splash your face with cool water or use a facial soap if you prefer not to leave grease on your skin.

Step 5

Dry your face and apply your face mask, leaving out the tender area round the eyes. Try to relax while the mask takes effect – from five to twenty minutes, depending on the type. You could massage in a little eye cream before you apply the mask and then that can be working round the eyes while the mask treats the rest of your face.

Step 6

Rinse off mask and pat skin with toner or splash with cold water.

Step 7

Massage in your usual moisturizer.
Note: If your skin tends to broken veins you should *not* steam the face and should choose the very mildest of skin toners and masks, those made specifically for this skin type.

GROWING OLDER

It is important to emphasize the need for good habits and daily skin-care, because they are the only way to fight the advancing years. There are no miracle treatments for skin that has lost its youthful

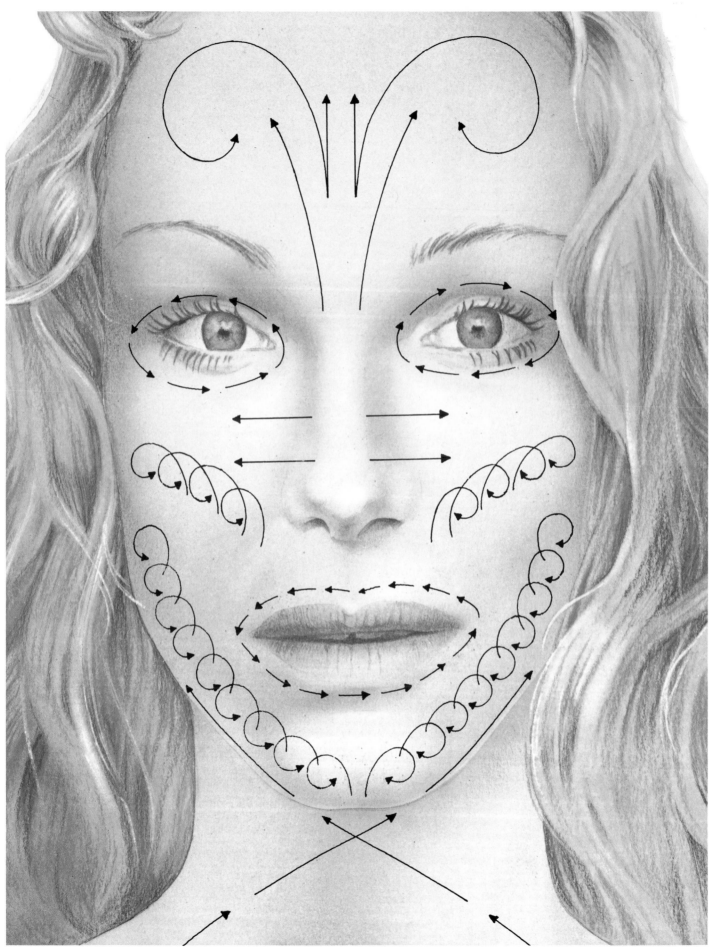

The arrowed lines marked on the face above indicate direction and flow of each massage movement described with hand positions opposite.

FACIAL MASSAGE

Get into the habit of giving yourself a daily face massage when you cleanse or apply nightly moisturizer or skin food. Massage relaxes tension in the face, stimulates the blood supply, and helps to keep skin elastic and young looking. Make sure there is enough cream under your fingers to prevent skin dragging. Massage movements should be in continuous flowing rhythm in an upward direction to counteract natural tendency of skin and muscles to droop.

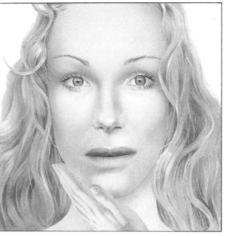

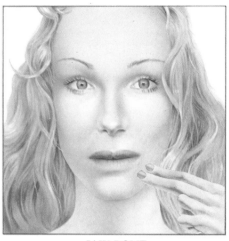

NECK AND CHIN
Always start with neck as this stimulates blood supply to face. Put left hand on right collar bone, then sweep hand up and across neck, then up side of face to left ear. Repeat with right hand on left collar bone.

JAW-BONE
With first two fingers of each hand, work up jaw-bone from chin to ears in a continuous upward spiralling movement. This helps to release tension built up around jaw line, which soon pulls down corners of mouth.

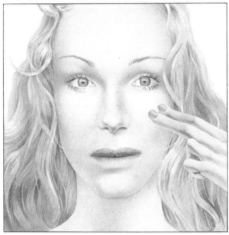

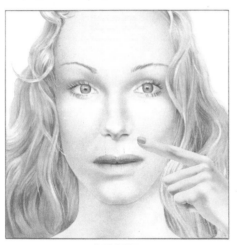

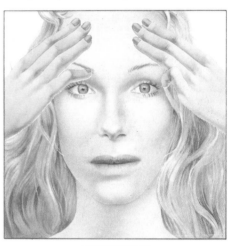

CHEEKS
With first two fingers of each hand, work from side of nose to upper corner of cheek-bone in a continuous upward spiralling movement, taking care not to drag skin near eyes. This helps to delay droop of lower cheek area.

MOUTH
Tiny lines often form along lip line. This stroke helps to keep lips supple and lines at bay. Using forefinger or middle finger, go round and round mouth in a circular movement, first in one direction and then in the other.

FOREHEAD
Massage up forehead from bridge of nose in curving lines to hair line and away from centre using first palm of hand and then flat of three fingers and alternate hands. This stroke helps to iron out frown lines.

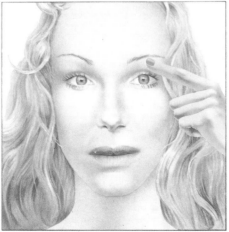

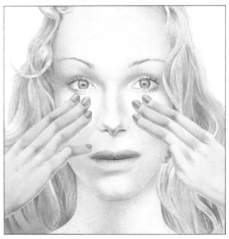

EYES
With forefinger, or third finger for lighter pressure, circle around eyes gently, with enough cream under fingers to slip easily over skin. Finish with tiny circles in indentations between outer corner of eye and hair line.

NOSE TO EARS
Starting with finger tips resting on nose, sweep gently across face, both hands together, from cheeks to ears. Repeat this in soft, stroking movements. This stroke smooths and lifts cheeks and eases tension across face.

bloom and elasticity except, finally, to have it lifted by plastic surgery.

No one knows what it is that signals our bodies to start ageing, but at a certain time, and this varies enormously from woman to woman, our cells' capacity to renew themselves slows down.

The downward path usually starts in the early thirties when small expression lines begin to show and the skin loses its firmness. At this stage regular skin-care is vital, for it really can slow down the ageing process.

As a woman approaches the age of menopause, from the middle forties to fifties, the fine lines start forming into wrinkles, the skin becomes crepey, loses its smoothness and springiness and starts to bag and sag. Again, skin-care can help a great deal. At this age the supply of the so-called 'female' hormone in the body, oestrogen,* is slowing down and it has been noted that women taking extra oestrogen to replace this loss, hormone replacement therapy (page 123), do tend to have younger-looking skins.

Beauty therapists all agree that the neglect or care that a skin receives over the years plays a part in how quickly it ages, but there are other factors involved: your general health, your diet, your environment and your hereditary characteristics; if your mother looked sixty when she was eighty, the chances are that you will, too.

You should always be on the look-out for changes in your skin which indicate that you should adjust the products you use. Greasy skins, for example, get much less greasy as they get older, and someone accustomed to using a fierce astringent may be doing more harm than good by the time they are in their thirties; the products you use in your twenties will not be the ones you use in your thirties or forties.

Always be gentle with your skin. Never drag it or pull it or squeeze it too hard, and never be afraid to seek professional advice at any stage, from a beauty therapist, a doctor or a store beautician.

When you are bored to death with your skin-care routine and tempted to abandon it, remember that there is *no cure* for wrinkles, but that your routine can delay them.

Crow's-feet and laugh lines can be positively attractive; actress Anne Bancroft has them and is stunning. Frown lines, however, are not endearing and frowning is often just a bad habit. One does it without thinking – in the office, reading, and especially when driving. Make sure you have a good pair of sunglasses if bright light makes you wrinkle your eyes or frown. Get two pairs and keep

one in the car, if necessary. Some women stick a tiny piece of Sellotape in the centre of their forehead before driving or working or at any time they might relapse into a frown without realizing. It may look silly, but it does remind you to stop. If you frown a great deal it could be a sign of eyestrain, so have your eyes checked regularly.

Simple facial exercises help to prevent a face stiffening and setting as it gets older, and will keep it more mobile and expressive – but only if you do them regularly. Include them in your daily exercise programme (see page 60).

Neck exercises are especially helpful. They will help your posture and remove tension and stiffness, aches and pains, from the neck and shoulders. We often stiffen up in that area without being aware of it. Neck exercises are particularly good after a long drive or a tiring stint at a desk or typewriter. Always do them gently, never force a movement.

There are muscle-exercising machines on sale for use at home, and similar machines are sometimes used in salon face treatments and slimming treatments. The basis of them all is an electrical impulse which makes your muscles contract and relax without you doing a thing. But unless you intend to have these treatments regularly, or to use your machine regularly, it is better to stick to the facial exercises on pages 65 and 75.

SUNTANNING

Wind, cold, a polluted atmosphere, central heating – all these are enemies of the skin which can be combated by your daily skin-care routine. It is sensible, if you know you are going to face especially rigorous weather conditions, say hiking, skiing or sailing, to protect your face with an extra layer of moisturizer, your lips with Vaseline or a special lip salve and, perhaps, your nose with a sun barrier cream.

Of all the skin's enemies, the sun is the most powerful. It drains the moisture from the skin, dehydrating it and helping to age it prematurely. It is obviously no use telling a sun-worshipper to give it up, but everyone should realize how harmful the sun can be, and take care to ensure that they get the benefits of a tan without its ill-effects.

The much-coveted suntan is simply the skin's natural response to, and defence against, the power of the sun. The ultra-violet rays of the sun prompt the skin to produce more of the pigment melanin, which gives our skin its colour, for this pigment acts as a natural sun-screen. The ultra-violet rays also have an almost immediate effect on the

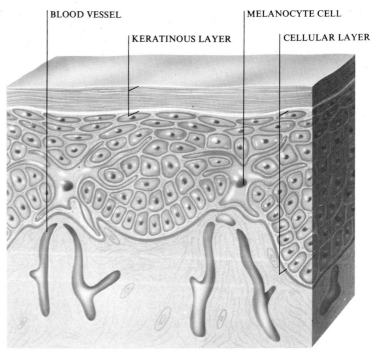

Untanned skin showing too little melanin pigmentation to protect it against the harmful ultra-violet rays of the sun.

surface of the skin, turning patches of pigment, such as freckles, dark brown. We all have a natural limit to the depth of our tan according to the amount of melanin we produce.

There is ample evidence that exposure to the powerful rays of the sun over many years can increase the chance of getting skin cancer, but normal holiday suntanning is quite safe in this respect. The danger applies particularly to fair skins which have less melanin to protect them from the sun. Negro skins and dark skins exposed for centuries to the sun have a natural immunity.

There are pre-sun tablets on the market that contain Vitamin A and calcium, for it is known that the ultra-violet rays of the sun diminish the level of Vitamin A in the body. Some people swear by these, others say they make little or no difference, so it is up to you to decide whether they work for you personally and help to protect you from burning.

Once on holiday you *must always* follow this often-repeated, boring advice:
1 Only sunbathe when your face and body are protected with a good suntan cream or lotion. Choose one made for *your* skin type and buy enough not to have to be mean with it.
2 Unless you are using a waterproof lotion, re-apply the suntan cream each time you have been in the sea, especially on the more vulnerable parts of your body: the shoulders, nose, chest,

tops of thighs, backs of knees.
3 Most important of all, ration your tanning-time sensibly. Eileen Ford, a top New York model agent, who cannot afford to have girls laid off because of sunburn, suggests the following routine. Take a kitchen-timer clock on to the beach with you and set it for between five and twenty minutes, depending on whether you are fair-skinned and burn easily, or dark-skinned and less vulnerable. Apply your tanning lotion and then lie in the sun until the timer goes off. Immediately splash your face and body with cool water, or swim or shower quickly, apply more suntan lotion and then go and sit in the shade for twenty minutes, after which you may go back into the sun and repeat the whole process. You can do this several times in a day, but never, never allow your skin to burn or you will spend the second week of your holiday watching the tan you rushed too quickly in the first week peeling off.

Remember that sunburn really is a *burn* and there is no cure – the after-sun creams and lotions only help to relieve the soreness and subsequent dryness. Cold tea can help take the sting out of sunburn and you can finish the treatment resting with the cold tea bags soothing your burnt eyelids! Always lavish your body with moisturizer or after-sun cream when you have finished sunbathing and at night. To keep a tan as long as possible you must prevent the skin from drying and

BLOOD VESSEL   MELANOCYTE CELL

KERATINOUS LAYER   CELLULAR LAYER

THREE STAGES IN THE TANNING PROCESS

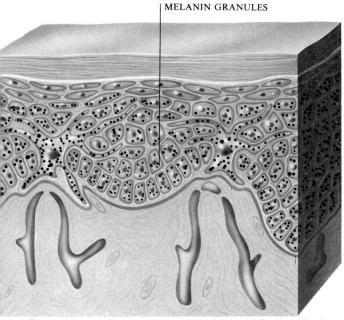

MELANIN GRANULES

After exposure to the sun, cells called melanocytes begin to divide and increase output of melanin granules. Skin may be pink and tender.

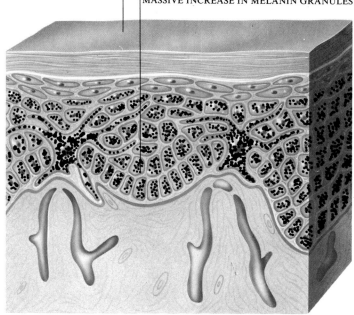

KERATINOUS LAYER DARKENED

MASSIVE INCREASE IN MELANIN GRANULES

Melanin pigment has infiltrated surface of skin, giving darker appearance. Skin is now well protected and sunbather has achieved a tan.

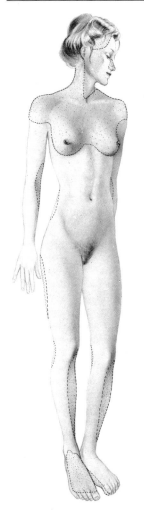

AREAS MOST VULNERABLE TO SUNBURN

flaking off quickly. Always use a bath oil, any vegetable oil such as olive or maize oil will do, when you have a tan; this will keep it smooth and gleaming and help it to last.

The sun will bring out freckles and darken any pale pigment patches you may have on your face and body. The only way to prevent this is to use a sun-block which prevents the skin tanning altogether.

Strap marks can spoil the whole effect of a smooth golden tan, so shrug off your straps or undo the back of your bikini before you sunbathe.

Sun-lamps, either used at home or in a beauty salon, can help to start off a tan before your holiday, but you must still be careful when you get out into the strong sun. They can also keep you lightly tanned and healthy-looking all the year round. If you decide to buy one, and they are temptingly priced these days, be sure to buy a reputable brand and never, never be foolish enough to use it for longer than specified in the instructions or without goggles to protect the eyes. Always use a body lotion or oil after a tanning treatment to prevent dryness.

The drying effects of the sun, so harmful to dry skins, can be very helpful to greasy skins, tightening the pores and smoothing them out. For this reason ultra-violet sun-lamp treatments are often recommended for those suffering from acne or excess oiliness of the skin.

Fake tanning by means of colourless creams or lotions is a harmless and popular way of making sure that you are not the whitest person on the beach. These creams and lotions simply dye the skin, they do not protect it, so you need to be just as careful in the sun as if you were lily-white.

Two or even three applications of these creams tend to give better results than one, as some of the streakiness overlaps and disappears. Fake tanning creams are quite difficult to apply, and you need time and patience to do it properly. Always follow the instructions given, and try to enlist the services of a friend so that you can each help the other with the inaccessible parts of the body. The dry and horny areas of the skin – elbows, knees, feet, palms, knuckles – sometimes take the dye more strongly, so go carefully in these places. It is less chancy, and less drying, not to use fake tanning creams on the face in case they streak unexpectedly; better to colour the face with a transparent gel make-up or a transparent stick make-up in a suntan shade.

Some beauty salons will apply a fake tanning lotion for you. This treatment is not cheap, but the results are usually better than you can achieve at home.

SKIN PROBLEMS

Acne

It seems so cruel that acne occurs in the teenage years when a young person has less confidence and is probably more preoccupied with

his or her appearance than at any other time. What hollow consolation it is at fifteen to be told that you will grow out of it! (In 90 per cent of cases, acne is gone by the age of twenty-five.) But acne occurs in adolescence because it is at puberty that the sebaceous or oil-producing glands in the skin start working and it is when this oil production first begins that the problems appear.

The distressing spots of teenage acne are brought about by oil clogging up the pores of the skin. Blackheads form first and then, if these become inflamed, red spots develop, followed by yellow pustules if the spots become infected. The oil blockage may be due to one of several irregularities: it could be that the skin has an excessive number of sebaceous glands; it could be because there are a normal number but they are over-producing oil; or it could be that the oil being produced has a high viscosity or thickness. Teenage skins can also suffer from the opposite: too little oil is produced, causing a very dry skin.

It has been suggested that acne is 'psychological' – caused by something like boyfriend or examination worries. According to experts, this could only be the case if the stress is so severe that it actually interferes with the normal oestrogen level in the body.

All sorts of treatments have been prescribed for acne, from lotions and medicated creams to the Pill, diet and ultra-violet sun-lamp treatments. These are discussed below.

1   Antibiotics. These are frequently prescribed to remove the bacteria that cause the skin infections. One of the side-effects of the antibiotic *oxytetracycline* is to reduce the viscosity or thickness of the oil being produced by the sebaceous glands. This in turn is effective in preventing new pore-blockages and dealing with the spots already present. Only oxytetracycline has this effect on oil, it is not a general property of all antibiotics. Only your doctor can prescribe antibiotics. If you find your doctor unhelpful when you consult him about acne, you can ask to be referred to a dermatologist.* Long-term, low-dose antibiotics are probably the best treatment for all but hormone-dependent acnes.

2   Beauty therapy. Many beauty therapists provide special acne treatments. These generally involve clearing the skin of blackheads by hand or by suction, steaming the face, perhaps with ozone, massage, either by hand or with an electrically-operated machine, and a face mask of some kind. Some treatments will also include ultra-violet sun-lamp sessions. Research seems to show that the latter have the best results, but *no* acne treatments achieve miracles, and all may take two or three months to show improvement. The therapist will usually sell you special creams and lotions to use at home, but only a doctor can prescribe a more radical course with hormones or antibiotics.

3   Diet. Nowadays, diet is not considered as important a factor in the treatment of acne as was once thought to be the case. However, a good diet, one that includes lots of fresh vegetables and fruit, meat, fish, milk, cheese, eggs, honey and wholemeal bread and cuts back on the 'rubbishy' foods such as crisps, chocolates and sweet or fizzy drinks, will keep you healthier and benefit skin and figure as well.

4   Hormones. The so-called 'female' hormone oestrogen tends to decrease the rate of oil production by the skin, meaning that the acne will be improved. This is why a woman's skin is often glowing and spot-free during pregnancy, when large amounts of oestrogen are being produced by the body. In the very small number of cases of acne which are hormone-dependent certain contraceptive pills may improve the condition of the skin, but you should ask your doctor's advice on this.

5   Skin-care. Keeping the skin

144

clean and as oil-free as possible must be the main aim of the acne sufferer. This can be done by washing night and morning with hot water and a facial soap or rinsable cleanser (use a medicated version of either of these if you can find one) and using a complexion brush, or a man's shaving brush, fairly regularly. You can wash with ordinary or medicated soap, but these might make your skin a little too dry and tender. During the day a clean-up with facial soap and water or an alcohol-based cleansing lotion applied with cotton wool is not a bad idea.

Acne sufferers should use a special acne lotion or a skin toner or astringent on the greasy areas of the face, and they should try to keep the skin clear of blackheads by squeezing the most obvious ones from time to time. Follow the instructions given under Blackheads below.

Red spots or white pustules should *not* be squeezed as this will only spread the bacteria further and make the problem worse. Dab these spots with a drying spot lotion, or surgical spirit, or bathe them with hot water.

If you suffer from acne you should try not to use any grease on your face, but this does not mean you may not use a grease-free moisturizer to keep the skin supple.

Pore grains rubbed into the greasiest areas when you wash or an oatmeal scrub from time to time might be helpful: take a little finely-ground oatmeal, mix it with some water to form a paste and massage into the skin. Rinse off with water. A regular home facial (described on page 139), once a week or so, would be a good idea. Both the steaming of the skin and the face mask are helpful in combating grease.

Make-up, preferably medicated or as grease-free as possible, can be used to disguise the spots, but it must be removed properly at night. Care of the skin, particularly the cleaning of it, is very important.

6   Ultra-violet treatment. The ultra-violet rays contained in both natural sunlight and the artificial sunlight that comes from an ultra-violet lamp help to melt the oil and dry out the excess in the skin. Both sun and sun-lamp treatments are valuable to acne sufferers. If you do buy an ultra-violet lamp you must be sure to follow the instructions and not be tempted to give yourself extra time. It is the regularity of the treatment that is more beneficial.

Acne sufferers are sometimes left with scars long after the spots themselves have disappeared. These can be removed – or at least improved – by scarification, or

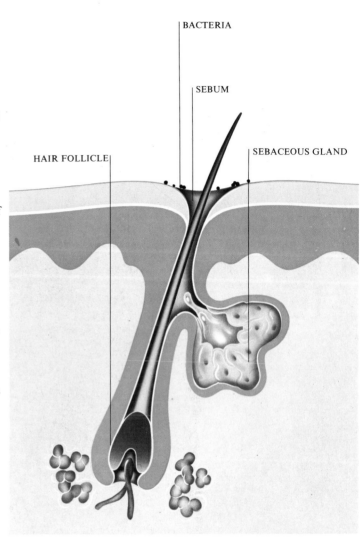

BACTERIA

SEBUM

HAIR FOLLICLE

SEBACEOUS GLAND

Hair follicle and sebaceous gland, known medically as a pilo-sebaceous unit. Above is shown healthy, normal growth from skin free from acne.

removal of the top layer of skin down to the level of the scar (see Skin peeling, page 139). In Britain, this treatment is available under the National Health Service but there may be a long waiting list. In other countries, you should also consult your doctor or dermatologist.

Allergies

An allergy can develop quite suddenly; in fact, you may have been using the product that has caused it for some time. It is not uncommon to develop an allergy to an eyeshadow or eyeliner; when the eyelids become red and sore and itchy, you slap on more make-up to cover them up and it gets worse and worse. If the skin becomes inflamed and sore on any part of your face, stop using *all* your beauty products. If the allergy goes away, in a day or two

you can reintroduce your cosmetics one by one until you track down which one it is that is causing the reaction. Or you can simply try another brand of make-up: if you are allergic to one eyeshadow it does not mean you will react to them all. In this case it would probably be sensible to switch to products from one of the hypo-allergenic ranges; these are made for women who tend to suffer from cosmetic allergies. If the allergy does not get better when you stop using cosmetics, see your doctor, as the allergy must be caused by something else.

Blackheads

These can be kept to a minimum in most cases by your regular skin-care routine and home facial. But on greasy skins they will keep recurring around the nose, chin, forehead and cheeks. Soften the

SKIN WITH ACNE

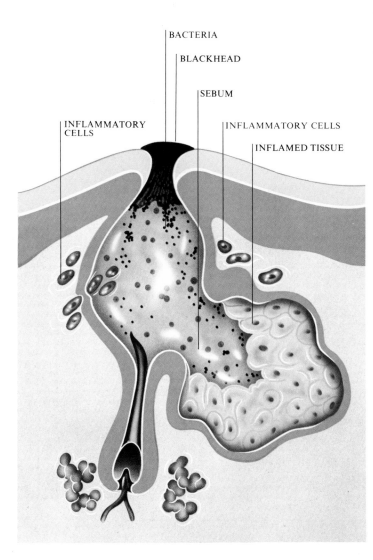

BACTERIA

BLACKHEAD

SEBUM

INFLAMMATORY CELLS

INFLAMMATORY CELLS

INFLAMED TISSUE

Pilo-sebaceous unit of acne patient. Build-up of keratinous debris in the duct hinders excretion of sebum from enlarged sebaceous gland.

area of the blackheads by warming with a sterile flannel wrung out in hot water, then squeeze each blackhead very gently between finger tips covered with clean tissues. Do not tackle any but the obvious blackheads as too much squeezing may damage the skin or cause a spot to form. When you have removed the blackheads, dab the area with astringent or surgical spirit to close the pores.

Crepey skin
This is simply caused by ageing. The skin loses its elasticity and resilience, begins to look loose and is marked with tiny criss-cross lines. Crepey skin shows first on the eyelids and on the neck. It can sometimes arrive prematurely, caused by crash diets or neglect of the skin. Be sure that your skin is cared for, that you are using your moisturizer, skin food or eye cream regularly. A blitz treatment of moisturizing, toning and stimulating by a beauty therapist may help.

Dark rings or bags under eyes
Bags and dark rings under the eyes may be caused by lack of sleep, bad diet or illness, or they may simply be a problem you have inherited. In this case there is very little you can do about them except disguise them with make-up or in the case of bags under the eyes, or drooping eyelids, have them removed by plastic surgery. This is usually a most successful operation (see page 208). The eyes heal quite quickly – it should take a month before you look absolutely normal again, but with dark glasses to disguise bruising and stitches, the patient can generally be out and about in a few days.

Freckles
Happily, we no longer consider freckles unattractive as the Victorians did, in fact quite the opposite. Freckles can be bleached with special creams, but since they will always reappear in sunlight, there is not much point. Keep out of the sun if you wish to keep your freckles to a minimum and prevent them running together. Otherwise, simply be glad that they usually go with striking colouring and are often the envy of others.

Puffy eyes
Puffy eyes may be caused by lack of sleep or high living, but they may be hereditary, too. Sometimes they are caused by putting on too much or too heavy an eye cream at night. If your eyes have become puffy since using an eye cream, change to a much lighter variety, use much less or give it up altogether. Splash the eyes several times with cold water in the mornings to reduce the swelling and puffiness.

In old age, when the skin loses its elasticity, puffy eyes may develop into drooping lids. These can be successfully treated, as for bags under the eyes. Always be very careful when applying or removing cream or make-up from the eye area: the skin is very delicate and it is important not to drag or stretch it.

Sallow skin
Your skin tone – sallow, fair or whatever it may be – is inherited, and there is little that you can do to change it. But you can help to change its appearance by stimulating the circulation and helping the skin to shed dead cells more quickly. Do this by concentrating on your nightly massage and toning treatment, and by using a complexion brush and, perhaps, an exfoliating cream occasionally (or an oatmeal scrub as described on page 139). A face mask to suit your skin type would also be useful. Any or all of these treatments would be equally suitable if your face is simply going through a temporary post-winter sallow phase.

Beauty treatments done by a therapist using an electrical massage machine to stimulate the skin may also be helpful, and make-up can help tremendously to 'lift' a sallow skin, especially the use of blusher.

Spots
Many women are prone to spots just before they menstruate, because the level of the hormone oestrogen is low in the body at that time. These are usually quite short-lived, and there is not much to be done about them. There are many antiseptic or drying lotions on the market that can be dabbed on to hasten the drying-up and disappearance of a spot, and some women use surgical spirit, applied repeatedly with a cotton bud. It is really most sensible not to squeeze spots – you can make them much worse or even spread them. Better to buy a cosmetic stick that hides blemishes of this kind. Some women get spots if they eat too rich a diet: chocolates, for instance, often make you spotty. Stick to a healthy diet, lots of water to drink, lots of fresh air and exercise and sleep. Any one spot which gives persistent trouble and lasts an abnormally long time must be shown to a doctor: it is possible that it could be a rodent ulcer* which must be caught and removed early before it spreads.

Whiteheads
These form when oil gets trapped in a 'blind' skin duct. Having no way to escape, the oil sits under the surface of the skin; it looks like a tiny white bead. Massage sometimes helps to disperse newly-formed whiteheads, but a persistent one has to be treated in the following way. A sterilized needle should be used to pierce gently the top of the whitehead, which can then be squeezed out through the opening you have made. Dab disinfectant or surgical spirit on to the area afterwards. For information about other skin problems, see page 219.

YOUR BODY
Whether out of guilt, thrift or laziness, a good many women seem to operate on the principle that what the eyes don't see the heart won't grieve over – in other words, they will spend time caring for their faces but neglect their bodies altogether.

Bodies show age just as quickly as faces and, like faces, they respond well to regular care. And if you need more persuading, just remember that there may come a time when the tired, slack skin on your body will give your age away however well cared for and lifted your face may be – and by that time it will be too late to do much about it. Care of the body, like care of the face, is based on a regular routine which can be as simple as this: a good diet (see page 38) and regular exercise (see page 55). With the basics right you just have to bath regularly with a few drops of bath oil or vegetable oil in the water. Regularly scrub your thighs, upper arms, chest and back with a bath mitt, brush or loofah. Regularly go over the horny parts of your skin – elbows, feet, fingers, knees – with the pumice stone. After the bath, rub a little body lotion into these same horny parts. But to get the most out of your bath, see page 125.

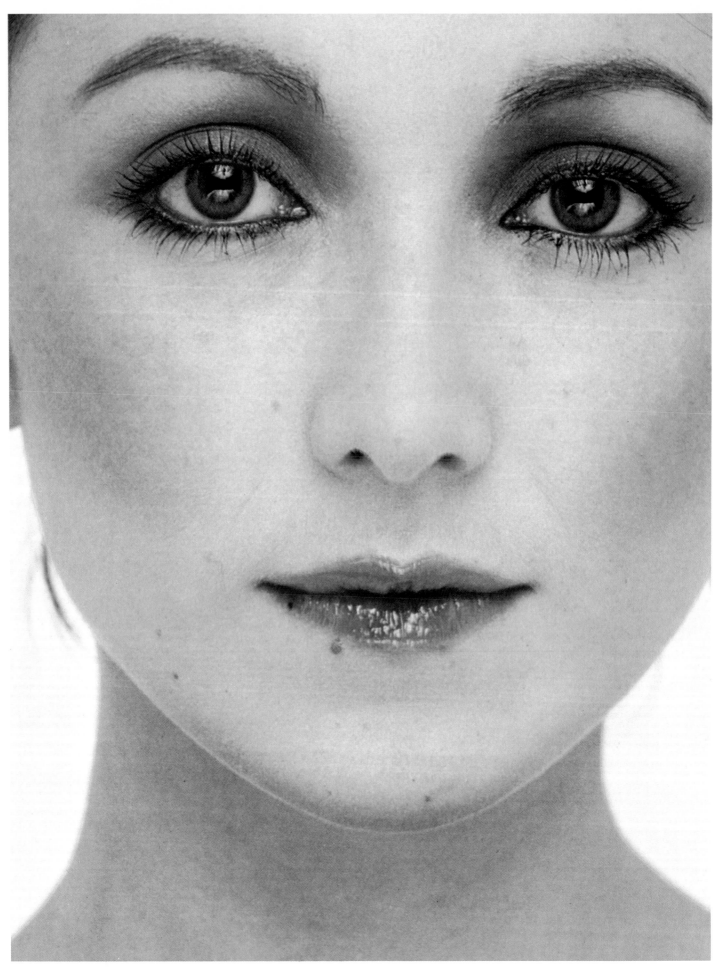

Make-up

In the days, not so very long ago, when a woman's face was her fortune, a great many of us would have found ourselves verging on the edge of bankruptcy. For a woman born with a plain face a hundred years ago had no way out of the cruel trap set for her by nature. Sometimes, one wonders if our sophisticated cosmetics are not one of the great gifts of science to women born in the twentieth century.

We are lucky enough these days to have a vast range of safe, subtle and effective products at our disposal. What most of us lack is know-how when it comes to choosing and using them. This chapter will steer you through the maze of bottles and jars and colours and tell you how to pick among them, how to assess your features and make cosmetics work to your advantage. This is not to

suggest that we should all be hiding behind thick masks of make-up pretending to be something other than we are. Rather the opposite. The great value of modern cosmetics is that a little goes a long way. It is the fashion today to wear much less make-up than we did ten years ago. Some women now despise cosmetics altogether, believing it wrong that we should be brainwashed into disguising our natural faces in order to make ourselves attractive or to conform to society's standards of beauty. Why should we when men don't, they argue quite reasonably.

The fact is that a touch of blusher, a brushful of mascara or a gloss of lipstick can bring a face alive, sharpening its personality and originality, and bringing confidence and reassurance to those who feel plain or plain ugly.

If make-up can be a crutch, it can also be a trap. Women often get 'set' at what they consider was their most attractive period. As their looks were clearly a success at that time, they lack the confidence to change them and the make-up or hairstyle that was once thought pretty becomes outdated and unsuitable. If you wear make-up, it is important to keep in touch with fashion.

Of course, it takes courage to start wearing a bright red lipstick when you have worn a pale one for years, and husbands and friends don't usually help much. However, before you can use cosmetics effectively you must know yourself and what you are aiming for. The way to do this is to look at your unmade-up face completely objectively, as though it were a drawing you were going to colour in. Try to visualize, rather as a painter would. where colour, shadow, highlighter or pencil emphasis would help. Would it be more flattering to put heavier make-up under the eye rather than above; should you be trying to make your eyes longer rather than rounder; would your blusher do more if it were placed higher, or lower; should you extend the line of your eyebrows, or use a redder lipstick? Another way is simply to decide which are your best features and concentrate on emphasizing those. Faults can also be worked on and turned to your advantage, giving your face originality and expression, though it takes a certain amount of experimenting, a bit of courage and a lot of style to play up an ugly feature successfully.

Juliette Greco emphasized her sallow looks by powdering her face white and using no other make-up except black around her eyes; Jenny Gaylor, a model with a long face and wide mouth, exaggerated these looks by using a shiny red lipstick. Study your face and try to develop a look which is all your own.

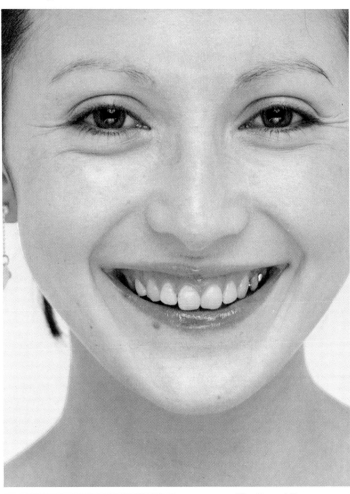

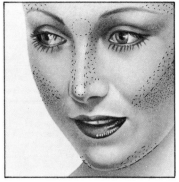

The Round Face
This is often a little plump around cheeks and jaw, hiding underlying bone structure. Shape by shading, one tone deeper than foundation, in a triangle under cheek-bones and either side of chin. Use blusher on cheek-bones and forehead from eyebrow out to hair line. Put dark colour on eyes taking shadow in towards nose, with highlighter on centre of lid. Shade nose either side with highlighter on bridge and tip. Keep lips pale and narrow. Completed make-up opposite.

SHAPING YOUR FACE

Apart from plastic surgery, there is nothing you can do to alter the basic shape and structure of your face or features. However, it is possible to fake good bones by shadowing and highlighting the face, but it *must* be done subtly or not at all. Walking around with a jaw shaded dark brown and a white streak down the centre of your nose is not going to fool anyone. The way you make up your eyes, where you put blusher, shader and highlighter, and even the colour of your lipstick are all simple ways of coping with facial faults. Barbra Streisand turns an aquiline Jewish nose into an asset by using dramatic eye make-up, while model Margaux Hemingway balances her strong jaw line by keeping her eyebrows dark and heavy.

On this and the following pages you will find descriptions of various face shapes and advice on make-up to emphasize the good points and disguise the bad. Do not feel that you have to follow the shading for your face shape religiously, but use it to achieve a better understanding of your face. Attractive faces come in all sorts of shapes, sizes and ages, most of them a long way from the classic oval which is supposed to be the perfect face shape. The first lesson is to learn to make the best of what you have, however imperfect it may seem to you. Small eyes can be made to twinkle like stars, a fat face can look charming, and a huge mouth can grin infectiously. Beauty is not just bone structure and skin, it is very much a question of vitality and expression as well. If only everyone could leaf through the books of photographic models that agencies send to likely clients, they would be immensely encouraged to see the extraordinary variety of faces that are considered attractive enough to earn their owners a good living.

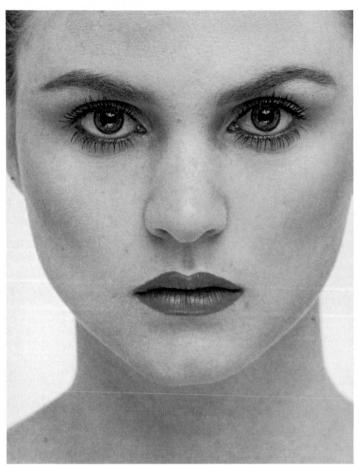

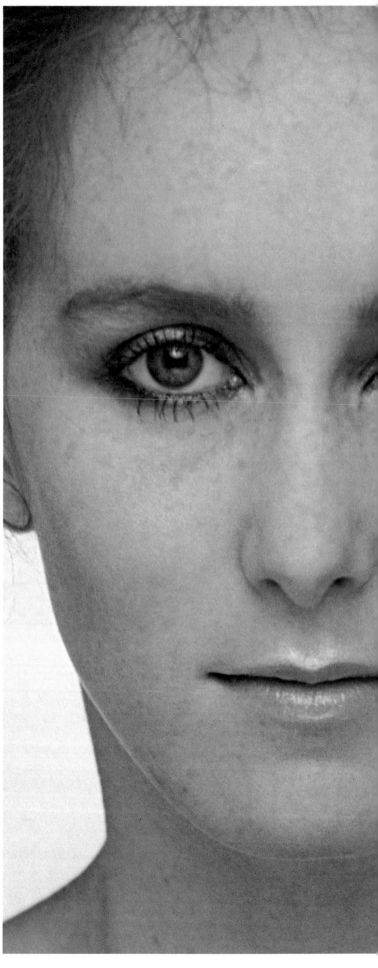

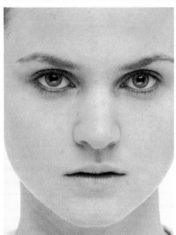

upwards to emphasize line. With a bright lipstick make top lip slightly pointed. This, with the light blusher, will help to make the chin appear more pointed. It is important that your make-up has no horizontal lines. All shaping and shading must lift to outer edges of face to give the illusion of lifting the jaw line. Because a square face can look rather heavy, make-up must be particularly well done. Although the lipstick and shadow used are dark in tone, the final effect of the whole make-up must be delicate, not harsh.

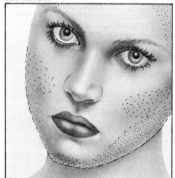

The Square Face
This face has wide cheek-bones and a strong, wide jaw line. Use shader, one tone darker than foundation, under cheek-bones, out to hair line and down to and under points of jaw. What you are trying to do is to soften the square edges and make your face appear longer and thinner. Shader blended from above temples to outer corners of forehead helps to narrow top of face. A light blusher on cheek-bones and chin will lift them. Use a dark eyeshadow under eye and on lid from inner point of eyebrow to outer edge, sweeping slightly upwards to outer line of brow. Blend highlighter under centre of brow to outer edge. Tidy under outer corner of eyebrow and brush

148

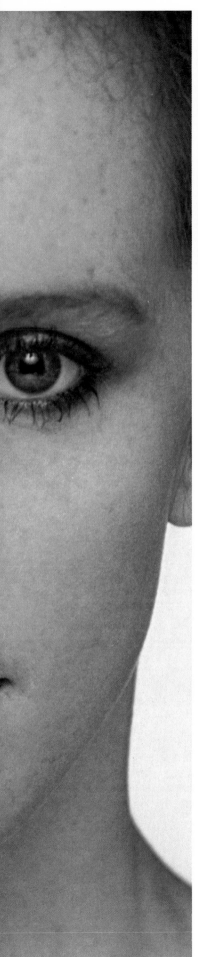

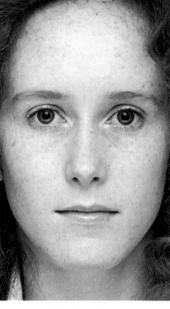

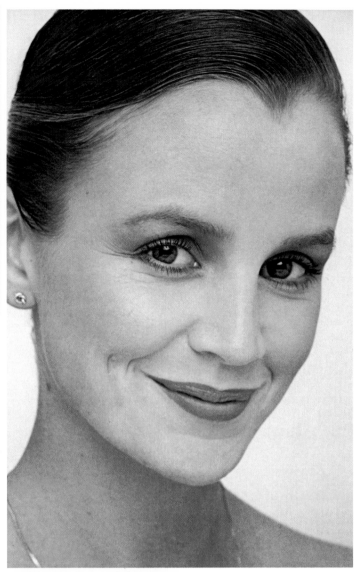

The Long Face

Very often, this is not an extra-ordinarily long face but one which appears long in proportion because it is thin and narrow. The object, therefore, is to round out the contours of the face and create width with blushers, highlighter and horizontal lines. A warm blusher above eyebrows, blended up to hair line, and on and under point of chin helps to reduce length. To achieve width across eyes, use a pale, silvery shadow along whole width of eyelid, blended to outer corner of brow, and mark socket line with softly smudged pencil. Under brow, blend highlighter out to full width. Use a pale eyeliner under eye from inner corner to middle and carefully blend with a softly smudged pencil under lower lashes, taken out to a slightly extended line which also helps to create the illusion of width. Use highlighter on and under cheek-bones and add blusher slightly lower on cheeks, blended across width of cheeks but not out to hair line. This will widen face across centre. Lips will also give width if you wear pale lipstick taken out to corners of mouth, with highlighter along line of top lip to emphasize the horizontal line.

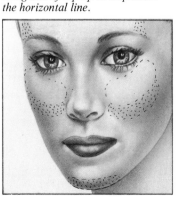

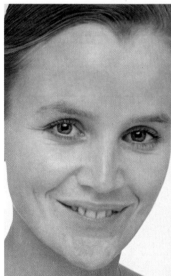

line with softly smudged brown pencil. Fill in area above socket line, from inner corner of eye to outer edge of brow, with a pretty pearly-pink eyeshadow. Use a clear blue kohl pencil along edge of eye above lower lashes to widen eyes and emphasize the colour and sharpen with the finest line of softly smudged pencil under lashes. Blend blusher on cheeks almost to hair line to emphasize face shape and give lips their full curve with rich, deep pink lipstick.

The Oval Face

This is generally considered to be the perfect face shape. All that the lucky owner has to do is to use make-up to emphasize the lovely bone structure; certainly no correction is needed. Use bronze shadow on eyelid and mark socket

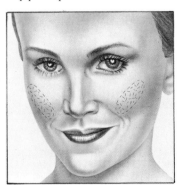

149

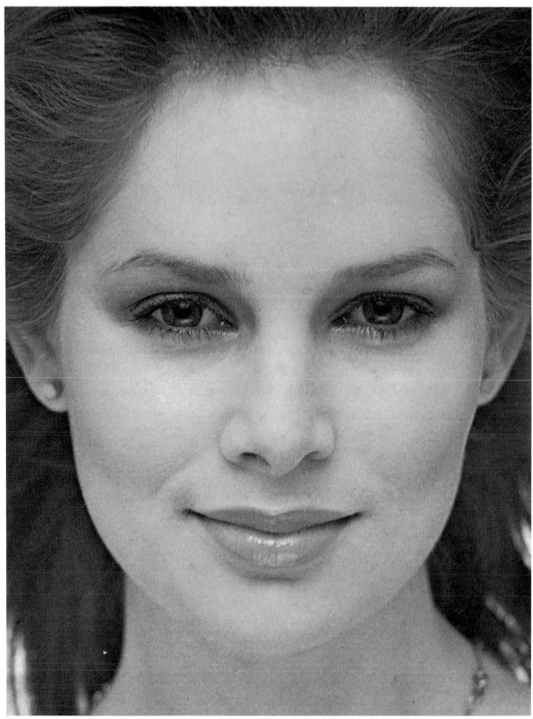

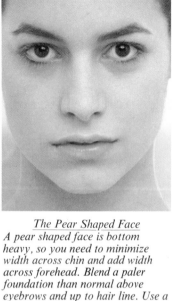

The Pear Shaped Face

A pear shaped face is bottom heavy, so you need to minimize width across chin and add width across forehead. Blend a paler foundation than normal above eyebrows and up to hair line. Use a lightish blusher on cheek-bones but do not take colour out as far as hair line, as this will have the effect of narrowing your face at the top. From under cheek-bones, blended down in a triangle shape to points of jaw, use a shader one tone darker than foundation. Lips should also be dark to minimize width across lower half of face. Eyes are strong and dramatic with dark shadow, but use lots of goldy highlighter, lifting up and out to eyebrow to increase width across brow line. Use a grey kohl pencil above lashes from middle of eyelid to outer corner and under bottom lashes along full width of eye.

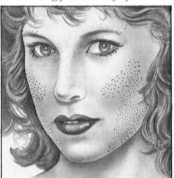

The Heart Shaped Face

This face is disproportionately wide across the top for the narrow, pointed chin. Make-up helps to redress the balance. Use blusher on cheek-bones and shader one tone darker than foundation, blended out to hair line, to pull in cheeks and give your face more shape at its widest point. Use goldy eye-shadow on lid, with smoky blue from inner corner up to brow and from under eye to outer corner of brow. Add highlighter under centre of brow and a line of blue-grey kohl under lower lashes, following upward line at outer corner. This helps to reduce width by bringing attention towards centre of face. Put a little blusher on chin, blend in highlighter on each side, and make mouth generously curved in a warm-toned, pale lipstick to round out chin and give width to lower part of face.

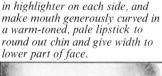

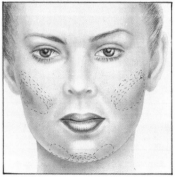

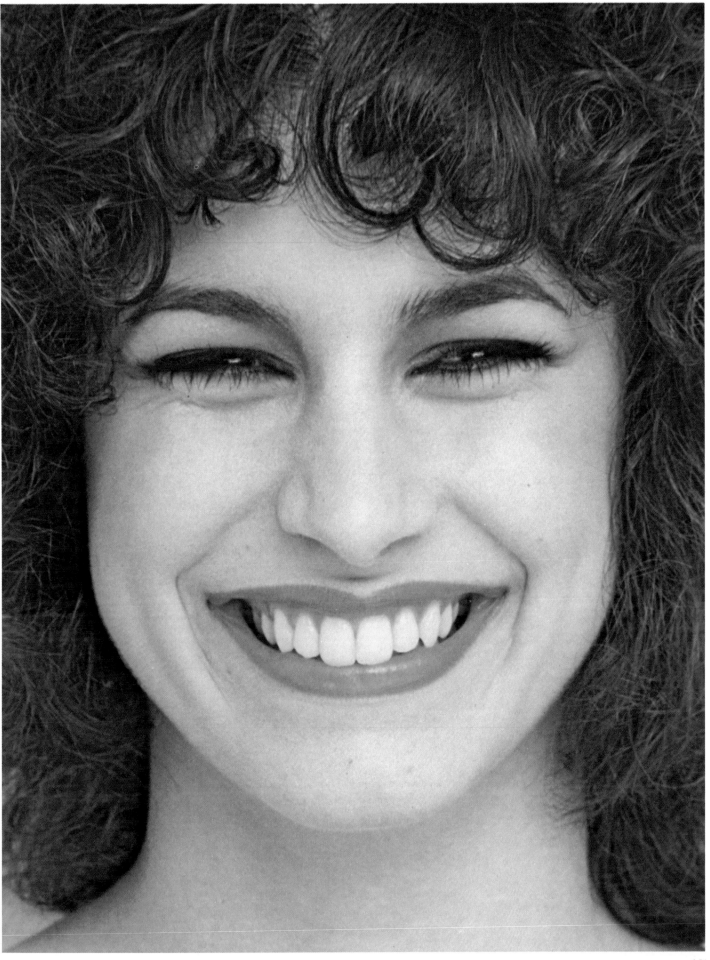

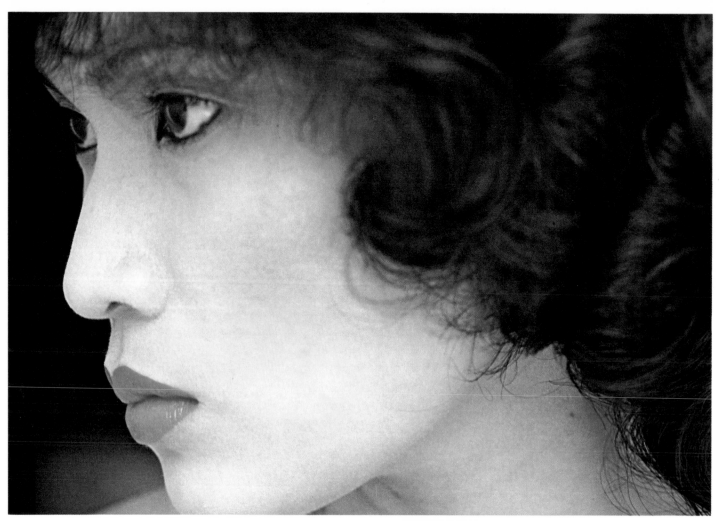

The basic composition of all skins is the same. We have an equal number of melanocyte cells, producing melanin pigment, which forms the skin's natural protection against the ultra-violet rays of the sun. The variations in skin tone are caused by the strength of the sun, which activates the cells to produce more or less melanin, and by genetic differences which also control the productivity of the melanocytes. However, whatever colour the skin, the same basic rules apply. You should choose your foundation to match your actual skin tone as exactly as possible. Anything lighter or darker will show as a mask with an unattractive ring around the jaw line, unless extreme care is taken to blend the foundation away perfectly. If the skin is in good condition, a tinted moisturizer is preferable for a more natural look. Colour and shape should be added in the form of blushers, shaders and high-lighters. A light dusting of translucent powder will eliminate shine without altering tone.

A creamy Mongolian skin can look a little flat and lifeless, but this can be played to dramatic advantage by going for a mono-chromatic look using masses of black kohl to outline the eye and

several layers of mascara, very well brushed through, to give a thick, velvety fringe of lashes. Highlighter can be applied high on cheek-bones, with shader just underneath on a neutral foundation base. The alternative is to use the creamy skin tone as background and add vivid pastel (see above) – a stunningly unusual effect.

Darker skins often have pale patches where there is a pigment deficiency. Special toning cover sticks are available and a foundation which exactly matches the skin will give a smooth finish. Each skin has its own peculiarities, but dark skins are often a little oily so it is advisable not to wear foundation unless absolutely necessary. Use a powder to blot shine on nose, chin and forehead only. Tinted moisturizer is the best foundation for this sort of skin if it is in good condition. Particular care should be taken to follow the advice for greasy skins on page 138, especially for negroid skins which are very delicate and scar easily if abused by over-zealous treatment of spots. A bonus of this sort of skin, however, is that it ages and wrinkles far slower than any other. Use blushers to give warmth to cheeks, and eye and lip colours can be as bright as you like.

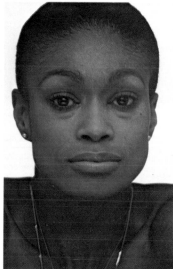

Above: Tinted moisturizer is used as base, with blusher to give colour on cheeks. Blue-violet eyeshadow is blended over whole of lid, up to inner point of brow and around inner corner of eye, to narrow bridge of nose. Pearly pink high-lighter under outer corner of brow also helps to push eye towards nose. Blue kohl along eye above lower lashes and shadow under lashes widen eyes and emphasize depth of colour. Mouth is vivid with clear red lipstick and gloss on lower lip.

Above: Flower-tinted make-up gives colour to rather flat skin tones. Creamy foundation base has lots of pink blusher under cheek-bones, blended up towards eye and out to hair line. Pearl highlighter on cheek-bones emphasizes high slanting lines. Leaving lid uncoloured, violet shadow circles eye in an echoing almond shape, filling to brow at inner corner. Highlighter under arch of brow lifts outer corner of eye. Black kohl rings eye inside lashes, lifting at outer corner and dipping towards nose to tilt eye even more. Lips are carefully outlined to give full shape and brilliantly coloured with petunia pink.
Right: Foundation matches skin tone to give smooth base, with warm pink blusher on cheeks lifting up to outer corner of eye. Translucent powder is used to blot away shine on nose, chin and forehead without changing foundation colour. Eyes are well shaped so make-up is to emphasize, not correct. Deeper-toned brown shadow is used around socket of eye and in towards bridge of nose. Lavender shadow on lid is taken finely round under eye to circle it with colour, with pink highlighter on centre of lid and highlighter under brow. Bright red lips are filled in to natural curve and well glossed.

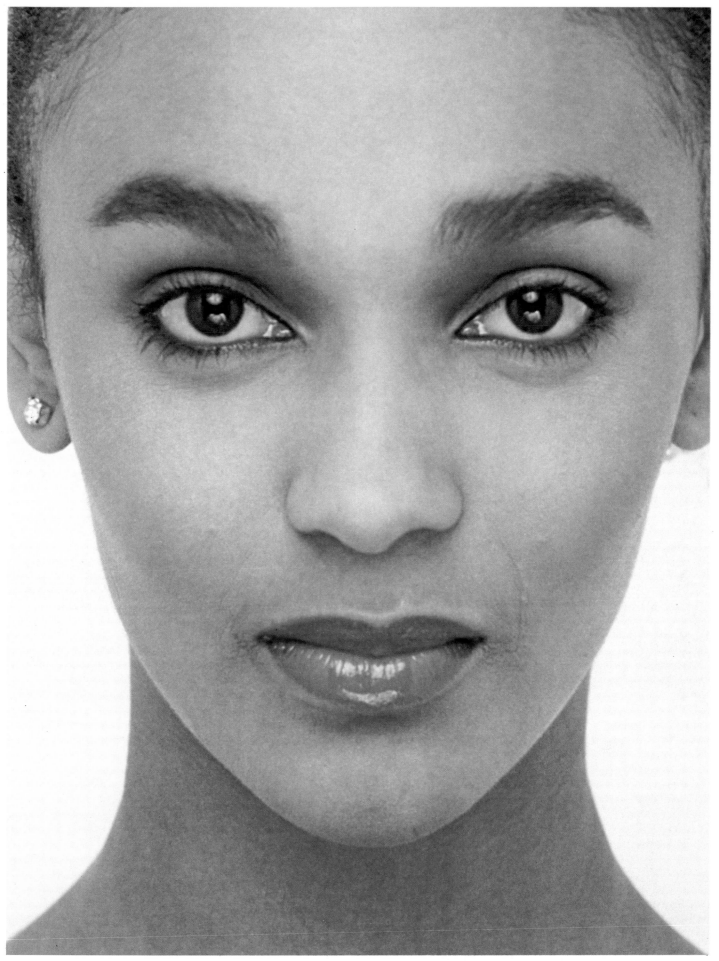

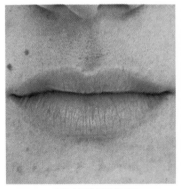

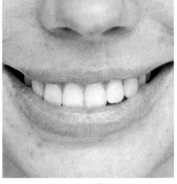

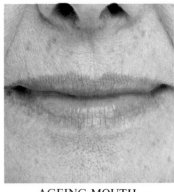

| FLAT MOUTH | THIN LIPS | WIDE MOUTH | AGEING MOUTH |

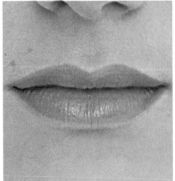

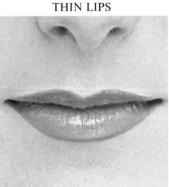

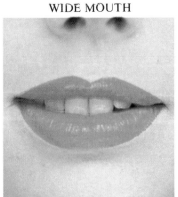

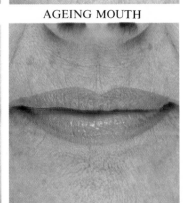

FACIAL FAULTS

The infinite variety of shape, size and position of features is what gives each face its unique identity. Heaven forbid that we should all correct, change and disguise our looks to meet some socially accepted idea of what is averagely beautiful! An unusual feature can give a face great strength and individuality or it can spoil facial balance. Wide apart eyes can have a touching naivety and a generously wide mouth great humour, but very close together eyes or a down-turned mouth can make a face appear misleadingly bad-tempered or sulky, to the great distress of the owner of the feature. What we are suggesting here is *not* that everyone should take to cosmetic camouflage, but that the following few pages – which show how to use make-up to correct problem eyes and lips – should be used to help you to handle your features with more confidence.

Study your face carefully. If you have features which worry you, look to see if they match up with any of those treated here and try the suggested make-up in good light and when you have plenty of time to spare. The particular colouring may not suit you, as it has been chosen for the actual features photographed, but the tonal quality is important. The make-up corrections are based on simple principles of optical illusion. Light tones enlarge areas, highlight them or bring them closer; darker tones make areas smaller, push them back or take the eye in the direction of the

colour used; dark shadow against light will have the effect of pushing the lighter area forwards. It is important to blend tones and lines softly where they meet, so that eye make-up in particular has no hard lines. Lips will usually show a prettier shape with a clear line on the top lip, although the bottom lip should be softer. Remember also that the way you tidy or brush your eyebrows can help the shape of your eyes. A heavy downward droop of the brow will push the line of your eye down, while brushing up the outer corner of the brow, not plucking it away, will help to lift a sleepy-looking eye. Mascara applied more thickly to outer lashes and brushed outwards will help to elongate the eye and to pull it away from the bridge of the nose. Try different techniques and products to see whether you get better results from eyeshadow and sponge or brush or eyeshadow stick, liquid eyeliner or soft eye pencil, lip brushes or lip pencils. Whatever you choose, keep pencils well sharpened and brushes clean.

Use the make-up suggestions on the following pages as a basis for experiment rather than as absolute rules. The proportions of every face are different and the individual balance of the features within the face shape is what really matters. If you have a problem feature and the make-up suggested makes you look better and feel more confident, incorporate it into your regular make-up routine. If the make-up feels wrong or unnatural on you,

try to simplify or modify it so that you feel more comfortable. On the other hand, if you are perfectly happy with your wayward feature, you might try using the reverse of the corrective make-up to exaggerate your looks and bring drama or humour to your face. Many people have done this very successfully, although it needs a lot of practice and a great deal of confidence to carry it off well. The important thing is to feel relaxed with your make-up and happy inside your face.

CORRECTING LIPS

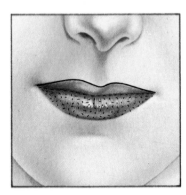

Flat Mouth
Lips may have a well-defined curve but are flat and lacking the soft, rounded shape which is so attractive. Darker lipstick is used at outer corners of mouth to push lips forwards. A paler tone is used towards middle of lips with highlighter at centre top and bottom to make them appear a little plumper.

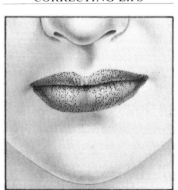

Thin Lips
Very narrow lips deprive a mouth of expression so curves need rounding out. Outline lips very softly with lip pencil just outside natural line, then smudge line so that it almost melts away. Fill in with a paler lipstick on top lip than the one used on lower lip, although neither should be too deep in tone. Be sure that lipstick covers lip line so that there are no hard edges.

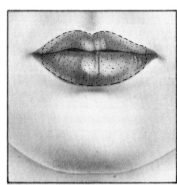

Wide Mouth
A big mouth can be attractive if lips are prettily shaped. Take

154

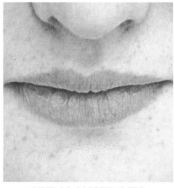

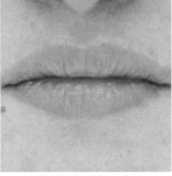

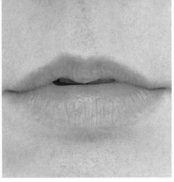

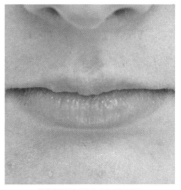

UNBALANCED LIPS DROOPING MOUTH UNEVEN LIPS BUTTON MOUTH

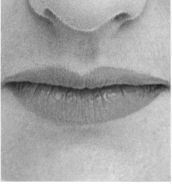

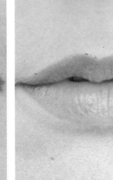

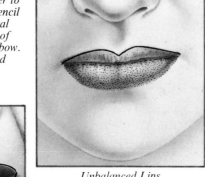

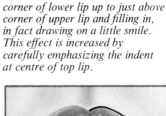

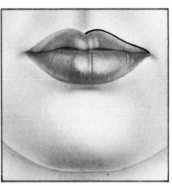

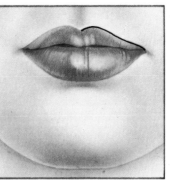

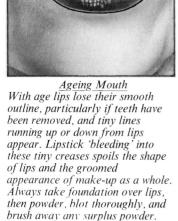

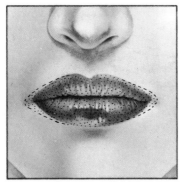

foundation over lips and powder to cover natural lines. With lip pencil draw in shape just inside natural line, stopping short of corners of mouth, making a neat cupid's bow. Always fill in with a dark-toned lipstick, which will reduce prominence of lips.

Ageing Mouth
With age lips lose their smooth outline, particularly if teeth have been removed, and tiny lines running up or down from lips appear. Lipstick 'bleeding' into these tiny creases spoils the shape of lips and the groomed appearance of make-up as a whole. Always take foundation over lips, then powder, blot thoroughly, and brush away any surplus powder. Carefully outline lips with dry-textured lip pencil, as it is important to avoid anything which might make lips greasy. With a tissue, soften lower edge of bottom lip, as a hard line here is very ageing. Fill in lips with medium-toned lipstick and blot. If gloss is used, it should be only in centre of bottom lip.

Unbalanced Lips
This is when one lip is thinner than the other. If top lip is too thin, extend lighter-toned lipstick outside natural line of lip and fill in lower lip with a darker tone to reduce thickness. If bottom lip is too thin, extend pale lipstick over natural line of lower lip and fill in top lip with darker tone.

Drooping Mouth
This gives a sad, downturned expression to the face, but it can easily be made more cheerful by taking a line with a lip pencil from

corner of lower lip up to just above corner of upper lip and filling in, in fact drawing on a little smile. This effect is increased by carefully emphasizing the indent at centre of top lip.

Uneven Lips
Sometimes one side of the lips does not match the other. This is particularly noticeable if it is the top lip. Use a lip pencil to outline top lip, rectifying the shape, then smudge line carefully to take away hard edge. Fill in new shape with medium-toned lipstick.

Button Mouth
This is usually neatly shaped but because it is small it can look a little mean or bad-tempered, so it needs to be given a rather more generous size. This can be done by extending natural line sideways just beyond natural corner of mouth. Take care not to increase height of mouth. If lips are not too thick you can afford to flatten out cupid's bow a little to increase horizontal effect and thus make mouth appear wider.

Sensitive Lips
It is impossible to achieve a smooth, glossy finish to lip make-up if lips are chapped, cracked or peeling.
   The skin of the lips is very sensitive and can react painfully to adverse weather conditions, both cold and hot. To protect lips, always use a moisturizer under your lipstick. A little petroleum jelly smoothed on to your finished lips will do a double job, giving glossy finish and effective protection. In hot sun, a special barrier cream is often necessary.
   If your lips are well protected but still crack, you may be allergic to your lipstick. Try switching to a different brand, preferably a hypo-allergenic* one with perfume and other known irritants screened out. If this does not help, see your doctor; the allergy may be caused by something quite different. An allergy to nail polish can cause a reaction on the lips if you touch your mouth frequently. If you find that your lipstick changes colour on your lips, try using the special barrier cream under your lipstick.

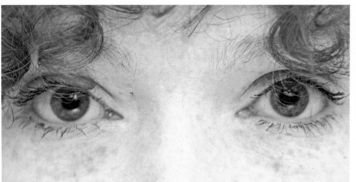
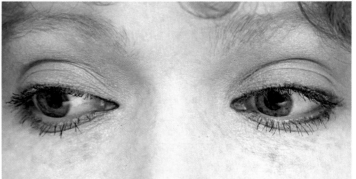

WIDE APART EYES

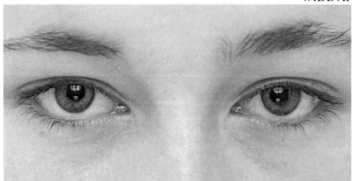
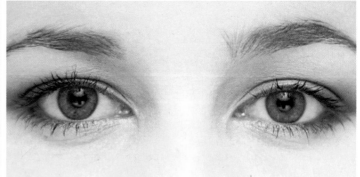

CLOSE TOGETHER EYES

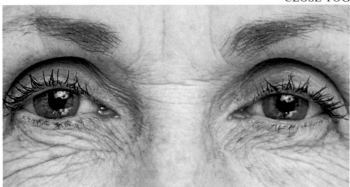
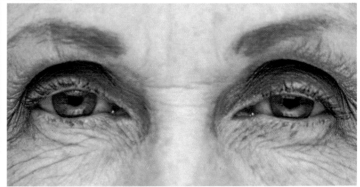

AGEING EYES

CORRECTING EYES

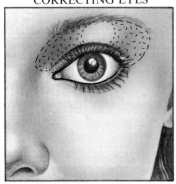

Wide Apart Eyes
Eyes set too wide apart flatten bridge of nose and take attention away from centre of face. Eyes can be drawn closer together by using deep-toned eyeshadow on lid and round inner corner of eye, with medium-toned shadow filling area between lid and brow, around eye towards bridge of nose and out to full width of brow. Highlighter in middle of upper lid keeps interest

in centre of eye. Bright kohl along eye above lower lashes and into inner corner pulls eye in towards nose. Softly smudged pencil above upper lashes from middle of lid to outer corner also helps to push eye in towards centre of face.

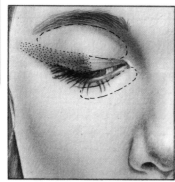

Close Together Eyes
Very pale eyeshadow under inner corner of eye and filling whole area between lid and brow helps

to lift eyes away from bridge of nose. Darker shadow from middle of lid, blended to outer corner of eyebrow, also helps to draw attention outwards and widens overall effect.

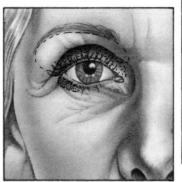

Ageing Eyes
Light-toned eyeshadow all round upper area of eye, above lid from inner corner of eye to full width of brow, opens and lifts eye. A deeper-toned shadow on lid with

highlighter in centre gives eyes more emphasis and sparkle. No hard lines must ever be used round the older eye and mascara should be light and well brushed through.

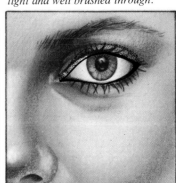

Protruding Eyes
Plenty of dark eyeliner around eye, inside lashes, reduces white of eyeball and thus diminishes bulging effect. Medium-toned shadow blended diagonally across lid from inner corner of eye, cutting across lid to outer corner,

156

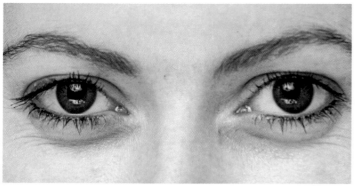 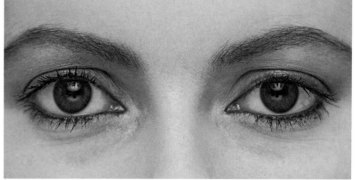

PROTRUDING EYES

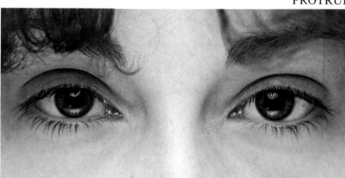 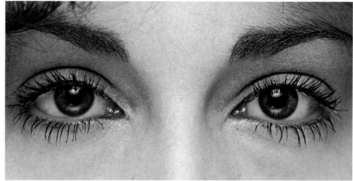

ELONGATED EYES

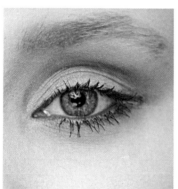 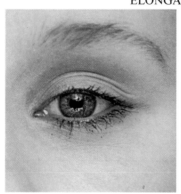 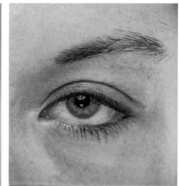 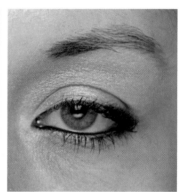

SMALL EYES   SLEEPY EYES

takes line outwards and disguises roundness and fullness.

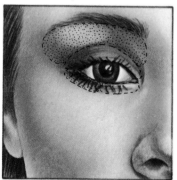

Small Eyes
Eyeshadow that gives an impression of lightness is used on lid and under inner corner of eye to enlarge eye and lift away from shadow of bridge of nose. No dark lines should be used around small eyes, but a line of pale kohl along eye above lower lashes helps to open and widen them. Deeper-toned shadow from slightly

above natural socket line blended up and out to full width of brow and just under outer corner of eye, emphasized with a little softly smudged pencil above outer corner, helps to bring eye forwards and give it more impact.

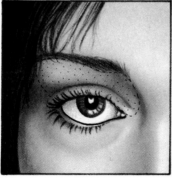

Elongated Eyes
No disguise is needed on these dramatically long and rather slanting eyes. Colour is used to emphasize their lovely line.

Pinky-beige shadow fills whole area above eye from inner corner along whole width of brow. A line of bright kohl along eye above lower lashes increases length. Drawing the kohl line down into inner corner of eye gives more emphasis to the slanting line.

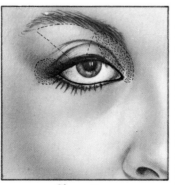

Sleepy Eyes
A light-toned shadow on centre of lid, blended up to brow line, helps to open up eye and deeper shade

round bridge of nose and at outer corner of eye reduces weight of upper lid and draws attention out. A line of black kohl along eye above lower lashes reduces droop of lower lid and kohl above outer corner of upper lashes, softly smudged up and out, also helps to lift eye.

Eyelashes
Lashes play an essential part in eye make-up. Straight lashes which do not show can be improved by using eyelash curlers. Sparse lashes can be augmented by properly applied false ones. Thick curtains of lashes are now usually confined to photography, but fine ones blend naturally with your own if trimmed and curled to match. Cover the fixing strip with eyeliner. Small strips of lashes can help corrective make-up: in the centre of your lashes they open eye wider; at the outer edge they elongate eye. Semi-permanent lashes applied individually look natural but don't usually last as long as supposed.

157

FACING YOUR FACE

The object of make-up is to make the very best of the face you were born with, not to change the way you look to become a poor copy of someone else. Your make-up should be as simple and natural as possible, so that you can relax and forget it and not have to do running repairs every few minutes.

The first thing to do is get to know your face, warts and all. You don't have to broadcast your imperfections to the world, but do be honest with yourself. Tie your hair back, remove every trace of make-up and look long and hard at your face in a good mirror in daylight. Study your face shape to see if the hints on pages 147–51 help you. Individual features could perhaps be improved with the corrective make-up on pages 154–57. Decide which are your best features and think how you can emphasize them. Armed with a good dose of honesty, you can then set aside some time to experiment with your make-up until you arrive at a formula which feels completely, comfortably, naturally *you*, which you can do quickly and efficiently as a daily routine. Remember that if your make-up is too complicated it will be skimped in the morning dash. Better to have a simplified version which you can do immaculately and leave the more elaborate ideas for parties or special occasions.

CHOOSING AND USING MAKE-UP

The enormous range of make-up products on the market can be fun to try and flattering to wear, or a terrible waste of money and a real source of anxiety. There is just so much choice, so many different types of make-up and methods of application, it is little wonder that many women simply don't know where to begin. Older women who started wearing make-up when cosmetics were less sophisticated often lack the courage to learn new techniques, preferring to keep to the routine they know. It is important to change your look from time to time, because nothing is more ageing than out-of-date make-up. Make-up which may have looked stunning when you first started wearing it can look positively grotesque a decade later. Fashions change, as do skin texture and face shape. Make-up needs to change accordingly.

Every face is completely individual, with unique planes, contours and creases, and your make-up should be similarly individual. Some people always wear powder, others never do; some use make-up pencils for all their make-up, others have a whole range of different gels. The important thing is to experiment until you find the type of make-up

which suits you, which gives the degree of colour and skin coverage you want, which doesn't clog your pores or need constant retouching. Remember that young skins are often greasy and afflicted with spots and need grease-free make-up. Older skins, lacking oestrogen,* can be dry and need to be kept supple with make-up which contains moisture and oil.

As faces and skins vary, so do our skills. Some nimble-fingered women can achieve marvellous results with paint brushes, others more fumble-fingered find different sized sponges easier to handle. Pencils can be simple and effective to use, as can a skilfully-wielded finger tip. The method of make-up application you adopt should be the one you find suits your skill and gives you the best results. Below is a list of the sort of products your make-up kit should contain and a few hints on choosing and using them.

Skin-care products
These are dealt with in detail earlier in the book (page 138), where you will find guidance on choosing the right products to suit your skin type.

Cleanser. Cream, lotion, rinsable cleanser, quick-cleaning pads for eyes or midday cleansing.

Toner. Astringent, toning lotion or skin freshener.

Moisturizer. Probably the most important item in your make-up drawer. Always put your make-up on over moisturizer; it will go on more smoothly, last longer and hold colour better.

Skin food Skin foods can contain any number of special ingredients, such as hormones,* vitamins or collagen. There is no proof that these do any more good than simpler skin foods, but the choice is yours; use them if they suit your skin, or try one of the skin food recipes on page 218, which will be far cheaper and probably just as good.

Foundation
Use the very lightest foundation you can get away with, disguising individual blemishes or broken veins* with a light covering stick. Choose a foundation exactly the same tone as your skin, neither pinker nor darker; put colour in afterwards with blusher and shader. When buying foundation, test on your face in daylight, not on your wrist under artificial light. Foundation may be in cream or lotion form and either matt or glossy. If it is liquid, always shake well before using. When applying foundation, put a little into the palm of your hand and blend with finger tips. It will be easier to judge how much you are using and it will go on much more smoothly. If you like a natural look, tinted moisturizer may be all you need.

Covering stick. Tinted to

blend with your skin to cover blemishes or dark rings under eyes; use lightly, taking care not to drag delicate skin around eyes.

Blusher, highlighter and shader
Use blusher to give your face colour, highlighter and shader – which should be one tone darker than foundation - to improve contours. Always put these cosmetics on in a good light to be sure you haven't been too heavy handed; they should be applied very subtly. You can buy powder, cream or glossy gel blushers. The cream version is usually used under powder; the powder, or pressed powder type, over powder; and the glosses should be left unpowdered for a natural sheen.

Powder
Wear as little as possible, always dusting off surplus thoroughly. Try using powder just on chin, nose and forehead to stop shine.

Loose powder. Either translucent for a very natural look or tinted, which should be one shade lighter than foundation.

Pressed powder. It is useful if used minimally to touch up make-up during the day, but not generally very effective as a regular powder as it tends to cake and clog pores.

Lipstick
Cream lipsticks, shiny transparent-looking gloss sticks, or pots of gloss; choose three or four lipsticks in different shades and textures so that you can switch around. The gloss lipsticks are pretty and natural looking, but eat off rather more quickly. Older women who have tiny creases along the lip line should choose the least greasy lipsticks, so that colour does not melt into little lines, spoiling the mouth shape.

Lip pencil. Useful to give a clear outline, especially if you wish to make any correction to lip shape. Choose a colour which blends naturally into lip colour.

Lip brush. Some people prefer to use a brush for outlining and also for filling in; it gives a good smooth finish to lip-colour.

Eye make-up
It is possible to buy excellent cheap brands of eye make-up to give a whole collection of eye looks. When applying eye make-up be bold, using too much rather than too little, then wipe off, blending as you go until you achieve the desired effect. Choose colours for fashion, for your clothes, or just because they look pretty, but don't feel bound by the colour of your eyes.

Eyeshadow. Comes in cream form to apply with brush or finger tip; loose or pressed powder to use with a brush or little sponge; sticks to apply direct to the eyelid and smooth in with finger tip; wands of liquid with a built-in brush; palettes of colours to use with water and brush; pots of

gloss to slick on with a finger tip; or soft pencils used on the lid with little strokes and then blended with the finger tip. The greasier forms of shadow will usually need setting with a light touch of powder and are not suitable for people with deep-set eyes, as they have a tendency to form lines in the eye socket. Easier to use are the powder shadows, but these are best avoided if you have dry skin.

Eyeliner. You need to be pretty expert to handle the liquid liners with brushes as they smudge so easily; soft pencils and kohl pencils are reasonably simple to apply, as is the cake form which is used with water and a fine brush. If you are running a line along inside your lashes, do it with a liner you have used often and can be sure will not cause irritation.

Mascara. Block mascara is the oldest and still one of the most popular and easy forms to use. Wands with spiral brushes are also effective; some contain fibres to build up the thickness of the lashes. Always apply two coats and brush lashes through afterwards. Unless your lashes are really black, a dark brown or brownish black mascara will give a more natural look.

Lash curlers. Well worth having. Lashes look thicker if they sweep upwards rather than forwards in a straight line.

False eyelashes. Rather obviously false if used in a strip, quite effective if cut into small pieces and used to thicken certain parts of natural lashes. Pretty fiddly to use, but worth a try if you are dedicated.

Extras
These are the odds and ends which make your make-up routine easier. Spend a few minutes each week to make sure pencils are sharpened and brushes and sponges washed.

Tissues. For removing make-up, many models carry a roll of toilet paper; it does just as well and is more economical.

Cotton wool. Easier to use in balls, but cheaper in a roll.

Cotton-wool buds. The type used for babies, very useful for blending in make-up on eyelids.

Pencil sharpener. An absolute necessity to keep all make-up pencils in good condition; choose one which will take the larger eyeshadow pencils as well as the normal size.

Tweezers. Keep handy for a quick tidy up.

Brushes. As many and as varied as you can muster. Keep any left in good condition when mascara or eyeshadow is finished; paint brushes and old toothbrushes are also useful. Keep well washed.

Sponges. Keep any left over from finished make-up. Sponges are good for applying foundation smoothly and the tiny ones on sticks are useful for eye make-up.

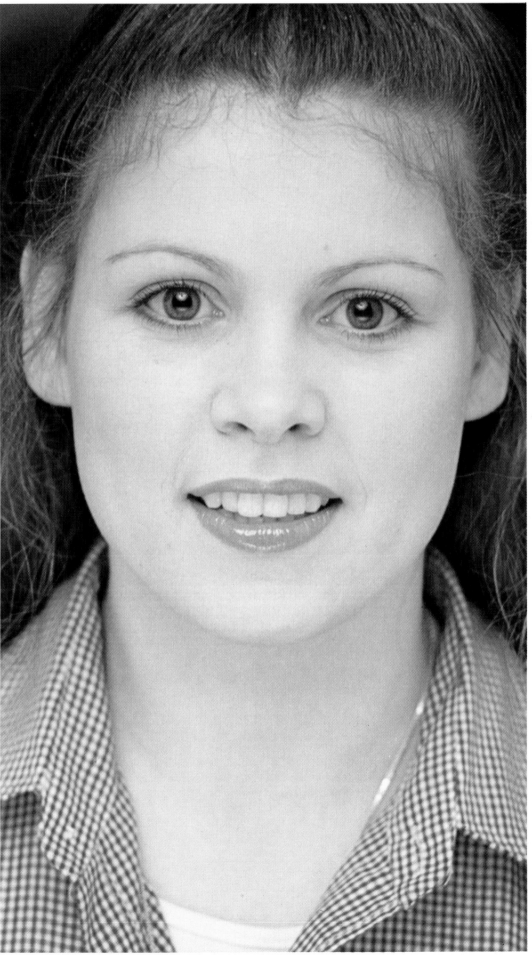

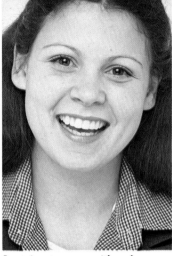

Irene is a teenager with a plump round face and lovely brown eyes. She wore very little make-up, just a dab of blue eyeshadow and a little mascara, not from choice but because with so many products on the market she did not know where to start, what would suit her, or how to apply the different products. At the age of sixteen make-up should not be ageing, but pretty and natural, giving emphasis to the face. With one or two spots and some fine broken veins* already showing on her cheeks, it was important that Irene paid careful attention to handling her fine, sensitive skin straight away. She needed a mild cleanser, gentle rosewater for freshening and a slightly stronger toning lotion on nose and chin to absorb oiliness and close the pores, and moisturizer for day and night. For Irene's make-up a tinted moisturizer was used instead of a foundation, to give a natural-looking warmth to her skin tone. A medicated cover-stick dealt with the few blemishes, and a light touch of translucent powder on the nose and chin took away shine. A soft, natural-looking blusher blended up and out from the middle of her cheeks to the hair line gave Irene's round face more shape. To emphasize and widen her eyes, a pretty pinky-beige shadow was used on the lids with highlighter under the brow. A softly smudged line of blue-grey kohl under the bottom lashes made her eyes look much bigger. The lashes were given two thin coats of mascara and were well brushed through. Irene's well-defined brows just needed a touch of brownish pencil and a little Vaseline was brushed on to give them sheen. A soft, browny-toned, glossy lipstick gave emphasis to Irene's well-shaped mouth, and the final effect looked natural and healthy.

159

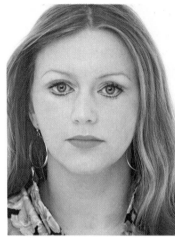

Josephine has just entered her thirties and for the last eight years she has been wearing her make-up much the same way, so the look was a little dated. The aim was to soften the rather hard and spiky effect caused by the pencilled brows, heavy socket shadow, black eyeliner and too much mascara. The first step was to apply a very light, warmer-toned foundation, which gave a glow to Josephine's skin. Blusher was then placed slightly lower on the cheeks than usual, to give more shape to Josephine's rather round face. The blusher was smoothed up and out to the hair line at eye level to lift the lines of Josephine's features, which have a tendency to slant down. Greeny-grey eyeshadow was blended from the inner corner of the eye, dipping across the eyelid and lifting right up to the outer corner of the brow to lift the droop of the eyes. Highlighter applied under the centre of the brow also helped. Soft grey eye pencil was carefully smudged under the lower lashes from the middle of the eye, lifting slightly at the outer corner. Dark brown mascara, well brushed through, looked much less hard than the black which Josephine had previously used and softly smudged brown eye pencil emphasized her very well-shaped brows. Josephine had always rounded out her lips over the natural line which gave a pretty, if rather sulky, pout. Her own lip shape was good and well defined, so this was lightly outlined and filled in with a misty pink lipstick, and a little gloss was added to the lower lip to give sheen. The finished look was softer and very much more feminine than before, but Josephine said that she honestly felt more 'herself' with the look that she was used to.

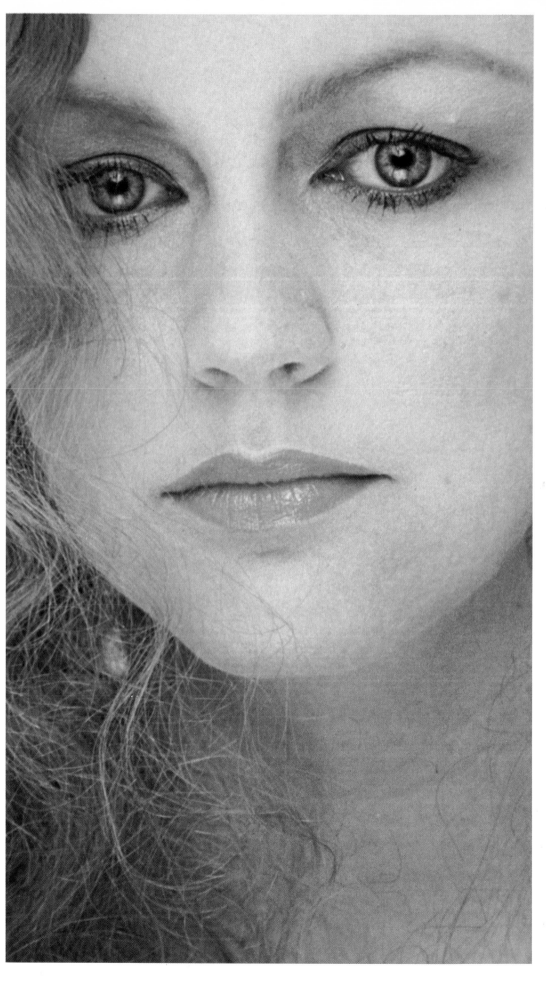

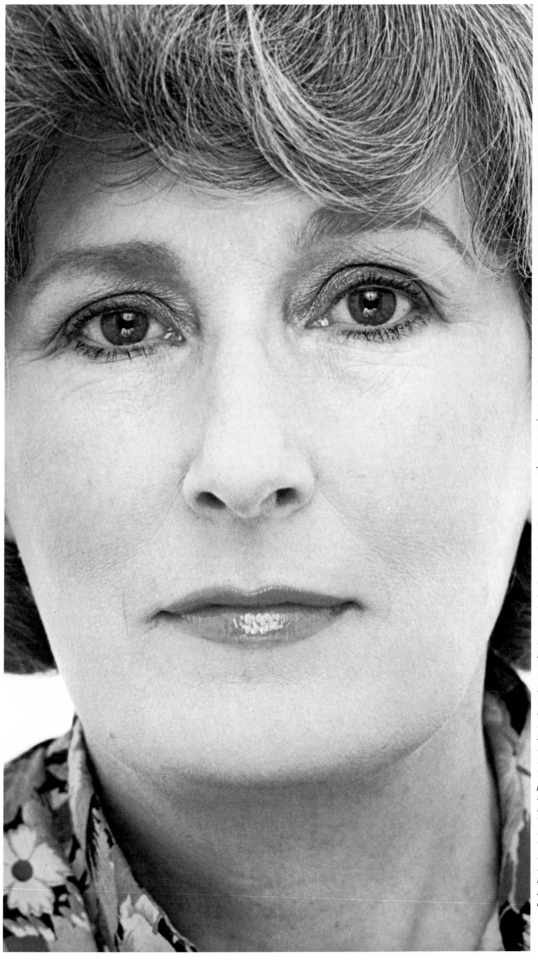

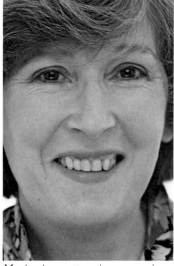

Marion is an attractive woman in her fifties. She has good features, but because she wore the very minimum of make-up her face lacked emphasis and the combination of the make-up which she did wear and her high colouring looked harsh. Marion's face was well moisturized first to smooth out tiny criss-cross lines, especially around the eyes. A very fine, beige foundation was used to tone down her high colouring and to cover the tiny broken veins on her cheeks. Creamy blusher, well blended in from the cheek-bones up and out to the hair line, gave shape and lift to Marion's face. A little translucent powder was applied to take away shine, carefully avoiding the area around the eyes. Marion had always used blue eyeshadow, believing it to be the only colour which would suit her, but her eyes are a lovely mixture of blue, green and brown and a silvery-brown shadow on the lids and highlighter blended from the inner corner of the eye up and out to the brow lifted Marion's eyes and was much more subtle. A fine, soft line of grey kohl was smudged under the lower lashes to widen the eyes and the lashes were given two coats of mascara, well brushed through. Marion's eyebrows needed tidying and were then given a touch of brown pencil and brushed into shape. Before applying lipstick, her lips were well powdered to help the lipstick to hold. The outline was then drawn in with a dryish lip pencil, and the lower line was smudged with a tissue to avoid any hard edges. Soft pink lipstick was well blotted and a little gloss was added to give sheen, but Marion was told to omit the gloss if it ran into the tiny creases around her lips. The soft, subtle tones of the make-up were very flattering, and made the best of Marion's excellent features.

STEP-BY-STEP MAKE-UP ROUTINE

Although your make-up will vary from time to time, it makes sense to have a regular routine to save time at the mirror each day. This simple system should take only ten minutes when you have put in some practice.

Points to remember

1 Make up where the light will fall directly on to your face and not cast shadows.

2 Pin your hair back so that you can make up right to your hair line. Your face does not need a white frame.

3 Be very careful to blend in make-up with finger tip, tissue or cotton bud, especially around eyes, cheeks and neck line. If foundation forms a line on your neck, blend it out with moisturizer.

4 You are often seen sideways.

5 Keep a supply of cotton-wool balls, tissues, cotton buds, clean paint brushes, old toothbrushes, eyelash brushes, and well-sharpened eye and lip pencils.

6 If short of time, do not skip through this routine and do it badly. Moisturizer, blusher and mascara are your three most important ·cosmetics, so just apply those well.

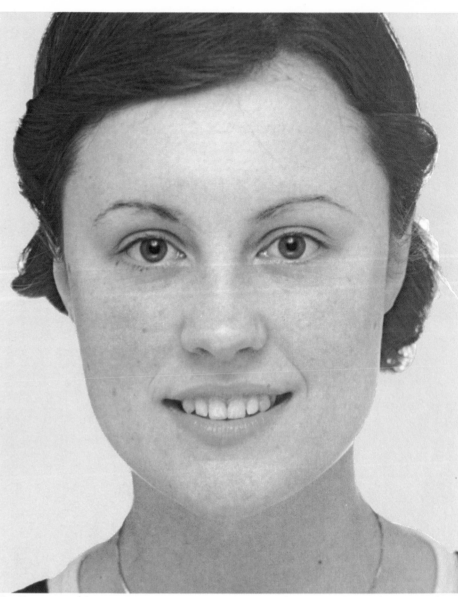

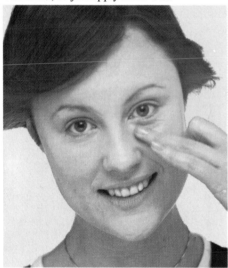

2 To disguise shadows under your eyes or hide blemishes, dot on eraser cream and smooth with little finger taking care not to stretch the fine skin under eyes.

1 Always put make-up on over a moisturizer, well massaged in all over face and neck. Besides doing your skin good, make-up – especially eye make-up – will go on more easily, last longer and look smoother. It is also less likely to change tone. If you prefer to use tinted moisturizer instead of foundation, follow instructions for stage 3, using non-tinted moisturizer on your neck.

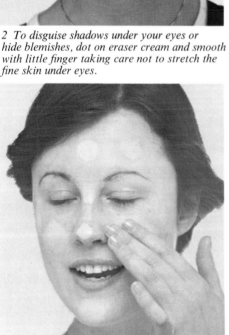

3 Apply foundation sparingly. Dot lightly all over face, but not neck, and smooth meticulously out to hair line and under jaw line to avoid any hard lines.

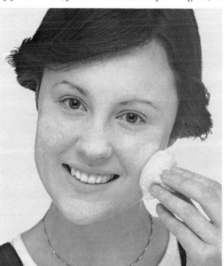

4 If you want to use powder, dust face or simply shiny patches on nose, chin and forehead with translucent powder on clean cotton-wool ball. Brush off surplus.

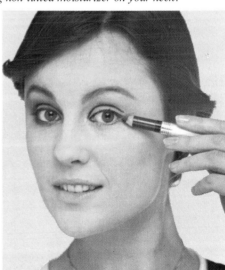

5 Outline eye and draw socket line with kohl or soft eye pencil. Smudge line with cotton bud. Pencils are easier to use as liquid eyeliner is difficult to smudge.

162

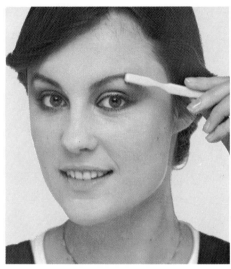

8 Brush eyebrows upwards and along length to tidy and give a nice shape. An old tooth-brush does this job well. Add shine with a little Vaseline on the brush.

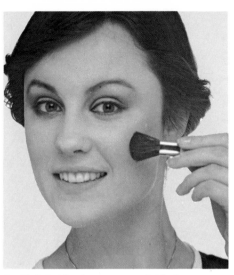

9 Lightly blend in just enough blusher to give cheeks a glow. Place blusher according to advice given on shading for your face shape. Smooth in carefully.

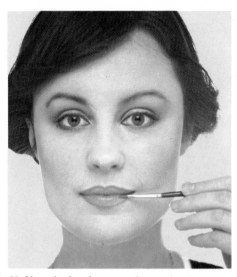

10 Use a lip brush or pencil to outline lips, softening for bottom lip. Apply lipstick. Add gloss or Vaseline on bottom lip to give sheen and prevent chapping.

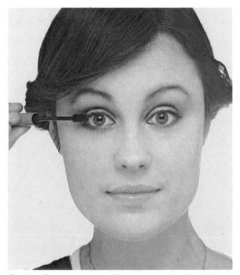

7 Apply two coats of mascara to lashes from base to tip, top and bottom, allowing each coat to dry. Separate lashes by brushing with a clean mascara brush.

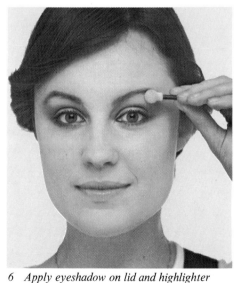

6 Apply eyeshadow on lid and highlighter under brow. Use too much shadow rather than too little so that you can see what you are doing. Smooth off surplus and edges.

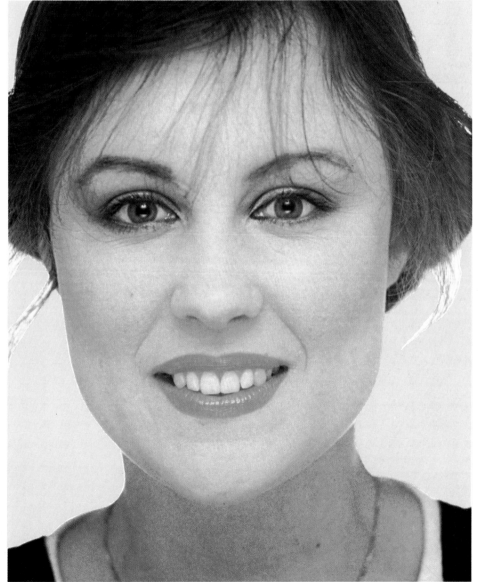

11 Your finished face should have no hard edges of make-up and should look and feel completely natural. Make-up done quickly and efficiently looks much more natural than a face which has been laboured over too long. If you keep your routine simple, you are more likely to follow it each day. More elaborate make-up can be fun, but keep it for special occasions.

A COLLECTION OF EYES AND LIPS

There is nothing more dating than wearing the same make-up year after year. Women who say 'I can't wear blue eyeshadow with my brown eyes,' or 'I wouldn't be seen dead in bright red lipstick', usually mean 'I haven't tried it and therefore I feel safer in what I have always worn.' Make-up should be used to enhance your features and make you feel more confident, but it is also for fun, to help you break out of routine, to give others around you a jolt and teach them not to take you for granted.

Fashion goes in cycles and although looks are never the same twice, much of the original remains. The Cleopatra eye, the Hollywood mouth, the Garbo look are with us at regular intervals. On the following pages you will find instructions on how to achieve these and a whole collection of other pretty looks. If you want to try something daring, make sure you give it the full treatment; nothing is sillier than wearing a new look without conviction. If you are going to giggle self-consciously, or apologize if anyone mentions it, your effort will be in vain and you aren't going to impress anyone. Also, make sure that your whole face fits. Don't wear a Hollywood smile with naive unmade-up eyes or the top half of your face will disappear. Similarly, face and clothes should work together: Cleopatra eyes aren't at their best with muddy boots and dungarees. Take your time, experiment with your face and wardrobe, and amongst this selection of looks you should find something to flatter or amuse you. Who knows, you may even find the 'you' you've been searching for.

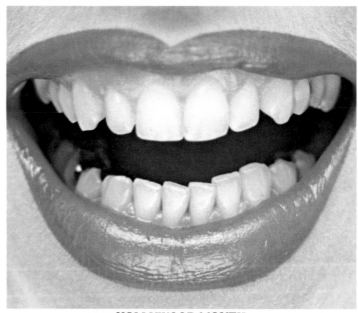
HOLLYWOOD MOUTH

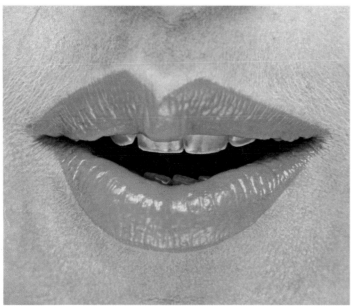
CUPID'S BOW

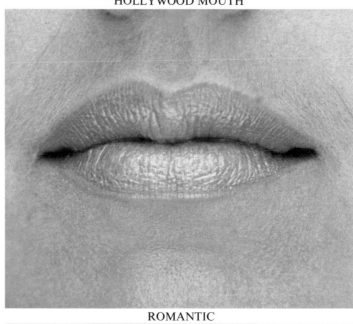
ROMANTIC

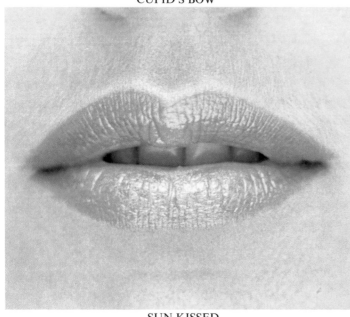
SUN KISSED

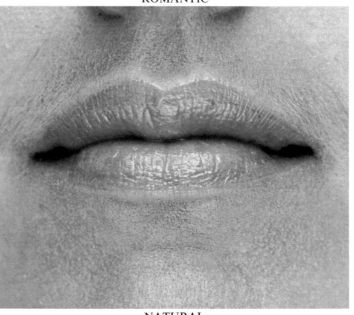
NATURAL

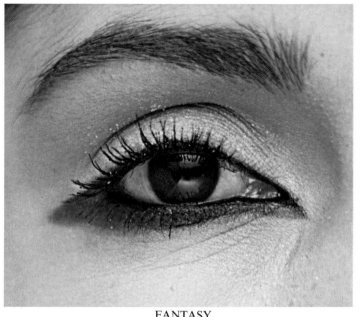

FANTASY

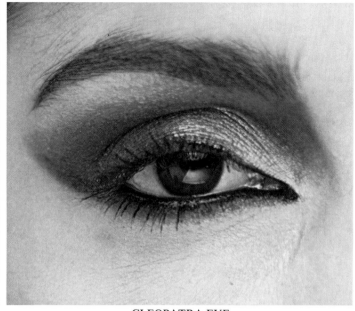

CLEOPATRA EYE

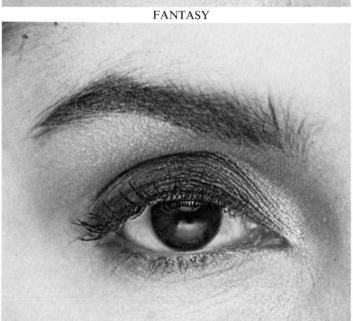

GARBO LOOK

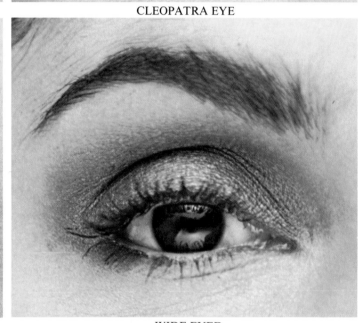

WIDE EYED

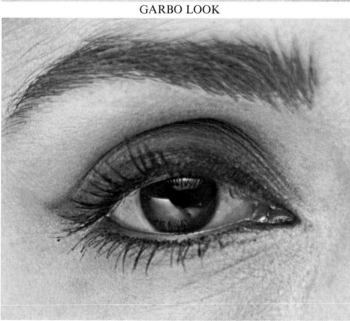

FIFTIES LOOK

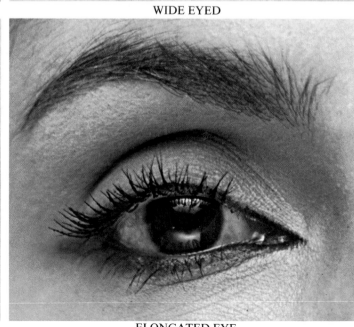

ELONGATED EYE

MAKE-UP FOR EYES AND LIPS

Never be half-hearted in your approach to make-up. Eye and lip make-up especially should always be definite and meticulously applied; if you use lines and colours, always make them clear and strong. Experiment with these make-up ideas when you have a little spare time, never just before an outing when you may be in a panic and without enough time to get used to your new look. Try each make-up several times, until you have selected your favourites, and modify them to suit yourself. This way you will feel really confident that you look your best when you test them out in public.

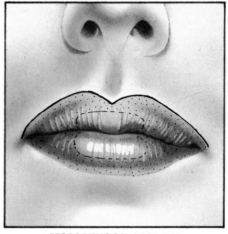

HOLLYWOOD MOUTH

No half measures are allowed with this look: it is big, brash and brightly coloured. Round out and exaggerate your natural lip shape with vibrant shocking-pink lipstick, using a lip pencil to draw in a clear curve on top lip if your lip shape is not strong enough. Place a blue highlighter in centre of both upper and lower lips and finish with a slick of gloss. If you decide to try this lip look, the rest of your face must of course live up to it – natural eyes would be completely overwhelmed. You could perhaps try one of the eye looks opposite. Your clothes should also complement your make-up.

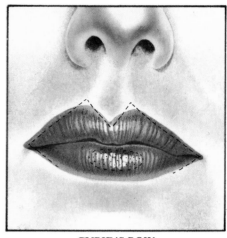

CUPID'S BOW

This is a humorous version of the 'It' girl mouth. Take foundation thinly over centre of upper lip to cover your natural lip line and draw a clear shape with lip pencil, bringing centre bow up to two definite points. Take upper lip line straight down to corners of mouth in a neat, well-defined shape; do not curve out top lip at all. Fill in bright red lipstick on top and bottom lip and put a dab of gloss in centre of bottom lip only.

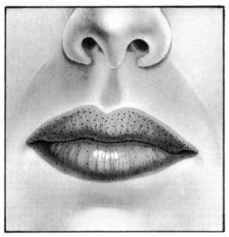

ROMANTIC

This mouth is young and vulnerable. Use clear pink frosted lipstick on top lip and one shade paler on bottom lip, to soften and plump it out. Your lip shape should be rounded and natural, so do not outline mouth with lip pencil. Lipstick can be slightly smudged along outer edges with little finger.

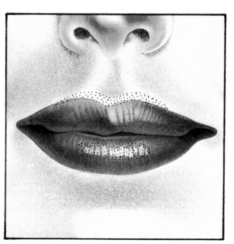

SUN KISSED

Here is a golden, glamorous look for summer. Apply gold stick make-up or gold glitter dust along centre of upper lip above cupid's bow. Fill in whole mouth generously with honey coloured lipstick and put more gold on middle of bottom lip. Cover lower lip with a thin layer of clear gloss. Although this is a very pretty lip look, anyone who has a tendency to react allergically to make-up should avoid it, as the gold dust could prove an irritant. A barrier cream applied to lips before make-up might help a little.

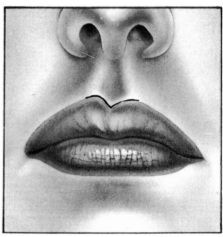

NATURAL

This is a simple and summery look, young and very natural. Outline centre curve of top lip with a soft brown pencil and smudge line carefully. Fill in lips with a pretty peach-tinted gloss, applied with your little finger. You will find the gloss has to be reapplied fairly regularly, but this is a good thing in the hot sun as it protects your lips and keeps them moist.

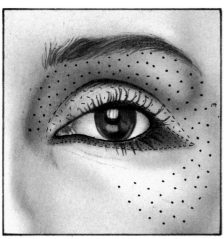

FANTASY

Place a pearly pink highlighter on cheek-bones and blend clear pink rouge from cheeks, under highlighter, to circle outer corner of eye, up to brow line and over eye to fill area between inner corner of eye and nose. Apply pearly pink shadow and a little glitter to eyelid. With a soft black kohl pencil, draw a fine line all round eye inside lashes, dipping down at inner corner of eye. Extend kohl out in a straight line from lower lashes and bring another line from centre of upper lashes out and down to meet it. Softly fill in entire area between these lines and eye. Add lots of mascara, well brushed through, to emphasize the dark frame.

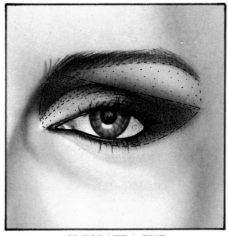

CLEOPATRA EYE

This is a strong, exotic, cat-like look. With a soft black kohl pencil, draw a line all round eye inside lashes, extending and dipping down at inner corner. Use black kohl again to draw a soft line up from inner corner of eye, alongside nose, to inner point of eyebrow; take it in a straight line across lid to beyond and above outer corner of eye. Draw line out in a straight line from lower lashes to meet it. Use gold shadow on actual eyelid, taking it no further than socket line, and-fill in whole area between lid and extended lines with softly smudged kohl. Put gold highlighter under outer arch of brow to lift line. Add masses of black mascara to give a sooty fringe.

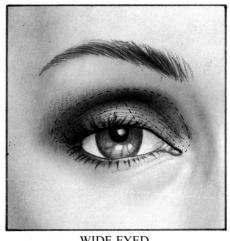

WIDE EYED

Use coloured eyeshadow to give a round-eyed, innocent look. Choose any colour you like; it is not necessary to try to match or blend with the actual colour of your eyes. Draw a fine, soft line around eye outside lashes, keeping eye neat and small; this is obviously not a look for someone who is already conscious of having small eyes. Using colour, strongly cover lid and blend up softly to brow, but not out beyond corner of eye. Place a small triangle of pearly blue highlighter at centre of lid to lift and round out shape.

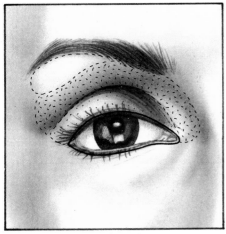

GARBO LOOK

This make-up gives a sleepy, heavy-lidded look by emphasizing and deepening the socket line. Draw soft lines with black kohl around outside of lashes to meet in a slightly extended shape at outer and inner corners of eye. Gold shadow exactly covers eyelid and copper shadow rises from inner corner of eye, alongside nose to inner edge of brow, and then fills round socket line to outer corner of eye giving a deeply hooded effect. Ivory-gold highlighter lifts from under arch to outside outer width of brow, emphasizing depth of eye even more.

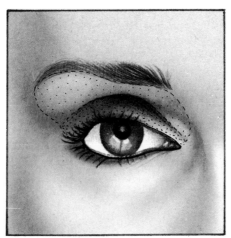

ELONGATED EYE

With a soft dark green pencil, draw a thickish straight line at base of lower lashes, extending it at inner and outer corners as you wish. Take a fine line around outside of top lashes to meet extended line. Brown eyeshadow covers lid, softly blended into socket line. With cream highlighter, fill up to brow line and beyond and above outer corner of brow to echo extended eye line.

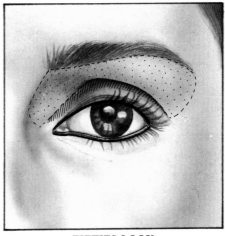

FIFTIES LOOK

Here is a gentle, deep-lidded eye, similar to the Garbo look but infinitely softer. Draw a fine, soft line with black kohl around whole of eye, making it thicken and lift slightly at outer corner. Using pale pink pencil, draw another line above lashes along bottom eyelid, to open eyes wide. Beige-brown shadow covers lid only and soft brown pencil is used to smudge along socket line to give it subtle depth. Cream highlighter fills whole area above socket line up to arch and out above outer corner of brow, to emphasize hollow line of socket.

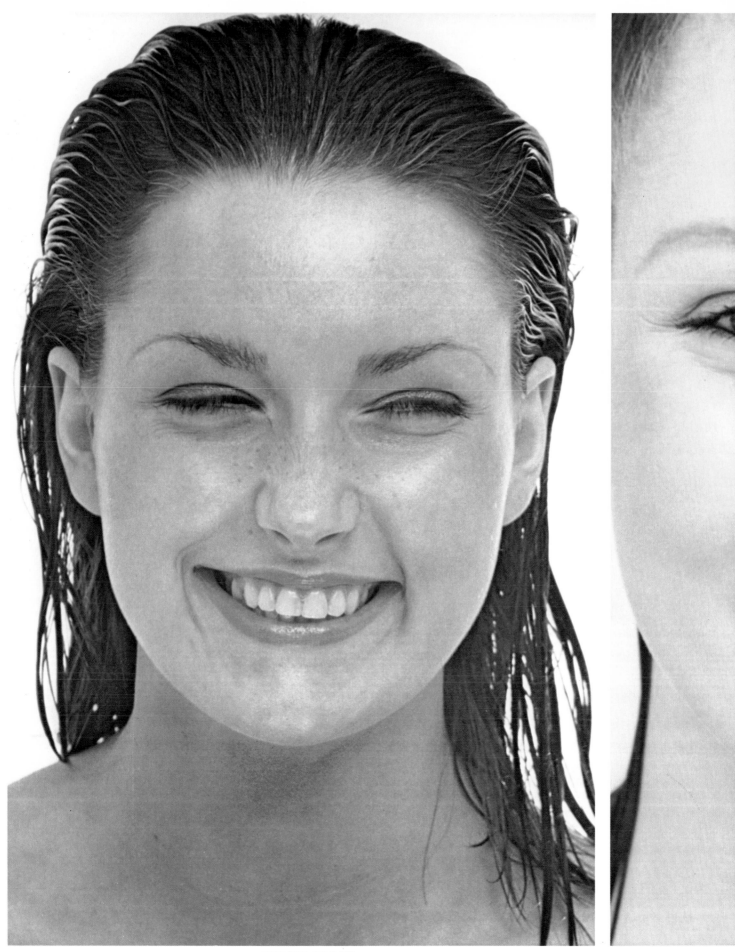

HOLIDAY FACE

168

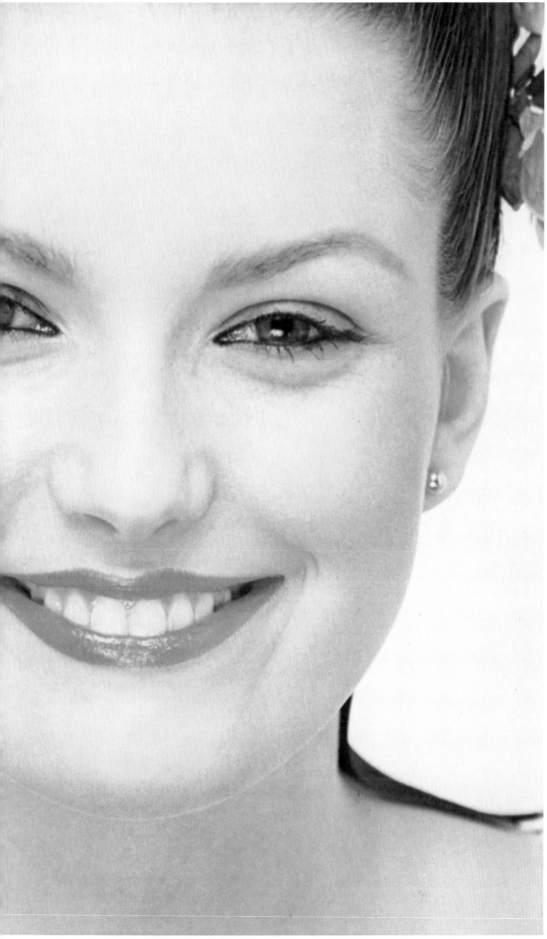

FRESH DAYTIME FACE

Once you feel confident about your basic make-up it is a good idea to make regular changes for different seasons and occasions, partly because it prevents you getting into a rut and partly because light changes quality from summer to winter and from daylight to artificial light and this affects the tone of your cosmetics. Never try a new make-up just before going somewhere special. You will probably be nervous and short of time and will finish in tears, not even liking the final effect. Experiment when you have the right light and plenty of time to concentrate.

Holiday Face

Skin tone is warmed by natural tan or tan-tinted moisturizer and copper-toned glosser on cheeks. Bronze eyeshadow on lids looks natural and sunny. Sun-tipped lashes can look very attractive, but if eyes need definition use water-proof mascara very well brushed through. Better still, have lashes dyed before the holiday. The dye looks completely natural, is water-proof and lasts about six weeks. Add copper gloss lipstick and a few freckles lightly dotted on with eye pencil and softly smudged.

Fresh Daytime Face

Natural pearly-tint foundation is used with soft pink blusher on cheeks for shape and colour. Silvery-pink shadow on lids with highlighter under brows widens eyes. Thin coats of mascara, carefully brushed through, and very fine eye-liner drawn inside lashes gives eyes definition. Shiny red lipstick makes a pretty smily shape.

Dramatic Evening Face

The foundation is pearly pale with a warm rosy blusher for shape blended out and up beyond eye level, lightly dusted over with translucent powder. Eyes are given strong emphasis and cleverly tilted by blending bronzed purple eyeshadow on lid and up to brow at inner corner only and lightly under lower lashes. Highlighter lifts outer curve of brow. Strong smudged lines of kohl circle eye, dipping down at inner corner and slightly up at outer corner. Several coats of mascara add to shadowy looks. Lips are strongly shaped with deep red lipstick.

Fun Face

A simple, natural-toned foundation and blusher form the base of this make-up. Lips are strongly defined in red but all the emphasis is on eyes. Gold eyeshadow stick coats lids, with a copper-toned shadow blended just above and highlighter under brow. Eyeliner circles eye inside lashes, which are given generous coats of mascara. Gold shadow stick is used to draw long, curving lines up face and forehead to continue on to hair, each line ending in a gold star fixed with a tiny dab of eyelash glue.

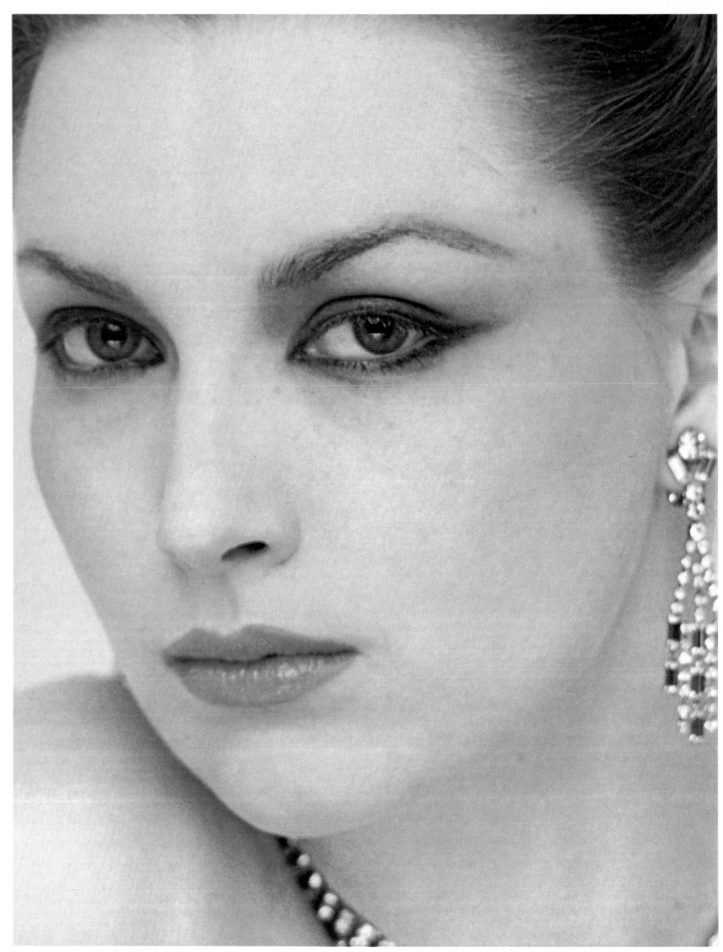

DRAMATIC EVENING FACE

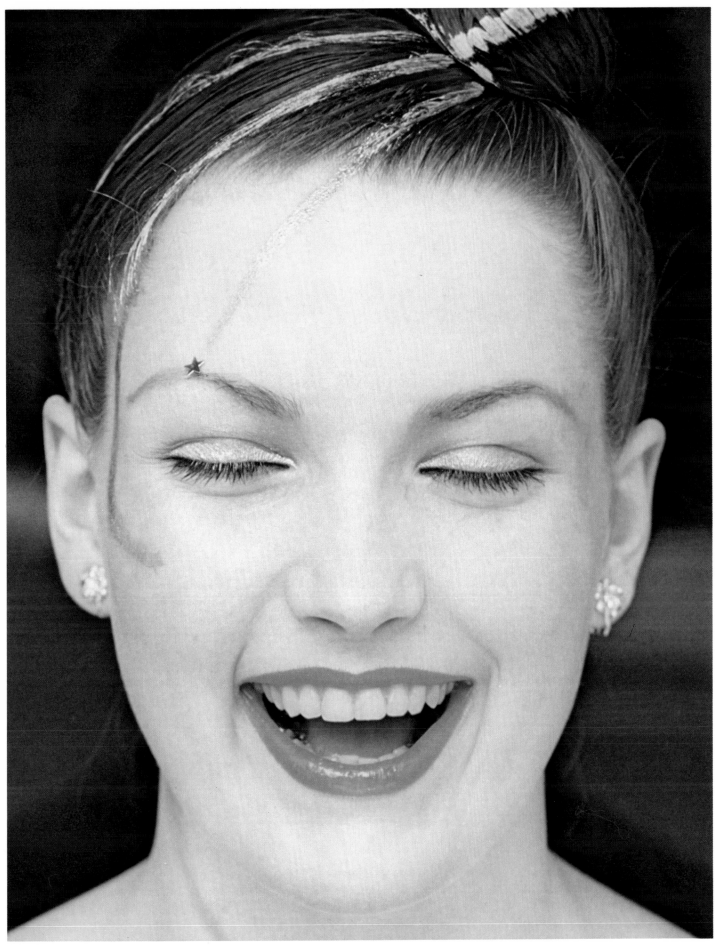

FUN FACE

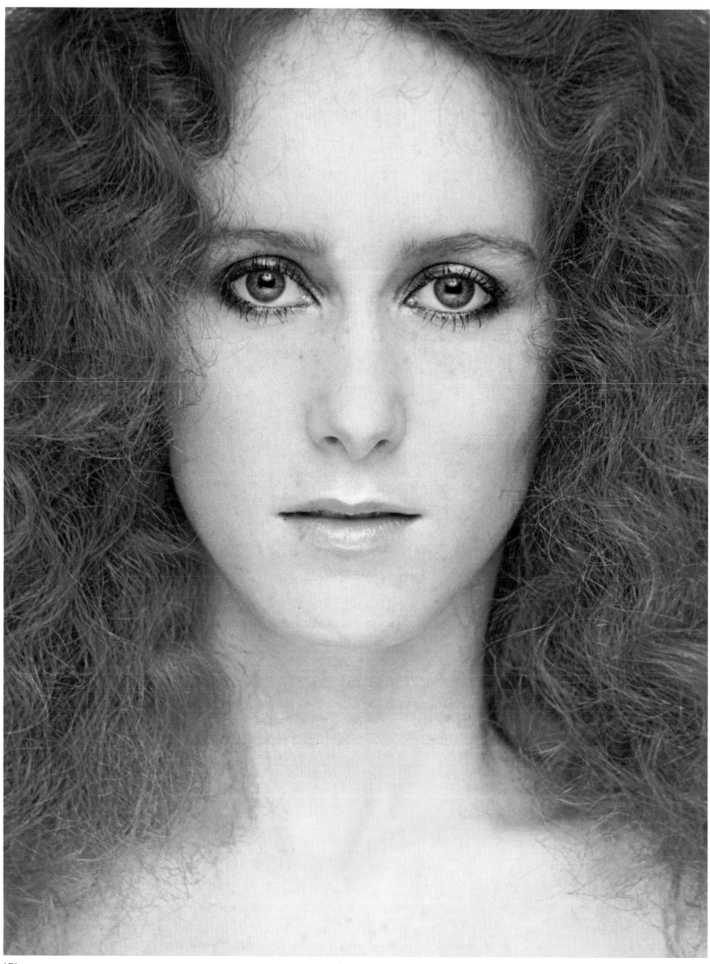

Hair

Hair is the great confidence giver. It is a scrap of inanimate material which can plunge us into despair or make the day for us. Can you count the number of times you have felt elated because your hair has changed mood? The change need not be dramatic – a comb, a ribbon or a new-fangled plait can give a fresh twist to your hair and a lift to your spirits in seconds. A change of hairdresser can sometimes make all the difference to the way you see yourself and a new hairstyle, if it's right, is the best of all morale-boosters.

Hair in top condition is marvellous stuff, and the word stuff is just right. For although it is a part of your body, hair behaves like an adaptable, amenable and very beautiful material. Together with the nails, it is the one part of the body you can touch without sensation, which

is surely why it is so abused.

The health of your hair goes up and down with your general health, and as the food you eat has everything to do with the well-being of your hair and scalp, these are often the first parts of you to show signs of strain when you have been ill or are dieting. Hair also behaves differently according to climate and age.

Your hair is the most changeable part of your appearance and for something like six thousand years has been regarded as a high fashion accessory. As with clothes, fashions in hairstyles reflect the state of society. The hey-day of the elaborate coiffure was in the reign of Elizabeth I, when there was unlimited time and money at court. Conversely, hairstyles were reduced to their simplest during the two world wars.

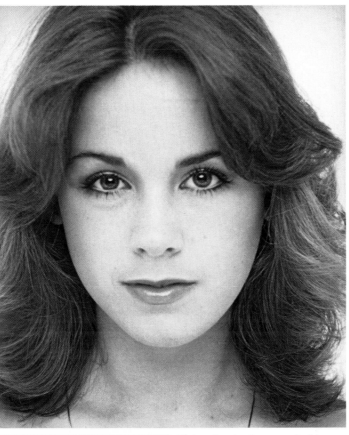

It is only in the last fifteen to twenty years that hair health has become synonymous with good hairdressing. The geometrical cuts of the Sixties taught us that hair was beautiful in itself, that it could look its best shining, simple and unadorned with curls. The revelation was so devastating that for a time many women wore their hair just as it grew, long and free and untouched by a curler or a stylist's scissors. Today, the natural look is still with us, but the means by which we achieve it are far from natural. The curls we fought in the days of the smooth bob are encouraged, or put in by complicated cutting and perming.

What we often forget is how much fashion dictates our way of thinking. It is very desirable, for example, to have shiny hair, but 'not nice' for it to be shiny with oil. But shiny hair is simply hair that has good light refraction, so the straightest hair is the shiniest. Very curly or negroid hair is so shaped that good light refraction is impossible. The pundits say that shine equals health, but that's far from the sum total. Much has been written about the problems of greasy hair, caused by an excess of sebum (oil). But what is an excess? Natural oils are an essential ingredient of hair health. We call hair greasy if it displays more oils than are acceptable in our society at this point in our fashion history – although, irrationally, it is perfectly all right to slick back a short haircut with pomade, which is only a nice name for a type of grease.

Cleanliness, and an absence of visible oils, has become so important that washing one's hair is viewed as a cure for all ills. 'I'm going to wash that man right out of my hair' goes the song, and in countless homes all over the world the ritual goes on, as a release from heartache, problems, stress or loneliness. Shampoo is as universal as toothpaste. We all use it and hope that life will be a

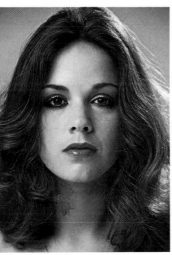

Hair colouring has seen the biggest change in hairdressing in the last few years. The many new products and techniques give scope for a whole range of possibilities. Very few are born with the splendour of natural hair colour, in marvellous condition, and blending perfectly with eye and skin tones (far left). Man-made colouring needs care in choosing and execution and make-up must be adapted to blend.
Left: Pretty hair can look dense and heavy without natural lights. Lowlights, a mild form of bleaching in strands, will transform it to a look of sunny lightness.
Above: Hair has been given lowlights at crown and forehead and is layered to frame face.

little better afterwards. And in a way it is better. Try buying new clothes when your hair needs washing and you rarely buy anything. Getting your hair looking right is one of the most vital preparations for any important appointment.

More time and money are spent on hair products than any other aspect of body beauty. When our hair pleases us we are, mentally and physically, a long way towards feeling, and therefore being, beautiful.

THE STRUCTURE OF HAIR

The discovery of the exact chemical composition of hair is very recent indeed. It was in the 1930s, in the course of research into permanent waving solutions, that the molecular structure was accidentally revealed. In comparing hair with natural fibres such as sheep's wool, the brothers William and Hugh MacDonald established that the principal constituent of hair (97 per cent) is a protein called keratin.*

Hair, like nails, is an appendage of the skin and similar in composition to the epidermis, the outer layer of skin. The point from which all hair is nourished and produced is the papilla, situated at the base of the follicle, a tube, or pocket of skin, from which the hair emerges.

The hair itself is made up of three layers. The outer layer, the cuticle, is a collection of overlapping flat scales. These scales can have as many as seven overlapping strata, or as few as three, bound together with a putty-like substance. The cuticle protects the cortex, which must always be reached if chemical changes such as colouring, bleaching or permanent waving are required. The cortex gives the hair its characteristic strength, texture and elasticity and stores the majority of the pigment, melanin, which determines hair colouring. The innermost layer is the medulla. It

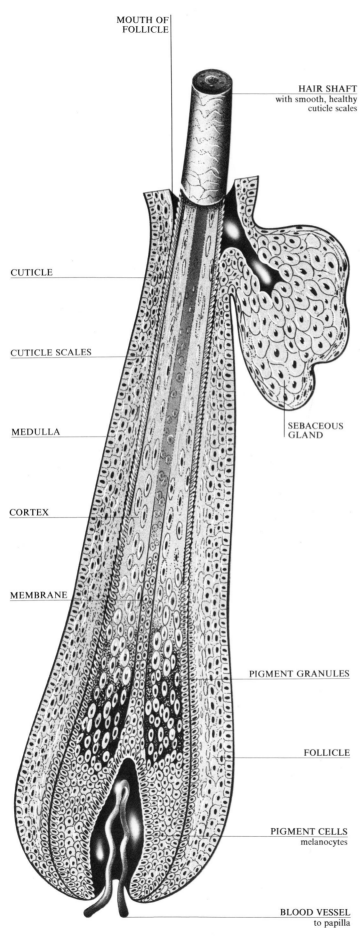

MOUTH OF
FOLLICLE

HAIR SHAFT
with smooth, healthy
cuticle scales

CUTICLE

CUTICLE SCALES

MEDULLA

CORTEX

MEMBRANE

SEBACEOUS
GLAND

PIGMENT GRANULES

FOLLICLE

PIGMENT CELLS
melanocytes

BLOOD VESSEL
to papilla

CROSS-SECTION OF HAIR AND FOLLICLE

is largely made up of air spaces with fragments of pigment. The medulla is often absent, though as this does not seem to affect the condition of the hair its function is something of a mystery.

The scalp and the epidermal layers beneath it are just as important as the hair itself, since the follicle and papilla, the living portions of the hair, are situated in it. It also carries the sebaceous glands* which supply sebum to lubricate the hair shaft and the arrector pili muscle which makes your hair stand on end, as it contracts under the influence of cold, stress, fear and pleasure.

HAIR GROWTH

Hair is the most rapidly developing cellular structure in the entire body, with the possible exception of bone marrow. It grows on average about $\frac{1}{2}$ in (1.25 cm) a month, faster in summer than in winter and more at night than in the daytime. Length depends on a growing cycle. The growing phase, anagen, can last for up to six years. Then comes the degenerating phase, catagen, when the hair follicle stops growing and then shrinks, and the papilla moves into a state of rest, the phase known as telogen. The resting stage lasts only a few weeks – unless the follicle fails to come out of the telogen phase, in which case baldness is the result. Hairs go through this cycle in an over-lapping sequence, so a normal, healthy scalp always has about the same number of hairs; there is no growing or moulting season as with animals. Some women can grow very long hair because they have a combination of a quick growth rate and a relatively long life span for each hair. Hair that will only survive a matter of months will only reach shoulder-length. The growth rate slows down as we get older, and as the individual hairs get older.

Fifty to a hundred hairs are shed every day. This is not a cause for worry, as the total number of hairs on your head varies from 90,000 to 140,000.

Hair becomes very elastic when wet and will stretch one-quarter of its length, returning to normal when dry. This enables hairdressers to set hair into a particular style which will last until the next time the hair is wet.

KNOWING YOUR HAIR

Start with a lock of hair, feel it, pick it up from the crown of your head and run it through your fingers. Does it run through unchecked, or do you feel rough prickles, especially at the ends? These are signs of dryness and damage. Smoothness depends on a light coating of sebum, a fatty substance which is the natural lubricant of hair and skin. An

excess of sebum shows in sticky hair which needs frequent washing. Wind the lock round your fingers to test the degree of curl. Very straight hair will spring back immediately, a wavy strand will hold shape, and very curly hair will either wind tightly around your finger or refuse to wrap round at all.

Density, texture, movement, colour and condition – these are the five characteristics which determine the look of your hair. The first four are a result of heredity. The fifth is a result of how you care for or abuse your natural material. Together these five characteristics influence choice and success of a hairstyle as much, if not more, than the shape of your face.

Density
Whether your hair is thick or thin depends on the number of hair follicles you are born with. Blondes have the most, then brunettes, and redheads the least.

Texture
Coarse or fine refers to the dimension of each hair shaft.
Fine: Silky usually shiny. Soft and slippery. Springs out of rollers. Dries slowly if thick and abundant. Drops quickly out of set.
Coarse: Springy, usually thick. Strong, sometimes glossy but often wiry and lacking sheen. Usually sets well, but wants its own way. Dries quickly.
Some hair may be a mixture of fine and coarse hairs, but usually one or other dominates.

Movement
This is determined by the growth pattern in the papilla, which defines the shape of the hair shaft.
Straight: Smooth and strong, can be fine or coarse. Lies flat when wet. Hates to curl, resists setting. Falls quickly into partings.
Wavy: Has lots of movement, more when short than long. Can be fine or coarse. Waves more when wet. Holds set well.
Curly: Springy, usually coarse and strong. Difficult to set. Tendency to frizz.

Colour
The natural colouring of your hair is due to pigment called melanin which is present in the cortex. The difference in hair colour is determined by the percentage of the four natural pigments – black, brown, red and yellow – and the number of air spaces in the cortex of the hair.

HAIR CONDITION

The condition of your hair is largely up to you, because general health and state of the scalp usually dictate strength and health of hair. Much damage is self-inflicted in the interests of fashion and most hair is damaged to some degree. Below are descriptions of different hair conditions, so that you can identify the state of your hair, and methods of treatment.

Healthy hair. Pliant and smooth-surfaced. Has a faint coating of sebum. Remains smooth when wet. Tangles little. Scalp free of flakes, slightly oily.

Dry and strawlike. Poor, brittle hair, split at ends and sometimes throughout its length. Hair lacks elasticity, breaking off when stretched. Scalp could have dry, powdery flakes. Often associated with dry skin types. The main causes are: natural, wear and tear and mechanical damage, and chemical damage. Natural: The usual culprit is an insufficient moisture level in the cortex. Another factor can be a lack of sebum flow along the hair shaft. Since each hair naturally contains water, if there is a lack of sebum to prevent evaporation much of this moisture is lost, causing the hair to dry out. This can be a hereditary tendency, or part of the ageing process. As a symptom of poor health, dry hair and perhaps dry scalp could result from hormonal imbalance, for example after pregnancy, or from emotional problems or poor diet. Some dry hair problems are really scalp disorders and may be accompanied by dandruff (see page 176).

Wear and tear and mechanical damage: This is so commonplace as to be the accepted norm. Many of us injure our hair simply by washing it wrongly (see page 177 for how to shampoo). The correct shampoo to prevent damage should be a mild one. If you like to wash your hair frequently it will do no harm provided you only shampoo once. Harsh objects such as spiky, heated or brush rollers, metal combs and plastic brushes will cause further damage to hair. Never use elastic bands as they tear the hair; a length of string or a pipe-cleaner is preferable. Limit the damage done by heated rollers, even if they do contain conditioner, by wrapping thin foam rubber around them. Electric tongs are drying and can burn ends badly. Never iron or tong your hair to straighten it. Central heating, sun, sea water and chlorinated water are also drying.

Chemical damage: This causes the protective cuticle to rupture, and sometimes to disappear altogether. It comes about when hair is carelessly or too frequently bleached, tinted, permed or straightened. It produces a symptom known as over-porosity, in which the cells of the hair shaft break down and become very soft and stretchy (see Test for porosity, page 178). Hair tangles easily and may have brassy or green tones from over-bleaching or incorrect colouring.

Dry and damaged hair should be conditioned regularly, but if used excessively or

unnecessarily, conditioner can make hair greasy and lank. First of all, if hair is habitually tangled after shampooing check that you are rinsing sufficiently. Some perfectly healthy just-washed hair is inclined to be fly-away and attracts static electricity, even if by the end of the week it has a healthy helping of sebum. Control this sort of hair with a very small blob of pomade-type conditioner, the sort you can use between shampoos. Rub it between palms to soften, then smooth on to hair sparingly and brush in. Rough, tangled hair needs a conditioner straight after washing. This is usually rinsed through to ensure an even spread; it makes combing much easier and adds body and shine. If the cause of damage to your hair is chemical, an organic protein reconditioner will be necessary. For dry hair, pre-shampoo treatments with natural oils may help (see page 215). But if the problem is getting the better of you and your hair is showing no sign of improvement, check your general health with your doctor and consult your hairdressing salon if they are strong on hair care, or find a trichologist.*

Greasy hair. Becomes oily a day or two after washing. Often accompanied by spots on forehead and nose. Oily scalp. Hair needs natural oils for health and gloss, but if sebaceous glands are over-active hair becomes lank after a

day or two. The cause is often glandular, and the condition is prevalent in adolescence when excess oil may well be seen round the nose and on the forehead and could partner a spotty skin. Other causes are pregnancy, climatic change, too rich a diet and nervous upsets. Baby-fine hair tends to look greasy quickly - but it should not be treated as such, just washed fairly often.

You can't alter the glands which are the cause of excess grease, but you can keep your hair clean. It is a myth that too-frequent shampooing will increase the output of sebum on to the scalp. Wash your hair as often as it needs but shampoo only once, using a mild, preferably non-detergent shampoo. You can remove oil from the scalp between shampoos by using eau-de-Cologne on a pad of cotton wool. Dab this all over the head between partings. To lift oil from the hair put Cologne-soaked cotton wool between the tufts of your hairbrush and brush lightly but thoroughly in all directions.

Diet plays an important part in caring for greasy hair. Fatty foods, spicy dishes and hot, strong tea and coffee, which are stimulants, all increase the activity of the sebaceous glands. Choose protein foods such as meat, eggs and fish, with plenty of fresh fruit and vegetables, and you will probably end up in much better shape altogether.

Keep a cool head always - heat on the scalp will encourage perspiration. Wash hair in warm water, never hot, and keep hair-dryers on warm or cool. Avoid the temptation to wear a hat to cover greasy hair problems - a loosely-tied scarf would be better if absolutely necessary. Brush hair lightly and little, taking care not to brush scalp. Greasy hair accompanied by dandruff is a common scalp problem (see page 176).

Split ends. The most common condition of all, caused by harsh colouring or perming solutions, straightening, too much sun, poor health, wrong shampooing, ill-treatment such as brushing hair when wet, damage from heated hair rollers or tongs, or using a hair-dryer too hot or too near your hair. Generally a dry hair condition, the cuticle is split at the end of the hair forming a Y-shape because the hair ends are deprived of sebum. The further away the ends are from the source of sebum the drier they become, and even greasy hair can have split ends.

Split ends are very common and though not curable are easily remedied, provided that the cause of splitting is also treated. The split ends should be snipped off with a clean club-cut movement of the scissors at fortnightly intervals, until all the split ends have grown down and been cut off. Split ends that are not removed

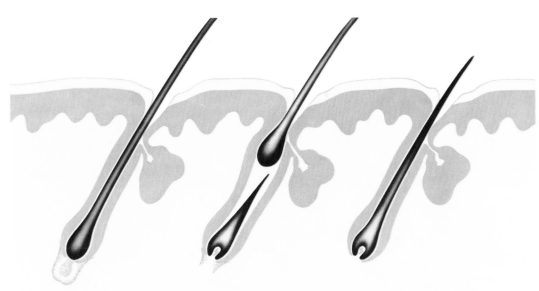

Catagen stage: Hair stops growing, root forms club shape, travels up follicle and is shed naturally.

Telogen stage: Old hair is shed, follicle goes into resting phase until new hair starts to form.

Anagen stage: Hair stays in active growth phase for greatest part of life, sometimes as long as six years.

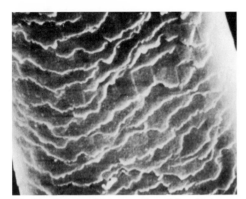
Healthy hair, cuticles smooth and flat. Hair should always be in this condition.

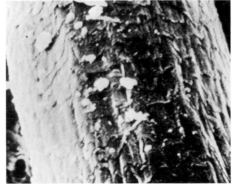
Hair shaft roughened, cuticles raised, caused by washing hair with over-alkaline shampoo.

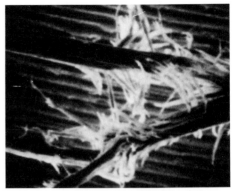
Ends of hair split and torn, caused by over-exposure to sun and chemical damage.

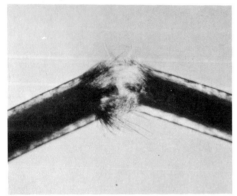
Hair broken, caused by using tight perm rods, heated rollers or metal grips on dry, brittle hair.

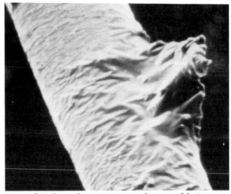
Superficial conditioner coats damaged hair, masking but not repairing ruptured surface.

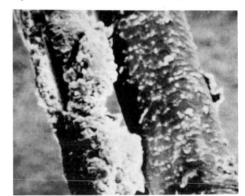
Build-up of chemical hair spray or setting lotion coating hair and causing it to dry out further.

can travel up the hair, causing breakage at different lengths. Ragged ends that cannot be removed can be smoothed over temporarily with a conditioner applied to ends only.

Greying hair. Grey hair is not properly grey, but a mixture of white and darker hair which gives a grey impression. White hair occurs when the melanin is not formed in the papilla and no colour pigment is present in the cortex. It is just as strong as coloured hair but takes on a different texture.
Greying of single hairs can start quite early, between twenty and thirty years of age. Cases of premature greying, which can start as early as adolescence, are hereditary and quite rare.

Other causes of greying can be worry, shock or severe illness. White hairs appear prominent and noticeable because they tend to be more wiry. Removing the odd one won't hurt – it is a myth that two grow when one is pulled out. You can't restore colour once it has gone, but a rinse on grey can often be more interesting than the original colour. Grey hair can be marred by unsightly yellowing streaks, particularly round the hair line and at the tips, at its worst if the hair is dry and porous. This yellowing can be caused through smoking or working in stuffy conditions. It is easily covered by a temporary colourant (see page 178). Greying hair

should be cut, conditioned and cared for meticulously to preserve gloss on the hair and so that its tendency to wiriness doesn't make it look unkempt and straggly.

SCALP DISORDERS

Dandruff. The general term for any type of visible flaking of the scalp. Shedding of dead skin all over the body is perfectly normal, it is only when this becomes excessive on the scalp that it is referred to as dandruff. It is noticeable first as small, white flakes which show up on shoulders.
a) Dry dandruff goes with dry hair and is associated with dry skin types. Dry, powdery flakes are present on hair and scalp. As this is a dry skin condition, the sufferer will probably have patches of dry skin elsewhere on the body. The hair, too, will be dry, and the scalp may be rather itchy. It is usually a hereditary tendency, but can be a sign of poor health or a vitamin deficiency, especially Vitamin B12. It can be aggravated by harsh brushing or combing, scratching or irritating chemicals. The worst thing you can do for this type of dandruff is to rush for the nearest bottle of anti-dandruff or medicated shampoo. These are strong shampoos designed for the oily type of dandruff and may well aggravate the condition. First, follow the rules laid down for dry hair and keep flakes away by washing with a mild shampoo. If the problem persists, see your

doctor or a trichologist, who may suggest shampoos containing zinc pyrithione or selenium sulphide. They should be used in moderation, as excessive use will cause the hair to go dull, lifeless and greasy. The occasional use of these shampoos and washing the hair with a mild shampoo the rest of the time should reduce flaking to a minimum. Keep hair and scalp meticulously clean, washing as often as necessary and conditioning carefully.
b) Oily dandruff is associated with oily skin types and often accompanied by spots on face, neck and shoulders. The sebaceous glands have become hyper-active, causing excess oiliness, and the flakes in this condition are yellow, greasy and soft to touch. The scalp, which is also greasy, can be red and sore. If the condition becomes severe, it is known as seborrhoeic dermatitis, a chronic scaling eruption usually with inflammation. Any such condition is prone to secondary infection; complications can result if the scalp is scratched and other hairy parts of the body, such as eyebrows and pubic hair, can also become infected.

During adolescence, the entire glandular system becomes more active and this can stimulate increased activity in the sebaceous glands. This leads to oily skin, particularly around nostrils, behind the ears and on the forehead, where spots may occur,

followed by spots on the shoulders or trunk. The spots are caused because excess oil traps dust and dead skin cells in the pores, which become inflamed and infected.

Other contributory factors could be an over-rich diet or one too high in animal fats. The condition often gets worse before menstruation, or when tired or nervous. Some experts think that stress is one of the prime causes of this type of dandruff.

A mild case can be kept in check by frequent washing with a gentle shampoo such as Castile and olive oil, with the occasional use of a stronger medicated or anti-dandruff shampoo containing zinc pyrithione or selenium sulphide, as mentioned under dry dandruff. If the chronic condition takes hold, consult your doctor or a trichologist, who will probably recommend the following treatment. The scalp must be thoroughly washed and then a cream or lotion that removes the scaly deposits must be directly applied. These preparations should contain one or other of the chemicals mentioned above. Follow instructions for use of the products very carefully and while the trouble persists avoid perming or colouring the hair.

Falling hair. A heavy hair loss or large tufts coming out at once, most noticeable when washing. The most common causes are hormonal, particularly after pregnancy and during the meno-pause. It can also occur when a woman stops taking the contraceptive pill, when there is a sudden reduction in the oestrogen* level. Excessive hair loss can also be caused by anxiety, shock, some drugs, radiotherapy, high fevers and crash diets. In most cases it will right itself when the body recovers. But, while your hair is in trouble, you will certainly need the moral support and advice of a qualified trichologist.

Bald patches. This is a distressing condition, nearly always with a medical cause. There are many types of alopecia, which literally means loss of hair. It *always* needs to be seen by a doctor and possibly a trichologist as well. Alopecia totalis, when all the hair falls, is very rare. The more common alopecia areata is first noticed in a white circular patch of baldness; the hair may appear to be otherwise quite healthy. Very short, bristly hairs surround the bald patch.

In middle age, hair may become less plentiful or begin to recede from the temples. This is a hereditary tendency. A change of hairstyle is the easiest solution; it may be that you still have a style suitable for more plentiful hair.

Do not massage or comb thinning or falling hair, brush gently into style. Wigs and false pieces, which could inhibit new growth, should be reserved for special occasions. Pink, flat patches of baldness, surrounded by stubs of hair, should be seen at once by a doctor. They could be signs of ringworm,* which is highly infectious. Advice on the treatment of ringworm can be found on page 219. And for information on how to eradicate head lice, see page 214.

HAIR PRODUCTS

Shampoo
A shampoo is simply a cleansing agent. This may seem to be a statement of the obvious, but it is easy to lose sight of this fact with such a wealth of products on the market, many claiming almost magical properties. The basic requirements of a shampoo are that it should remove dirt and grease efficiently, be easily removed by rinsing, not dry the hair by stripping it of its vital moisture content, and leave it shiny and manageable. The product should mix well with both oil and water and it helps if it has good, but not excessive, foaming qualities because dirt is lifted off the hair into the foam and is more easily rinsed out.

All shampoos have detergent properties, since the word detergent simply describes the ability to remove dirt from any material, including hair. What is frequently referred to as a 'non-detergent' shampoo is often simply a mild shampoo, probably with a low-lather action. In a hair salon, it would be a soft soap solution, which needs skilled application.

Which shampoo?
The tendency with modern shampoo technology and publicity is to blind us with science, and some selling points become very hard to fathom. The term 'pH balanced' refers to the chemical make-up of hair products, all of which are acid or alkaline. The extent of their acidity or alkalinity is measured on a scale of 1 to 14. The 'per hydrogen value' (pH) of hair and scalp is slightly acid, having a pH average of between 4 and 6. All soaps, on the other hand, are alkaline, so the good old-fashioned practice of a final acid rinse in vinegar or lemon juice counteracts the alkaline properties, leaving hair free of chalky residue and in its natural slightly acid state. Alkalis left on the hair, even in minute quantities, make the hair dull and can be harmful. Modern shampoos attempt to right this balance, and some are pH balanced to the hair, often without stating this on the label as a selling point.

Some shampoos sound more like something to eat than washing agents, with fruit, nut and herbal flavours and fragrances. These may give one a feeling of well-being, but their effect on the hair must be minimal, as all shampoo must be rinsed out of the hair thoroughly. There may well be certain brands that suit your hair better than others and you will probably discover these by trial and error. However, effective hair treatment comes *after* washing.

As a general rule, the best shampoos are the latest on the market, simply because research is improving them all the time. So don't stick to the same shampoo for years – but take exaggerated claims with a pinch of salt.

Soap shampoo. Usually
alkaline. Good shampoos will have a pH value of between 7 and 9. Poor shampoos would be above 9. Soap shampoos do not have a particularly good cleansing action and react with hard water when rinsing, leaving scum on the cuticle. They can be mass-produced easily, but are more expensive to make than soapless shampoos. However, they are not usually irritants and may be advisable for anyone whose scalp is sensitive or allergic to the synthetic shampoos. A final rinse of lemon juice or vinegar will help to remove scum and restore the acid balance.

Soapless shampoo. Made
from synthetic materials derived from petroleum by-products or from natural fats which have been chemically treated, these shampoos are cheap to produce, have excellent cleansing properties, are not affected by hard water, can be varied in strength to suit a specific need and can be rendered acidic without reducing their effectiveness. The disadvantages are that they are difficult to rinse out completely, they tend to strip hair of natural oils leaving it fly-away, and they can be irritants causing itchy, flaking scalps or dermatitis.* The pH value can vary between 4 and 9, depending on the quality of the product.

Dry shampoo. Usually in
the form of a powder or aerosol spray, these can be used as a stop-gap, an in-between remedy for greasy hair, or during illness. Dry shampoos absorb excess dirt and grease without wetting the hair. Puff the powder liberally on to the hair and scalp, leave for a few minutes and then brush out thoroughly. Do not leave any trace of powder in the hair or it will give a greyish appearance.

How to shampoo
Opinions vary considerably on how often you should wash your hair. Some hairdressers say it is all right to shampoo every day, others insist on not more than once a week. The best advice is to judge for yourself and see how your hair behaves. The stripping of natural oils from the hair may be a direct result of using excessive amounts of shampoo so use moderately and, if you are washing more than once a week, only shampoo once each time, unless your hair is in a highly greasy condition. Modern shampoos are very concentrated and the temptation is to use too much and to pour it straight on to the scalp. The best way is to use not more than a dessertspoonful dissolved in a tumbler of warm water. Apply half the solution to well-wetted hair and massage with finger tips, not finger nails. There will be little lather. Rinse with warm water and then apply the rest of the shampoo and massage into a good lather. Ideally, rinse using a shower attachment until the hair squeaks between the fingers and all shampoo is gone. Without a shower attachment, at least six large jugs of water are required. If you need only one shampoo use just a teaspoonful of the lotion, also dissolved in water, and massage thoroughly, rinsing as above. A final rinse with a mild acid such as lemon juice or vinegar in water will remove all traces of scum and restore the hair's natural acid balance.

Rinses
A lemon rinse, used regularly, helps to keep blonde hair from fading in winter. But don't use lemon if you have a sore scalp or any spots or rashes on the face or neck as it will sting. Use two teaspoonsful of lemon juice to 1 pt (600 ml) of warm water.

A vinegar rinse takes one tablespoonful of vinegar to 1 pt (600 ml) of warm water. The malt in malt vinegar is a good setting agent so it gives you double value.

The ideal method of drying your hair is to pat well with a good absorbent towel, remove tangles by running fingers through to loosen, then comb through gently and allow to dry naturally. Unfortunately for most of us this isn't practical and we turn to mechanical aids. If using a dryer-hood, hair should be left slightly damp and the roller-set allowed to finish drying naturally.

The temptation with blow-drying is to hurry things along. Very fine or chemically treated hair can be slow drying and the blow-dryer can be held so close as to burn: a good handspan away is quite close enough. The best routine is to half-dry hair naturally first, then finish it off with the dryer and styling brush.

Tangles must be carefully and gently removed with a comb before drying. Wet hair tangles easily, especially when it is out of condition. Tangles should be coaxed out from the hair tip. Never attempt to remove tangles by starting at the scalp and *never* use a brush on wet hair.

Conditioners
Hair conditioners, or 'instant conditioners' as they are some-times called, coat the cuticle of the hair, rather like a fabric conditioner. Some conditioners, more properly called recon-ditioners, contain hydrolysed protein which, because the weight of its molecular structure is similar to that of hair, joins the structure of the hair by 'salt-bonds'.* These penetrate to the cortex and temporarily strengthen the bulk of the hair. This kind of conditioner should only be used about once a month as a special treatment.

Some damage to hair is inevitable: it is normal for only the first $\frac{1}{2}$ in (1.25 cm) of newly grown hair nearest to the scalp to be anything like perfect. When hair is damaged it is the cuticle, or outer skin, which suffers first. The scales of the cuticle begin to lift exposing the cortex. In extreme cases there could be little or no cuticle left. A conditioner repairs this damage cosmetically. It literally paints over the cracks giving the hair body and smooth-ness, making it easier to comb and giving a superficial sheen. Used in moderation conditioners are excellent; used in excess they make the hair greasy and sticky. The effects last until the next wash.

Setting agents
Most setting agents are combed through hair after washing and help the set to last longer. Recently developed lotions help to give fine hair more body and others are for use when blow-drying.

Natural hairstyles are usually best set with the lighter lotions, often in spray-on form. Most are based on plastic polymers. The spirit-based lotions will help hair to dry faster and, though excellent for greasy hair, are not recommended for dry or damaged hair. The heavier gels are translucent mixtures of oil and gelatine and are only for unruly, resistant hair. Hair, especially very curly hair, sets best when wet. However, setting lotions take firmer hold when not watered down, so blot hair with a towel before applying the lotion.

'Natural' setting agents, such as beer, are effective and cheap. When using beer, choose a light or pale ale; it can be applied neat to the hair for a strong hold or rinsed through with water.

Hair sprays

These used to be known as lacquers and earned a bad reputation for the effect they had on hair. Much was blamed on the content, but the real damage resulted from their use – or misuse. Inept hairdressers often used quantities of lacquer to create a hairstyle they couldn't achieve by cutting and setting; the hair was virtually cemented into shape until the next shampooing.

Modern hairsprays are much lighter than the original lacquers and are usually adapted to suit the climate of the country in which they are sold. Their only real function nowadays is to protect your hairstyle against the elements. They are invaluable in wet or windy weather, especially for fine or fly-away hair. Hold the can a good handspan away from the head and always keep it moving. If you are not getting enough 'hold' this way, switch to a different product, don't try to achieve what you want by using more and more. Spray should be removed each night by brushing.

HAIR COLOURING

All hair colouring and bleaching involves chemicals and any permanent colour change will alter the structure of your hair. Effects depend on the natural colour and condition of your hair. It is obviously best to have colouring done by an experienced professional who can assess what will suit you and who has the technical skill to do the job properly. If, however, you want to try your hand at home, it is vital that you read the instructions on the packet very carefully and that you carry out the following tests.

Skin test

All permanent colourants and some semi-permanent colourants have a toxic base which is a para compound.* Because of the toxic element some people will be allergic to these dyes. The effects of a para reaction will usually

arise a few hours after application. The first signs are a blotchy appearance and itchy skin on face and neck. In severe cases the sufferer can become extremely ill. Luckily, reaction to a para dye is rare – perhaps one woman in a thousand will be affected. Manufacturers must print a warning and instructions with their products, and a hairdresser is legally obliged to carry out a skin test in all cases.

How to do a skin test: Cleanse a small patch of skin behind the ear with white (surgical) spirit or alcohol. Mix a small quantity of the tint as directed and apply to skin. Leave to dry undisturbed for forty-eight hours. If no irritation or inflammation occurs, it is safe to go ahead. The skin test on its own will do no harm.

Test for porosity
Over-porous hair is in a dry and damaged state. It will not hold colour, or will colour patchily due to degeneration of the hair shaft. To test, take a few strands of hair and slide your fingers upwards towards the roots. If the hair is rough, it is probably porous. Now test when wet. If the hair is unnaturally soft, like cotton wool, and very stretchy, it is porous and unsuitable for colouring.

Strand test
This is the one sure way of knowing the effect of colouring on your hair. To test, cut a few hairs, preferably from two or three different parts of your head. Mix a little of the tint (this can be done at the same time as the skin test). Apply to the hairs, carefully noting the development time. Rinse and check sample for condition in its wet state. Check especially the degree of elasticity. Dry sample completely before checking colour.

Temporary colourants
The mildest form of hair colourant, also known as water rinses, these temporarily coat hair with colour which will wash off at the next shampoo. It may come off gradually anyhow, on hairbrushes, in the rain or a swimming-pool, and will fade as the days go by. Temporaries which are combined with a setting lotion, as most are, have more staying power. When using the shampoo type for the first time, wash your hair first with your usual shampoo, and use the colourant for the second application. You can be more daring next time if you like the effect.

When to use. Temporaries are the ideal colourant for greying hair, as this is porous and often delicate. They are also good for masking yellow tones in white hair. Temporaries are a safe way to tone down yellow or brassy shades that frequently spoil bleached hair, but as bleached hair is more porous, particularly at hair tips, it can colour unevenly,

and it is important to care for the condition first. A temporary will show up as highlights on light brown hair, but will have little effect on dark brown or black.

Semi-permanents
These penetrate the cuticle of the hair and adhere to the outer layer of the cortex but do not chemically alter the hair structure or the natural pigment. A semi-permanent should last for between six and eight shampoos, fading gradually. Some are foamed in after washing, others are combined with a shampoo. Most manufacturers attempt to guide you in the result you can expect from a colour choice, but remember you are only adding colour to your own natural colour, so these semi-permanent colourants are best used only as colour refreshers.

Warning. Some wrongly named semi-permanents *do* contain peroxide. If the product claims to alter the shade of your hair, making it either lighter or darker, this *must* be the case, so read the package carefully. One or two products also contain the para compounds usually associated with permanent colourants. Read all the small print and, if necessary, do a skin test.

When to use. Because of the colour-on-colour principle, semi-permanents are at their most effective giving warm gold, russet or chestnut tones on brown hair; any shade from pale mouse to near black will benefit. Some products are specially developed to put softer, more subtle tones into drab blonde or bleached hair which all too often goes brassy. Semi-permanents are only partially effective on grey hair and will not cover white streaks, so they are not recommended if more than 5 per cent of your hair is white.

Permanent colourants
Here is a product upon which hang two very divided views, both of them valid. Any self-respecting hairdresser will advise you never to use a permanent tint at home, not because he wants the lion's share in this more expensive side of hairdressing, but because he knows that to apply it well needs a great deal of expertise. In many salons a specially trained colourist will deal with this aspect of hairdressing only.

The other side of the coin is that there has been a huge boom in the sale of do-it-yourself permanent colourants; they are the most widely-used products for hair colour change. The public clearly want them and manufacturers have greatly improved the composition and the method of application. Packets are carefully labelled and instructions detailed; every help is given to get the best possible result under home conditions. These para-

compound dyes are often known as oxidation dyes because of the use of hydrogen peroxide to activate them. They penetrate the cuticle, then react with the hydrogen peroxide and the natural pigmentation within the cortex to form the new colour which becomes permanently 'locked' in. When this happens hair is chemically changed. The strength (volume) of hydrogen peroxide depends on the job it has to do. A low-volume peroxide is mild, will not bleach, and is used when hair is to be coloured darker, a similar shade, or for covering grey hair. A higher volume peroxide is necessary if hair is to become lighter. It is said to 'lift' colour, as it removes pigment.

In a hair salon, the permanent tint is usually applied to dry, unwashed hair by dividing the hair into partings. This sectioning method gives the best control as some parts of the hair take colour more quickly than others. This method is the best choice at home also, although it is very fiddly to do unaided. The product usually comes in two bottles which are mixed together to form a cream or gel, which is applied to the sectioned hair with a brush. Much easier to apply are the shampoo-type permanents which are foamed on all at once. Unfortunately, however, it is much more difficult to achieve an even colour with these. It is worth remembering that heat accelerates the development time of a permanent colourant, so a tint will take more quickly in a hot climate or a warm, steamy atmosphere.

Root retouching
No new colour looks good if dark roots show through, so a four- or six-weekly routine of root retouching is a must. It needs a very steady hand and lots of patience. The process can take as long, if not longer, than a first application, since great care must be taken not to overlap on to pre-coloured hair. Some consumer products claim that no root retouching is necessary, and that a complete head tint can be applied every time roots show. However, this can give uneven colour as there are different development times between new and previously coloured hair.

Remember also that frequent use of chemicals on your hair *must* cause damage and lead to poor condition unless you take great care of it.

Rules for home-permanent colouring
1 Never colour unhealthy hair.
2 Do not colour
- if skin or scalp has abrasions or a rash
- if bleaches or other colourants, such as henna, or the liquids which claim to restore colour to grey hair have been used

- if hair has been permed or straightened within two weeks
- without asking advice on colour
- before you have done the three tests on page 178.
3 Do not colour until
- you have plenty of time
- you have read the instructions
- you have laid out all required equipment
      contents of colourant pack
      rubber gloves
      cotton wool
      old towel and/or T-shirt
      watch or timer
      non-metallic bowl
- you have applied a layer of cream to hair line to prevent staining.
4 After colouring your hair
- use a mild shampoo; strong shampoos, especially medicated ones, can drastically 'lift' colour, i.e. intensify it
- keep hair in good condition
- don't use further chemicals at the colouring session, especially a permanent wave which can strip colour; perm at least two weeks before you colour
- throw away any unused mixture; it will not keep and could be harmful to children
- if bowl is used wash thoroughly, immediately
- check that make-up and clothes blend with your new colour.

Henna
Henna is a non-toxic dye made from the leaves of the tropical Lawsonia plant; the strength of pigment varies according to the area from which it comes in Africa or Asia. Because henna does not change the hair chemically, the condition of your hair is enhanced rather than damaged by its use. Although people think of henna as a permanent colourant it does fade gradually, and its use is limited as it comes only in red or brownish red tones – the dye itself is green, as it is made from leaves. As henna is variable in colour it is not possible to standardize results and development time could vary from five minutes to an hour or more, depending on the henna, your hair and the desired result. The henna is mixed with hot water to form a smooth, workable paste and is applied to the hair in sections with a brush, as with permanent colourants. Sometimes black coffee or lemon juice are added to increase depth or richness of tone.

When to use. Henna gives marvellous richness to black and brunette hair. There is a fifty-fifty chance of good results on mousy hair, depending on the texture; it could be very hectic or very disappointing. Henna is not advisable on a natural blonde and is positively bizarre on a bleached blonde. It is *not* for grey hair, as it could turn it a vibrant orange!

Henna hazards
As colour is unpredictable, don't

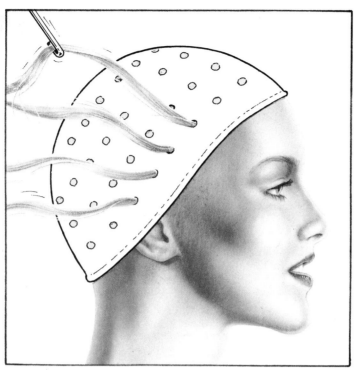

Home highlighting is easiest using swimcap, although results are not as fine as salon method. Tight-fitting plastic cap is well punctured, pulled on to head, and hairs to be bleached eased through with crochet hook.

colour your whole head without doing a strand test first (page 178). If your hair has been chemically treated by perming, straightening or colouring, don't try henna at home – let a hairdresser advise you as the results could be disastrous. Compound hennas which are mixed with other, usually metal, substances can be very risky. It is much better to stick to pure henna if possible.

Bleaching
Bleaching or lightening of hair can be done in two ways:
1 A colourant which is made up of the same ingredients as a permanent tint, i.e. a para dye plus hydrogen peroxide, can be applied. To remove pigment, the peroxide volume is higher to give more 'lift'. The deeper your natural colour, the stronger the mixture and the longer the development time required. A bleach will reduce colour in stages from red, orange, through to yellow, until almost all colour goes. But the longer a bleach is left on, the more damage it will do to hair.

To become blonde, a single application of bleach and toner combined in one product will lighten hair that is already light in tone. A darker natural colour will need two processes: a pre-bleach to remove pigment, then the new colourant. Pre-bleaching requires a great degree of technical skill and should be done by an expert, although you can buy products, made by reputable firms, to do this job at home if you are prepared to risk your hair.

2 A 'brightener', a mild bleach which keeps hair looking sunny throughout the year, can be used. It is usually incorporated in a shampoo or a setting lotion. These products are for hair which is already light in colour. They do not require root retouching if used only about every three months.

Highlighting
This is usually considered the most successful way to go blonde. It is the most expensive colouring process at a hairdressing salon, because it is the most time-consuming. Very fine strands of hair are 'lifted', and the cost and effect depend on how many highlights are put in.

If a great many highlights are put in the effect will be all-over blonde, while a few will give just a touch of sun. Experts may try special effects, such as 'tipping', which confines highlights to hair ends. Lowlights are another interesting way to brighten your hair. In this process, darker streaks are put into your hair by means of a tint. Unlike all-over colouring, highlights and lowlights grow out without showing a hard root line. They need renewing every six to nine months, although some hairdressers like to refresh partings and hair line in between.

The usual salon way to do highlights is by sectioning off fine strands of hair and bleaching them separately from the rest of the hair in strips of aluminium foil. A quicker method, introduced in America in the early 1960s, is the cap method. This is certainly easier to attempt at home, but the effects are never as fine as with the salon method. The hair is combed into place and a plastic swimcap is pulled on to the head, having first been punctured with tiny holes. The hair is lifted through in fine strands with a crochet hook. Bleach and peroxide are mixed into a paste and applied to the strands of hair outside the cap. Development time varies according to the lift required. The disadvantages of this method are that it is difficult to reach to the root, the cap can split causing bleach to seep through to other hair, and variable tones cannot be achieved. However, it is undoubtedly cheaper and quicker than the salon method. Before removing the cap, lather on shampoo all over it. This avoids pulling painfully and damaging the hair.

PERMANENT WAVING AND STRAIGHTENING
Permanent waving and hair-straightening are basically the same process. Both of them entail re-forming the hair shaft. In both cases a lotion softens the hair's structure; if curls are desired, hair is rolled or curled accordingly, while to straighten the hair and lotion is combed through and left to soften it, and then the hair is combed continuously for ten to twenty minutes. A second lotion, known as a neutralizer, is then applied to stabilize the process. In fact, this second solution does not neutralize or cancel out the effect of the first lotion since the hair has already been changed chemically. The second lotion fixes the hair into its new molecular structure by means of oxidation.

Perming can be done at home if you follow the instructions exactly. Wash hair first, as dirt or grease will inhibit the effect. Do test curls on strands at the nape of the neck: the larger the roller the looser the curl. If hair is grey, bleached or coloured curl will take more quickly, so check after half the recommended time. Do not perm if your hair has been coloured recently or if skin or scalp is blemished or in poor condition. Take great care and remember that you are chemically changing the structure of your hair; once damaged, you cannot put it right and have to wait until the perm grows out. Never attempt hair-straightening at home; ordinary perming lotions are not designed for it.

The frequency with which hair can be safely permed depends on its strength and condition. Some hair can be permed every three to four months, some less frequently, and some should not be permed at all. If you are in any doubt consult a good hairdresser, as perming requires great caution, particularly with difficult hair.

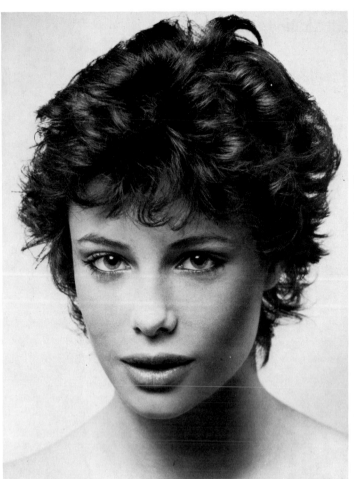

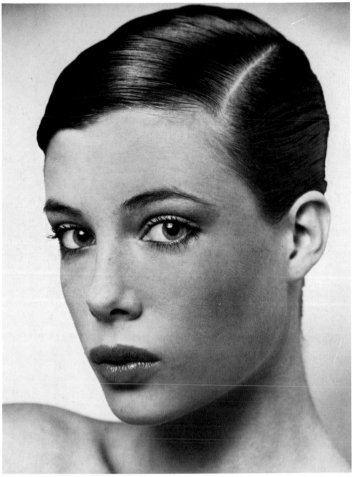

YOUR HAIRDRESSER

Trusting your hair to a new hair-dresser can be very worrying, simply because a mistake can take a long time to rectify. If your hair is cut too short or badly or the colour is wrong you will feel miserable, so do a little research first. Results speak for themselves, so look around your friends and neighbours, pick a pretty head, and ask for the name of their salon. If you are starting cold in a new area, a salon window will tell you a great deal. It should be clean and attractive and the price list should be clearly visible. If it's expensive, it doesn't mean that it is good, but indicates that the salon is aiming at an up-market clientele and probably has modern equipment.

The pictures in the window may not be styles created in that particular salon, often they are advertising showcards, but they will tell you the sort of work the salon admires. Be warned by this, because if the styles are high fashion that is what you are going to get. It is pointless going to the smartest hairdresser in town and paying the earth when their styling isn't going to suit you.

If the price list isn't in the window, go to the reception desk and ask to see it. Have a good look round. Check for cleanliness – a dirty salon can't be a good

one. The reception area can tell you a great deal. Are the staff busy or hanging about chatting? Is there a place for the clients' coats and a clean gown for everyone? Is the receptionist polite and well groomed and do you like her hairstyle?

Don't antagonize a new hairdresser by dictating to him. If he is good he will care about your hair as much as you do. However, it is helpful if you have a picture of a style you like. He may not agree that it would suit you or your hair, so be prepared to discuss it with him objectively. Tell him how your hair usually behaves and if it is coloured or permed; he *must* know what has been used on your hair, as horrible things can happen when chemicals are mixed.

Don't expect a miracle on the first visit. A hairdresser needs time to get to know how your hair responds and moves. He also has to take your face and figure into account, but a lot depends on your personality, so he has an advantage when he knows you better. He may persuade you to change your view of yourself. Nothing is more ageing than a hairstyle you chose ten years ago. Your face and hair line change, although you may not realize it. A good hairdresser will pick up your personal fashion look and

translate it into a hairstyle.

It is the expert in cutting who makes a top hairdresser. A basic training will teach methods and shapes, but to perfect the art takes years of practice. If the cut is poor, the hairstyle will be a disaster. If it is good, it should last until your next visit, be adaptable, and be easy to wash, set and maintain yourself.

Go for a wash and set on the first visit, and leave the cut until you are confident. Watch the stylists at work, and make sure they are doing the work which requires experience. A hard-pressed salon will delegate too many jobs to juniors. If you are thinking of having your hair coloured, talk to the colourist before your next appointment and check to see whether a junior is putting on colour. Most trainees are not up to this work and a mistake could be disastrous.

A popular stylist will not give of his best if he is rushed. Normally a salon's busiest time is the end of the week, Saturdays being the worst, so book earlier in the week.

Once you have found a good hairdresser stay with him or her; switching round does nothing for mutual confidence and rarely brings rewards for your hair either. For equipment to help you handle your hair at home, see page 214.

YOUR HAIRSTYLE

The hairstyles and their variations on these and the following pages were created by Leonard of Mayfair. A neat head in a very short hair-style has one essential starting point, a superb cut, so that even though hair is short it need not always look the same and can change mood by brushing. Here is an ideal style for springy, strong hair. It is also good for fine, straight hair which lacks body. A cut of this severity is at its best if facial bone structure is good, particularly chin line. A narrow nape of neck also improves the back view.
Above left: The basic style, a tumbled natural look. Hair is patted and rubbed vigorously with a towel, then allowed to dry naturally. In fine, straight hair, movement may need encouraging with careful use of curling tongs.
Above right: Eton crop achieved by a long side parting and a well-brushed shape, with hair taken behind ears. Sleekness comes from just-washed hair or a dab of pomade smoothed between palms of hands and slicked on.
Right: Individual flavour from clever Teddy-boy style brushing, a good cover for out-of-condition hair. When pomade is used on this style it should be massaged in well and combed through for a good sheen. Pomade should be washed out each night and applied fresh every day.

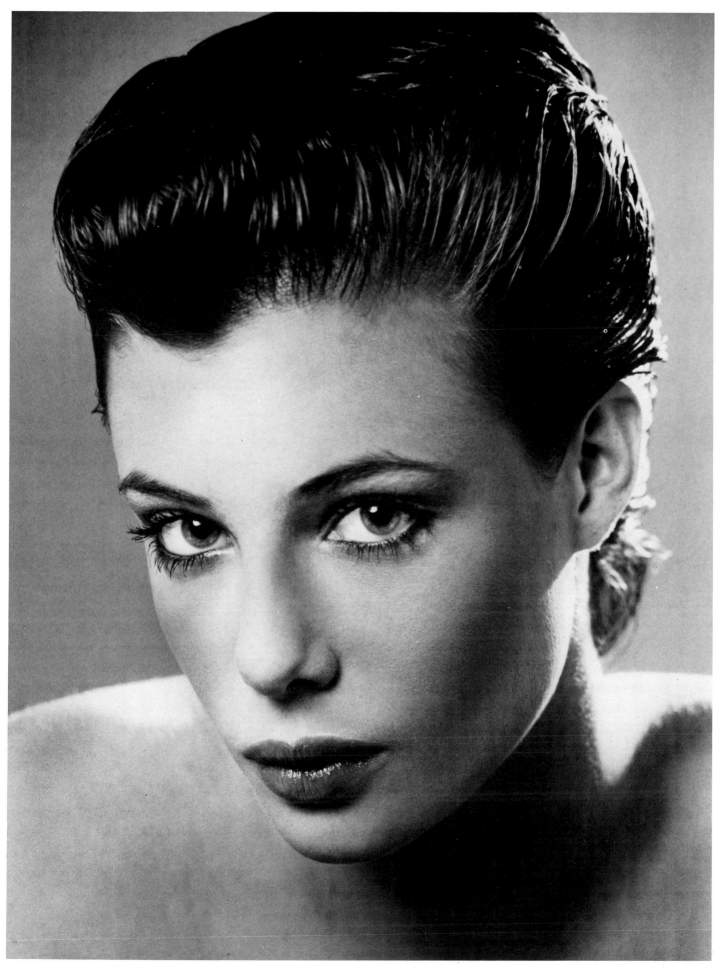

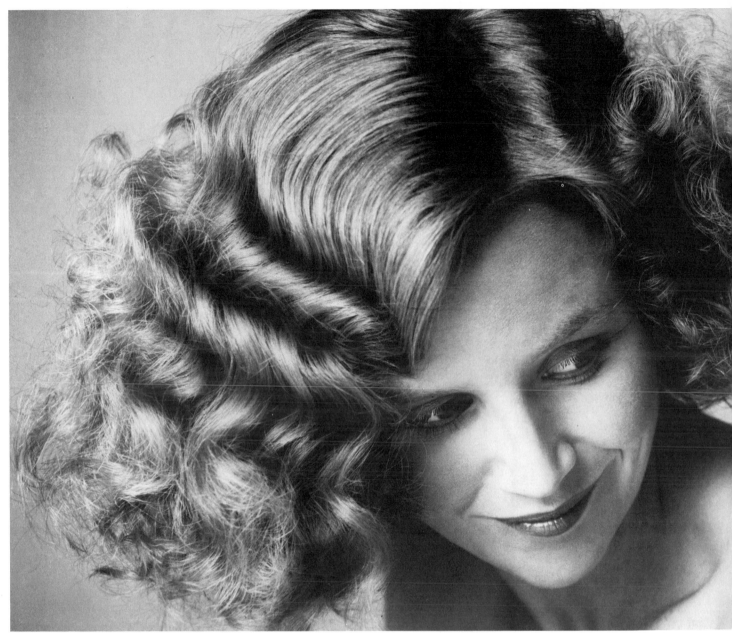

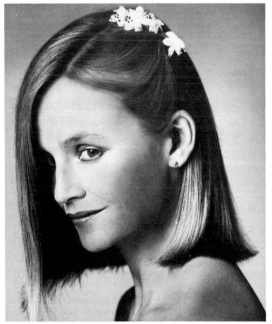

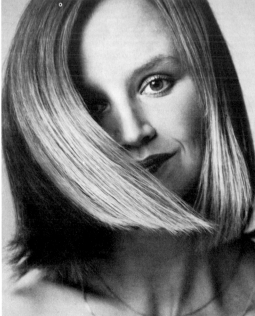

Typical Caucasian hair: fine, straight and fly-away. Here it is cut to one length to fall perfectly, for easy management. Like all ultra-simple styles, it calls for top condition with smooth, silky sheen.
Left: The basic style, straight, sleek and freshly washed to give a soft, natural swing which always falls back into place.
Far left: One side falling forwards, the other swept back in a comb. For slippery hair, a line of grips will hold brushed-back hair in place. Comb is slipped in afterwards.
Above: A tumble of ultra-feminine curls adds width to face and gives soft, casual lightness. Hair can be set after washing with small rollers, wound to within finger length of crown. The same effect could be achieved just for one night with heated rollers. A perm, again wound on small rollers, would give the style staying power if you wished to wear it regularly.

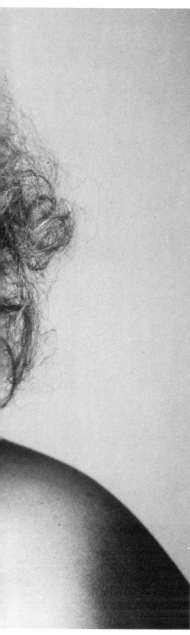

Right: A smooth and tailored twist for evening. From a side parting, front strand of hair on each side of head is twisted round, ends meeting at one side of crown. Ends are tucked away and secured with grips or pins (grips give a firmer hold). A decorated comb gives a finishing touch and hides under-pinning. On fine, light hair, comb alone holds securely. Another pretty version of this style is with a centre parting and two tiny plaits taken from temples to meet high up at centre back in a comb.

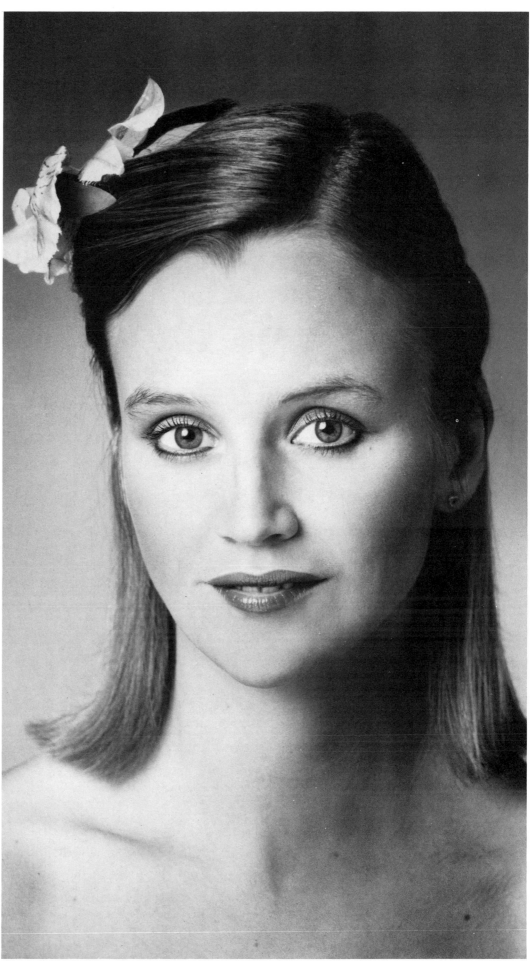

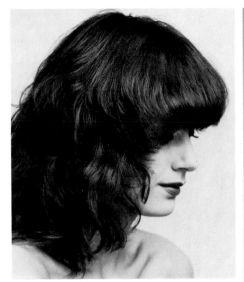

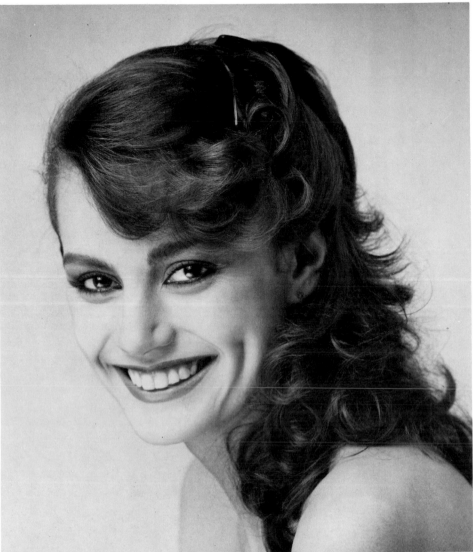

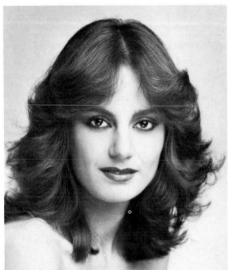

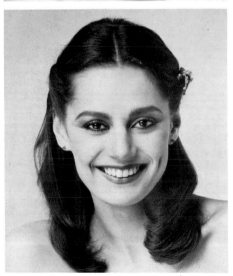

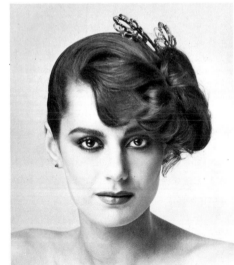

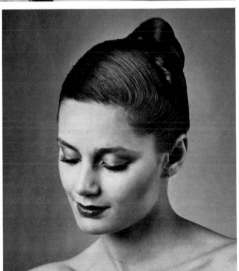

Very thick, fine hair with lots of natural movement.

Top left: The basic style is layer cut to add body, towel dried and brushed forwards. Fringe is straightened softly with brush and blow-dryer.

Centre left: Breezy softness framing face. From a centre parting, hair is curled naturally away from cheeks and neck by blow-drying, flicking hair up with fingers or styling brush as it dries. Style can be done with heated rollers, but effect would be more strongly curled and less natural.

Above left: Sleeker style, ideal for holidays when hair is wet or needs a wash. From a centre parting, hair from temples is rolled and twisted back into combs at each side of crown.

Above centre: Unusual evening style. Hair is brushed firmly through, then all swept over to one side. Swathe is bunched firmly with a band, then twisted and brushed into one large curl, secured with grips and pins. Finish off with a comb or flowers. Front fringe is curled on to forehead.

Above right: Top-speed top-knot, for a last minute solution when hair is wet or greasy (could be slicked with pomade for added brilliance). Hair is tightly wound round head and into a high bun, secured with band and pins.

Top right: Spanish style, perfect also for hair with a strong, natural wave. Hair is brushed through and firmly swept across back to one side. Two combs hold back in place, a third controls front crown hair.

184

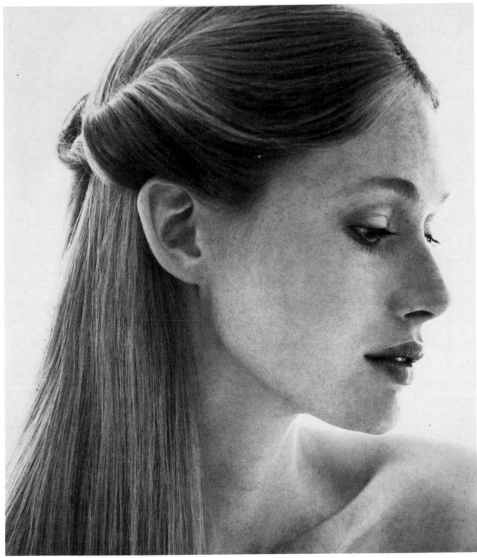

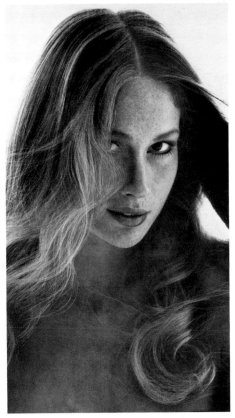

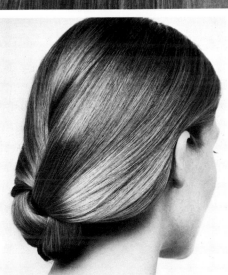

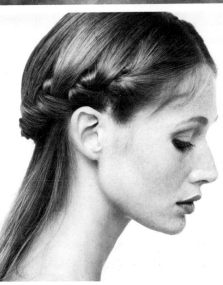

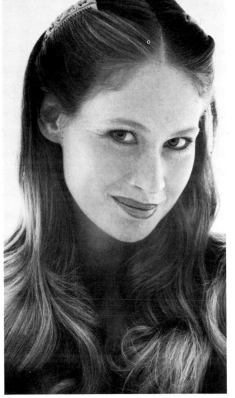

Very long hair, of a thick, abundant type with some natural wavy movement. Heavier texture hair needs firm handling when completing more complicated styles.
Top right: Flowing movement, brushed from a centre parting. Hair could be naturally wavy or curled at ends with large, heated rollers.
Bottom right: Off the face and easy. Brush temple hair up and back and finish each side with a comb. On heavy hair like this, arrangement is almost always in need of basic security. Before placing combs, slip a line of grips just beneath.
Above centre: Medieval lines formed by simple but rather fiddly plaiting, done more easily with a friend's help. This style would also add bulk to finer, thin hair. A narrow section is taken from front temple and plaited. After weaving a few times, next section of crown hair is brought in and plait continued; the process is then repeated. When plait reaches nape, having taken up all crown hair, end is secured temporarily and plait on other side completed. Nape hair is left loose, with ends softly curled. Plait ends are twisted into tiny bun high at back of neck.
Above left: Sculptured classic comes from a single, loosely woven plait, with ends banded and folded out of sight under hair line. Fix securely with pins.
Top left: Romantic twist, very straightforward. Hair is twisted back from each temple. Secure with grips and fix with one comb placed firmly at centre back.

185

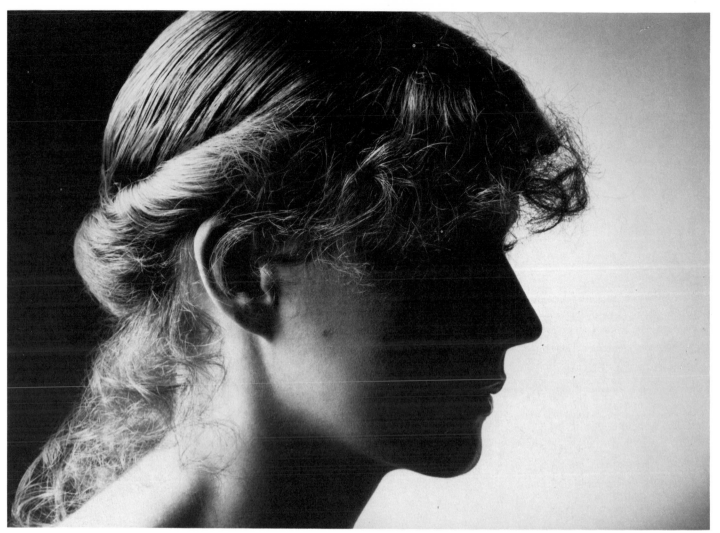

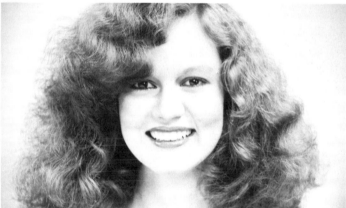

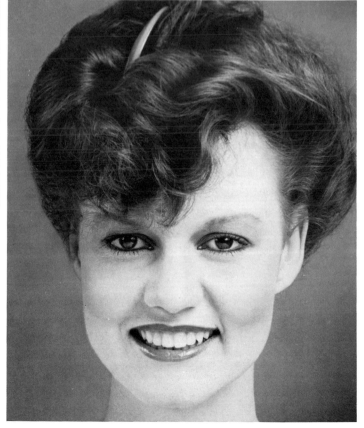

An abundance of thick, strong, wavy hair, often of Mediterranean origin, is easier to handle if cut conforms with direction of growth. Styles are limited, but sheer wealth of hair is rewarding.

Above: In its natural state. After washing, hair is lightly combed into shape and allowed to dry naturally. Fall over temple frames face.

Right: Combs work admirably in this type of hair and hold without slipping. Edwardian froth, shown here, is also adaptable for shorter and less wavy hair. To achieve, throw head forwards, brushing all hair towards face. Hold hair bunched together, while separating out a small section above each ear. Secure bunched hair close to crown with covered band, roll round, tuck in ends, and secure with grips. Now brush each side into centre, training ends over forehead, and finish with combs. Soft tendrils can be pulled out in front of ears.

Top: Elegant control for hard-to-tailor hair. Brush hair well, dampen, then comb to slick back. Divide hair between hands, then twist from sides to nape of neck, as for first stage of a knot. Pull out back tendrils. Bring two twists together, tuck in ends, roll hair up neatly, and pin securely into place.

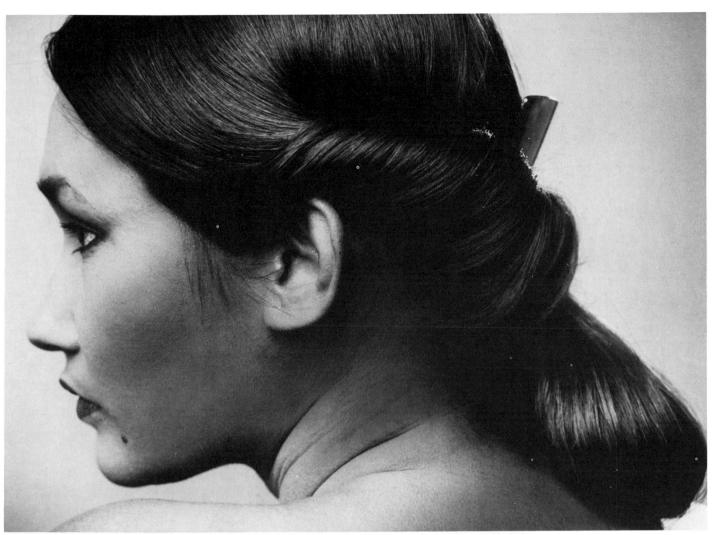

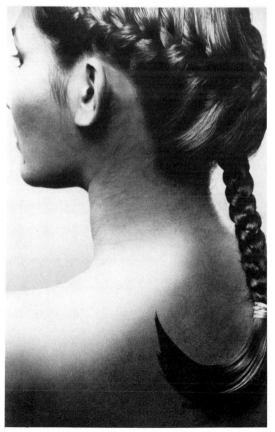

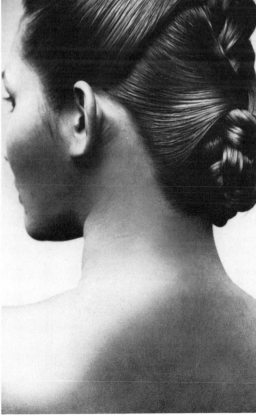

Eastern hair, thick and springy, is sometimes heavy to handle. By nature straight, shape and movement come with styling. *Above:* Basic swathing. Hair is divided into three sections. Two side sections are parted in centre and secured temporarily out of the way. Back section is brushed and folded under, ends are tucked in, and the whole is bunched with a band. Two side sections are rolled towards back, crossed, ends tucked in and pinned securely. Comb provides clasp and decoration. *Far left:* Grown-up plaits. Although style is simple, you may need help to achieve it as very arm-aching work is involved. Divide off narrow section of hair at temples and begin plaiting. After four or five folds, pick up next section of hair, blend into plait, and continue weaving. Repeat until all crown hair is taken up and secure ends temporarily. Complete second side in the same way. Finally, blend two side plaits into third from nape. *Left:* Fresh shape to plaiting. Make a huge parting from ear to ear across back crown and begin plaiting all crown hair. Blend two main side sections into plait, leaving nape hair free. Finally plait in nape section, tuck plait under hair line, and secure with grips.

187

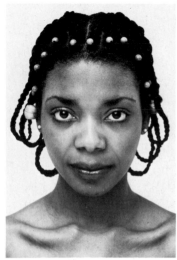

Classic African styles are achieved by using false hair, plaited into short hair. In this way, delicate negroid hair can be kept short and well conditioned while at the same time a variety of styles can be created.

Right: Scalp is squared off into divisions. False hair is woven into existing sections of hair by plaiting hair from root together with false hair. If natural hair is very short, some hair can be threaded into a large darning needle and sewn into plait to hold. Traditional beads are threaded or sewn on to ends.

Above: Scalp is divided as before. Beads are secured to short forehead hair by threading small sections of hair into a large needle and sewing beads in place. Looped false plaits are woven into real hair or darned in as before; ends are tucked in and secured with pins. This is fiddly and tiring work, easier if you have a friend to help. Hair is often more manageable if damped well or made pliable with gel.

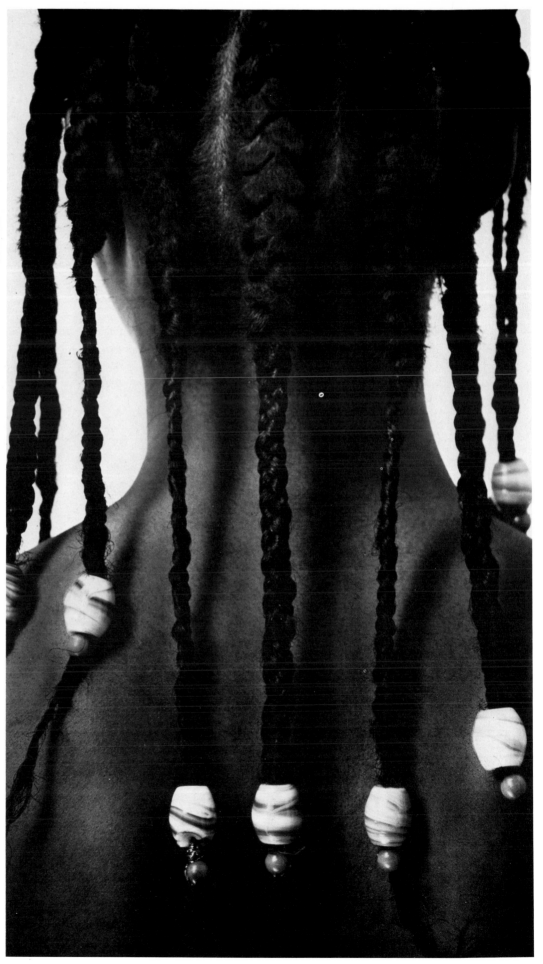

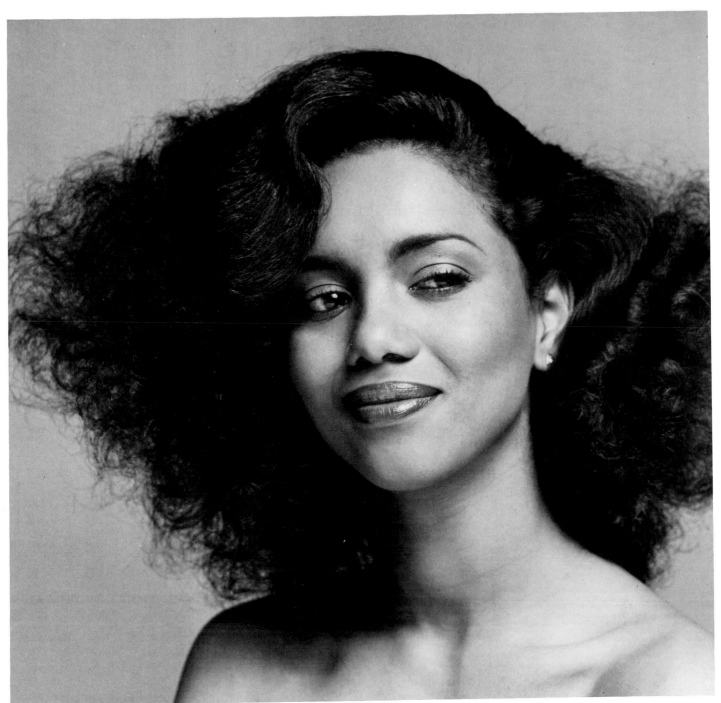

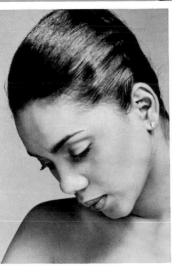

Fragile negroid hair needs to be carefully tended to maintain healthy, silky-soft condition. *Above:* Partially straightened by holding crown hair tightly when wet, then blow-drying. Rest of hair is left to dry naturally, then fluffed out with pronged comb and fingers. *Left:* Absolute control put in place by complicated plaiting. Enlist help of a friend unless you have put in plenty of practice. Hair is waxed, using strong gel, then combed backwards. A continuous plait winds from ear to ear. From a back parting, begin plait at ear level, weaving several times before blending in next batch of hair. Continue weaving and adding hair to plait until whole head is woven in and plait ends over other ear. Tuck ends under and pin securely.

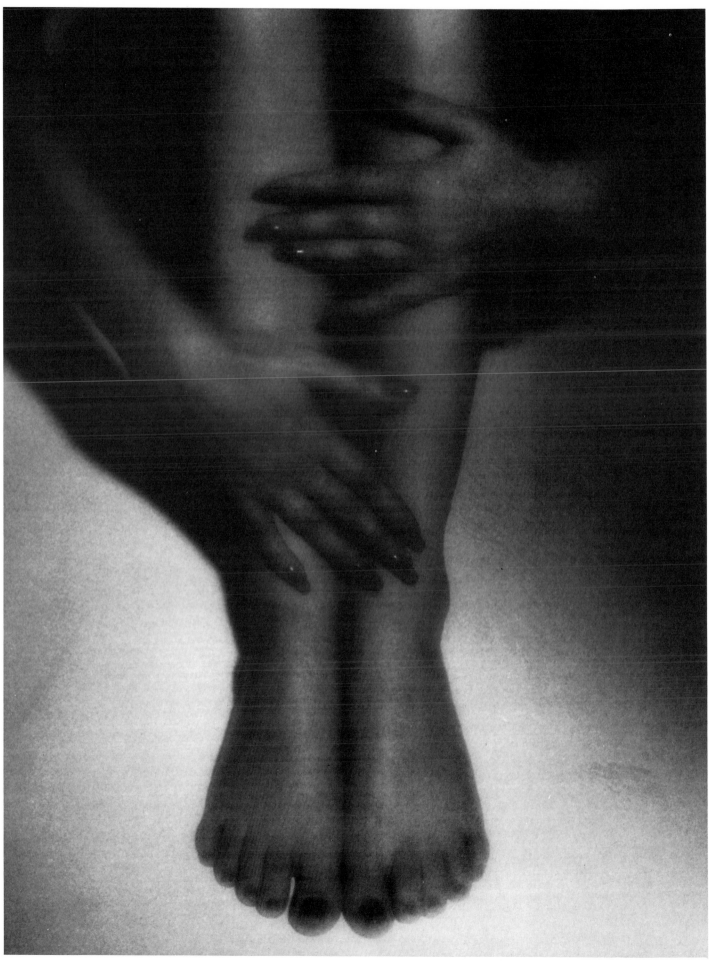

Hands and Feet

Our hands and feet get a regular battering in the course of our lives and yet we expect them not only to work efficiently but also to look good. We squeeze our feet into too-tight shoes and complain when they hurt or grow corns. We totter around on high heels that wreck the shock-absorbing and balancing systems that nature has engineered, and wonder why we are tired and headachy. We plunge our hands into oil-stripping detergents, we batter our nails against typewriter keys, we forget to wear gloves in the cold, and when we remember to smear on a dollop of hand cream we feel smug about it, and a little hurt that our hands still look rough and worn and not quite like those in the beauty pages. Beautiful hands are a tremendous advantage – women with fairly unremarkable faces and figures can have lovely hands that are almost hypnotically attractive to watch. Almost any pair of hands can look beautiful if they are cared for and manicured regularly, and our feet deserve similar attention. Aching feet can spoil our looks and make life a misery. Even if they don't hurt, how many of us could take off our shoes right now and show a pair of feet we don't have to apologize for? A monthly pedicure, massage with hand cream and some pretty polish could make going barefoot a pleasure.

Protecting the hands

Not so long ago, hands were thought to reveal your social status to the world – a 'lady's' hands were white and soft, showing that she did no manual work, and in order to keep them this way hand care was taken very seriously. It was quite accepted for a lady to sleep in gloves, put on over a thick coating of cream, so that all night the skin of the hands was being pampered and fed. It is astonishing how effective this treatment is; try rubbing in cream and then sleeping in short cotton gloves just once and you will be surprised at the softness of your hands next morning.

Gloves of all kinds are the first step to improving your hands. Rubber gloves are awkward to wear at first, but all experts agree that they are a habit worth cultivating. If you have time, rub a little hand cream into your hands before putting them on and make yourself wear them for all washing-up and cleaning jobs. A substitute for the sleep gloves is to smother your hands with cream and then pop on a pair of cotton gloves *under* the rubber gloves, but this is only worth doing if you plan to spend a couple of hours cleaning or washing. Buy rubber gloves that have their own built-in lining; they are much more comfortable. Keep them beside the sink so that you cannot forget to put them on. For finer, more intricate work such as cooking or hair washing, you can use thin surgical or hairdresser's gloves.

If you work in the garden, wear gardening gloves to save your hands. Put a barrier cream on underneath if you have particularly dry hands. Even ordinary wool or leather gloves are important for protecting your hands in cold weather. Think how chapped and painful and stinging your face can feel, and remember that unless your hands are covered they are suffering the drying effects of cold weather just as badly. For advice on how to cope with chapped hands and other problems, see page 219.

Cleaning

It may sound odd, but you can forget for days on end actually to clean your hands. You may *wash* them at odd moments during the day, but this is not the same thing. You are so busy cleaning your face, teeth and so on that your hands get left out.

Each night you should wash your hands with ordinary or facial soap, scrub the nails and cuticles* and knuckles, and, if you are dedicated, whizz over the hard bits of skin with a pumice stone. When drying your hands, develop the habit of pushing the cuticles back with the towel.

Stained fingers – either from vegetable or fruit juice or nicotine – can be coped with by rubbing with half a lemon. You may have to rub them with a pumice stone as well. Rinse well and cream.

Nourishing

Like skin-care products, hand creams are *not* necessarily better for being expensive. It is much more sensible to have several bottles of cheap lotion strategically placed around the house than one luxury bottle that you eke out nervously drop by drop.

Make the hand-cream habit easier for yourself by placing bottles in the places where you should remember to use cream: by your bed, by the sink, by the cloakroom basin, and so on. Last thing at night, after applying your moisturizer or night cream, massage in some hand cream. You don't have to spend long; just smooth on to the fronts and backs of the hands and massage each finger quickly. Bend the fingers backwards with the other hand and pull each finger gently to keep the joints flexible.

Lanolin is a good hand-softener, but it is also a little sticky, so use it only at night. It is excellent for the cuticles, so be sure to rub some in there, too. You can make your own hand cream from the recipe on page 218.

Dry, hard, dirt-engrained or neglected hands can have a special 'miracle wash' with sugar and vegetable oil. This unusual tip comes from a book on natural beauty by Clare Maxwell-Hudson (*The Natural Beauty Book*), and is very effective. Simply pour a little oil (maize, peanut or olive) into the palm of one hand and add a teaspoon or so of sugar. Rub the mixture all over the hands, really working it in, especially in the rougher areas. Rinse with warm water, dry and massage in a little hand cream.

Massage

After a manicure, or at night once in a while, give your hands a good massage.

1   Rub the cream into them thoroughly and then, one by one, massage each finger between the sides of the first finger and the thumb of the other hand, always working from the nail end towards the hand.

2   Now massage with the thumb in between the fingers, reaching over to rub the knuckles, too.

3   With the thumb tip of the other hand, massage each nail with a little lanolin or petroleum jelly.

Beauty treatment

You can give your hands a mask to improve the colour and texture of the skin, just as you do your face. If you use a commercial brand, choose a nourishing rather than a drying one, or make your own by mixing together:

1½ tbsp oatmeal
1   tbsp warm water
1   tsp olive oil
1   tsp lemon juice
1   tsp glycerine

Massage this mixture into the hands and leave for ten minutes, or overnight if you are prepared to wear sleep gloves.

Exercises

Exercising will stimulate the circulation of blood to the hands and encourage nail growth, and will keep the hands supple and flexible. As well as pressing back the fingers at night as suggested above, incorporate hand exercises into your regular daily exercise programme (see pages 64–65).

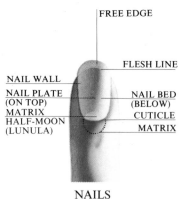

FREE EDGE

FLESH LINE

NAIL WALL
NAIL PLATE (ON TOP)
MATRIX
HALF-MOON (LUNULA)

NAIL BED (BELOW)
CUTICLE
MATRIX

NAILS

The most important part of the nail is the part we don't see – the matrix. The top of the matrix is sometimes visible as what we call a half-moon, but most of it lies below the cuticle. This is where the new nail cells are being built up and pushed forwards to become the nail plate, the horny part of the nail that we see. The nail plate consists of layers of hard, enamel-like substance, keratin,* which are held together by a small amount of moisture and fats. It takes from three to five months, depending on the individual, for the nail to grow all the way from the matrix to the tip. Consequently, and it is important to remember this, it will also take this long for any damage done to the nail while it was being formed in the matrix to grow out, or to see any improvement if you have started to condition your nails with a cuticle cream. Nails grow faster in summer than winter and faster on the right hand than the left. The rate of growth slows with age.

The nail bed lies under the pink part of the nail plate. The surface of the nail bed bears tiny parallel ridges which dovetail into similar ridges under the nail plate binding them firmly together. The nail plate and nail bed move forwards together as the nail grows. The free edge is the white part which is not attached to the nail bed; the nail walls are on either side of the nail plate; and the cuticle is the thin line of skin round the bottom of the nail protecting the matrix.

Foods and vitamins that encourage healthy nails
Nails need calcium, found in all dairy products: cheese, milk, yoghurt, and also in eggs. They need Vitamin B as well, found in yeast, in wheatgerm, cereal, wholemeal or rye bread.

It has been found that gelatine is particularly helpful to nails. One tablespoon of ordinary powdered gelatine taken once a day in water or fruit juice will make the nails stronger. It will take two or three months for the results to show, and you need to keep taking the gelatine as it is not a permanent 'cure'. For information on other nail problems, see page 216.

Manicure
Try to give yourself a manicure every week, whether you finish with polish or just a buffer; nails need looking after and a manicure does not have to take long. Collect everything in advance so that you do not have to keep fetching things and follow the diagrams and instructions. You will need:
bowl of soapy water or warmed oil
tissues
cotton wool
orange stick
cuticle clippers or scissors
oily polish remover
base coat
buffer
polish
sealer
nail repair kit.
Before starting, wash your hands and scrub your nails with a nail brush. Then you can settle down with a folded towel on the table and all that you need within reach.

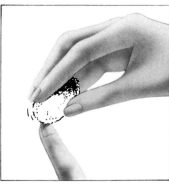

1 Remove old nail polish with cotton-wool balls and polish remover. Clean carefully especially round cuticle. Use an oily polish remover so that there is as little drying as possible and never be tempted to use acetone to save money: it will ruin your nails. Smudge-free remover makes the job easier and use enough cotton wool to prevent fingers staining.

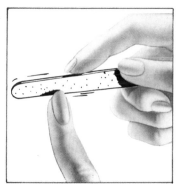

2 Using the fine side of an emery board, never a metal file, and holding it at an angle of 45° to the nail so that you are filing from just underneath, work from edges to middle in one direction only to prevent layers of nail plate separating. Never file right into corners of free edge of nail, as support is needed there to prevent nails breaking.

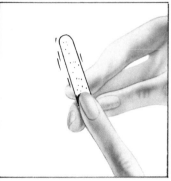

3 When the nail is filed into the shape you want, it is essential to bevel the edge. Bevelling is smoothing the edge of the nail by holding the emery board upright and brushing nail edge with light, downward strokes, using the fine side of the board and working in one direction only. This helps to seal the layers of the nail plate together and prevents layering.

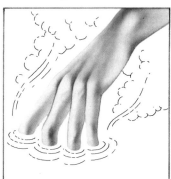

4 Rub a little cuticle oil into cuticles and soak nails for a few minutes in a bowl of warm, soapy water to soften cuticles, or do two jobs in one by soaking nails in a tiny bowl of warmed peanut or maize oil. Oil works as an inexpensive cuticle remover and is good for nails, too, as it keeps cuticles soft and supple. Dry nails and rub in hand cream.

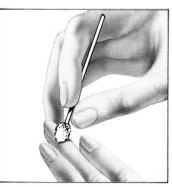

5 Wind a wisp of cotton wool around the pointed end of an orange stick and dip in cuticle remover or oil. Carefully work around cuticle to loosen it from nail plate and push back gently. If cuticle is stubborn, use the bare blunt end of the orange stick, taking care not to dig into the matrix or you will damage the growing nail and cause tiny white bruises on it.

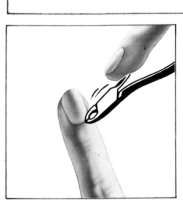

6 Clip away dead skin on cuticle or hangnail with cuticle clippers, taking care not to cut cuticle itself which can cause a painful infection and make cuticle tougher. Massage cuticle cream, lanolin or petroleum jelly into cuticles each night to keep them soft and detached from nail plate. Push cuticles gently back from nails with towel after your nightly bath or wash.

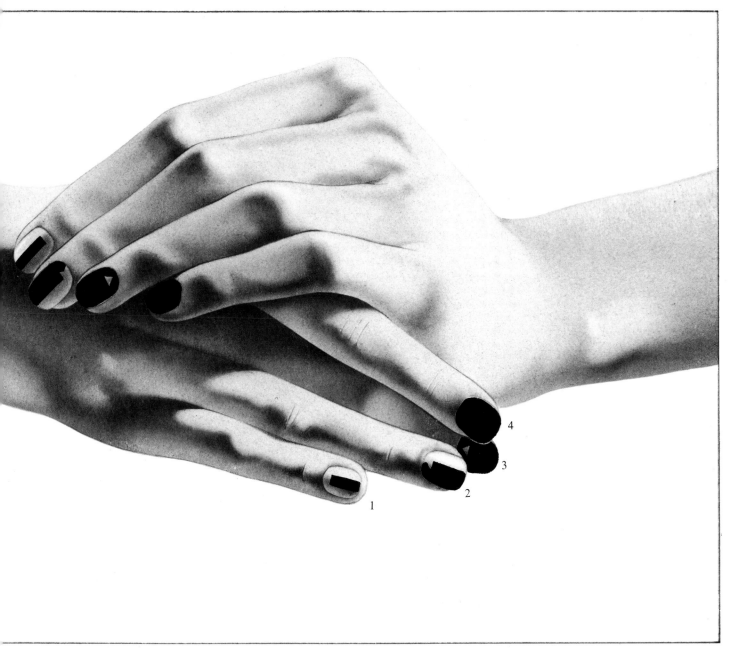

1
2
3
4

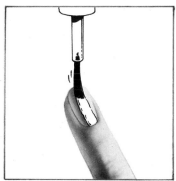

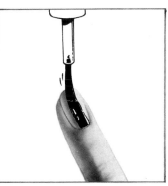

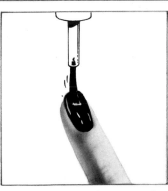

7 Wash off cuticle remover or tissue off as much surplus oil as possible. Polish will adhere without wiping nails with polish remover, which would undo the good of the oil soak. If you have a broken nail, wipe it with polish remover before applying patch (see overleaf). Apply base coat to nails before polish, to prevent staining and help protect polish from chipping.

8 All varnishes, nail enamels and nail-polish removers are drying to nails, but cream polish is marginally less harmful to weak and splitting nails than the frosted type. One, two or even three coats of nail polish can be applied on top of the base coat, using as few strokes as possible to prevent streaking, particularly with darker tones of polish.

9 A top coat or sealer on top of the coloured polish will take longer to dry but will help the manicure to last. When applying sealer, run brush along and under tip of nail to seal in polish and help prevent chipping. Dip a little cotton wool on an orange stick in polish remover and carefully clean off any spots of varnish around edges of cuticles or sides of nails.

For a perfect finish to your manicure, allow time to apply polish carefully. Make sure your hand is supported so that you are not aiming at a moving target. Put polish on with as few strokes as possible to prevent brush marks. Paint first stroke up middle of nail. Second and third strokes fill in underneath and up either side. Wide nails can be fined down by not taking polish to full width of nail. The fourth stroke is straight up the middle again to even out any brush marks. Add a second coat to get full colour of polish and to prevent streaking. Apply sealer coat and spray nails with quick-dry spray or stroke on a thin layer of oil once nails are no longer tacky. The surface of the nails will feel dry after ten to fifteen minutes but the layers will not be hard for several hours, so take great care not to scrape or dent them during this time.

Mending nails

The best method of mending a broken nail is to use a patch. Nail-patching kits are available which consist of special tissues and strong fixative or glue.

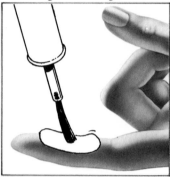

To mend break above flesh line. Tear tissue from pack provided; the jagged edge of a tear is less visible on nail than a cut edge. With thumb, hold tissue on forefinger and wet with nail glue.

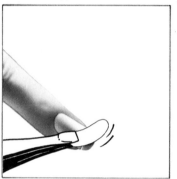

Using tweezers or orange stick, lay tissue on nail over break. Leave enough to tuck under edge of nail and cut off rest. A bad break may need a second tissue placed vertically over first.

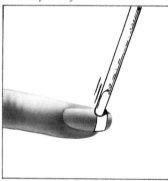

Wet underneath of nail with glue and tuck tissue under with orange stick. Smooth patch with a little solvent on finger tip. Apply more glue on top of patch and under nail. Allow to dry. Paint as usual.

   To mend break on flesh line.
Where tissue cannot be tucked under nail behind break, use a fine wisp of cotton wool wetted with nail glue. Smooth on to front of nail and thread through break, fixing firmly under top of nail. Apply patch on top of cotton wool and tuck behind nail to finish off repair neatly.

Natural nails

If you want to give your nails a rest from nail polish, here are two alternatives to try.

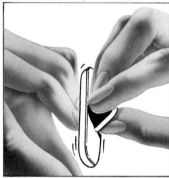

Buffing. A nail buffer is a pad covered with chamois leather or some other soft fabric with which you rub a shine on to the nails. It is a good treatment, stimulating the circulation and encouraging growth. You may use a nail buffing powder or paste or even a little oil with the buffer. The nails should be buffed in one direction only, preferably going from base to tip.

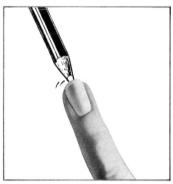

White pencil. Uncoloured nails sometimes look prettier if the tips are whitened by running a white pencil behind them. This enhances the natural look, but only works when the free edge is a good shape and of an even length on all ten fingers.

False nails

It is astonishing how many women, including models, television personalities and film actresses, wear false nails. There are two kinds: those that are glued on to your nails and those that are individually moulded on to your nails, using a type of cement and a shield-shaped mould. The stick-on kind are preferable, since the moulded nails are best done by a professional and can prove rather expensive.

Stick-on nails come in various sizes and shapes; buy those that best correspond to your own nail shape and size. Judge by width, and don't be put off if they are too long. The secret of effective-looking false nails is *preparation*. Each nail should be tried in place and then clipped and filed to the right length: don't have them too long or they will come off.

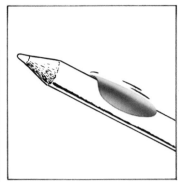

If angle across false nail is too shallow or too curved for your finger, soak nail in hot water and then either flatten out nail or curve it more deeply around pencil or orange stick. Take great care not to bend nail into too sharp an angle or it will crack. Prepare all ten nails in this way, as it is important that they fit properly in curve and length.

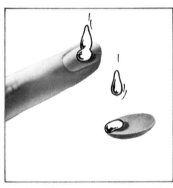

Apply nail glue to bottom half of each false nail. Allow to dry for at least half an hour or, even better, leave to dry overnight. Always keep nails in correct order to avoid confusion when it comes to sticking them on. Before applying false nails, loosen cuticles of your nails and apply nail glue to entire surface. Allow to dry for at least half an hour.

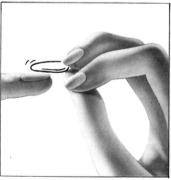

Taking great care not to damage either matrix or cuticle, carefully stick prepared nails on to your own, slipping bottom edge of false nail just under loosened cuticle. Press on firmly and your new nails will be very secure. Even so, always go out armed with a tube of nail glue in case of embarrassing accidents! Apply your nail polish as usual.

To remove stick-on nails, put a drop of the glue solvent provided in the pack into the side of each nail, or put your hands into hot water and peel the nails off when the glue has softened. You may find that if you have put the nails on really securely they take a bit of shifting, which is just as well: you don't want them coming loose every time you have a bath. Often, some glue is left adhering to the nail. You should be able to dissolve this with the glue solvent, provided you have some left – unfortunately, quantities are a bit mean. Usually the glue will rub off in a ball or can be picked off gently with a pin.

Cement nails are best applied by a professional, though there are home kits available. However, if they are applied by an unskilled and too-ruthless operator, they can be damaging to your nails. A professional will roughen the surface of your nails to help the cement adhere. Each nail is then individually moulded on to your own nail and trimmed and filed into shape when dry. The nails look extremely realistic, but there are 'growing out' problems when the lower edges of the false nails show on your own nails. The false nails must then be remoulded or filled. Some people find that after wearing cement nails for a while their own nails are weakened and may need a layer of mending patch while they toughen up.

Nail-biting

Hardened nail-biters can go through every supposed cure, from hypnosis to bitter aloes, without success. Often they only manage to stop biting their nails when they begin to take a pride and interest in them. Wearing false nails on and off can help by allowing the real nails to grow a little, so providing encouragement. The next step is to place emery boards wherever you might need them: in the kitchen, in your make-up bag, in your cardigan pocket, in the car, beside the bed, and in your office. When tempted by a snag or rough edge you can then immediately file it smooth. Manicure your nails every two days, no polish at this stage as they will be too short, and keep filing them down so that the torn, layered, jagged edges finally grow out into smooth and healthy nails. When long enough, coat them with opaque polish to disguise the fact that the free edges are much longer than most people's, and continue to manicure them frequently.

The rewards are positively intoxicating: no more extra-ordinary contortions of the hands in order to hold a glass or cigarette without your nails showing. You can now relax in other people's company.

FEET

Women in the Western world are not as foot-conscious as they are in many other places. Go to the hairdresser in the Far East and they may automatically whisk away your shoes and make you sit with your feet in a bowl of warm water, and then come and perform a thoroughly professional pedicure.

Most of our foot problems are our own fault, caused by total lack of care, or worse, by squashing our feet, which are highly complex systems of bone and muscle, into too-tight shoes or balancing them on too-high heels. Current fashions make it a little easier for us to be kind to our feet these days; the winkle-picker toes and stiletto heels that were once *de rigueur* have thankfully gone the way of many fashion fads. It is not as difficult nowadays to find shoes that combine elegance and style with comfort.

Pedicure

Whether you leave nails natural, buff them, use transparent polish, or sport toe nails to match finger nails, a regular pedicure will do marvels for the health and appearance of your feet. If you plan your pedicure after a bath, cuticles will be well softened; otherwise, you will need a bowl of warm, soapy water big enough to put your feet in without spilling. Put the bowl on the floor or a steady surface and lay a towel underneath. Collect everything you will need before you start:
nail-polish remover
cotton wool
nail brush
pumice stone
nail clippers
emery board
orange stick
oil and cuticle remover
hand cream
basecoat, varnish, sealer.

Rule 1

For healthy feet, buy shoes that really fit properly. Remember that many very painful foot problems can start with ill-fitting shoes. Never be persuaded by a bullying sales assistant; insist on shoes that feel comfortable in the shop. If they aren't comfortable there, they will be hell when you get them home. The best time to buy shoes is in the late morning or afternoon, when the trials and tribulations of the day have taken their toll and your feet are slightly larger than they were early in the morning.

Rule 2

Vary the height of the heels you wear. Very high heels throw the weight of the body off balance and can cause backache and even headaches. Try to spend *most* of your time in heels that are not more than 2 in (5 cm) high.

Rule 3

Go barefoot, or in thong or exercise sandals, as often as you can. Make it a habit, as the Japanese do, to slip out of your day shoes when you get home.

Rule 4

Exercise your bare feet as part of your daily exercise programme (see page 64). To give spring when walking the foot has two supporting arches: one lengthwise from the heel to the ball of the foot, the other running across the ball of the foot. In flat feet the weakened arches have fallen and much weight is carried on the sole of the foot, which is very tiring. Check the print of your foot from time to time by sprinkling talcum powder on the floor and making footprints. A healthy arch should show a good curve on the inside of the foot; a flat foot with a fallen arch will show a straight line. Exercise will help to strengthen the arches.

Rule 5

Massage your feet when they feel tired, preferably after a bath when they are clean and relaxed. Massage hand or body lotion all over the foot. Hold the foot in both hands and press the sole firmly with the thumbs along its length, especially on the ball of the foot. Massage each toe and between each toe. Pull the toes out gently. Massage round the Achilles tendon and ankle.

Rule 6

Give yourself a pedicure regularly – you will be surprised how much difference a little attention makes to the look and health of your feet. Don't neglect them just because they are not on show.

Rule 7

Visit the chiropodist once in a while for a good clean-up and scrape, and diagnosis of any serious problem (see page 212). *Always* go to the chiropodist if there is anything that particularly bothers you. It is silly to suffer when a visit to the expert could put the problem right.

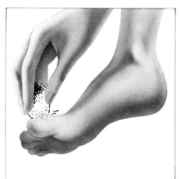

1 Remove old nail polish with polish remover and cotton wool. Take a few minutes to give feet a thorough check over for any dead skin, developing corns, moistness, cracked skin, or infection between toes. Check also that toe nails are the right length: if too short, feet will look blunt and unsightly; if too long, pressure from shoes will cause ridges to develop.

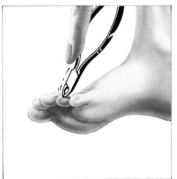

2 Trim nails to right length and shape with clippers. Never use scissors on tough toe nails as they can tear the whole nail tip off or crack it into the wrong shape. Smooth edges with an emery board and bevel as shown in manicure. Toe nails grow very slowly, taking ten to eighteen months to renew themselves, so if you cut weekly you will find little change.

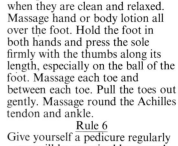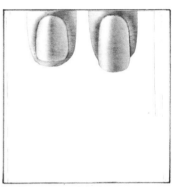

3 Be very careful always to cut toe nails straight across top. The right and wrong ways are shown in the illustration above. Do not shape nails down into corners of nail wall. This is one way of encouraging ingrowing toe nails, which can be extremely painful and difficult to reverse once they have become established in a wrong growing pattern, cutting into skin.

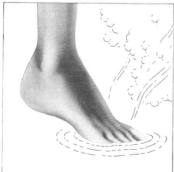

4 Soak feet in warm water for a few minutes, but no longer or you will remove natural oils. Scrub toes with nail brush. Tackle hard, dead skin under feet with pumice stone, special scraper or dead-skin removing cream. Push back softened cuticles with towel and dry feet thoroughly, especially in between toes where skin can easily crack and become infected.

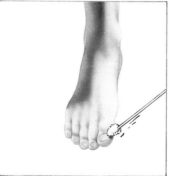

5 Go round each cuticle with cotton-wool-tipped orange stick dipped in oil or cuticle remover, cleaning underneath and down sides of nail. Loosen cuticle and push back gently from nail plate. Clip away dead skin with cuticle clippers. If using cuticle remover, scrub toe nails again with brush or tissue off excess oil. Push back softened cuticles with towel.

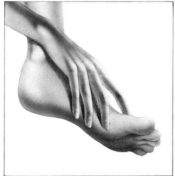

6 If skin between toes still feels a little moist, rub in talcum powder and brush off surplus. If you have a foot perspiration problem, spray foot with special anti-perspirant and allow to dry for a couple of minutes. Massage feet and ankles with hand cream, working upwards from foot to knee in direction of blood flow, with sweeping movements as shown on page 84.

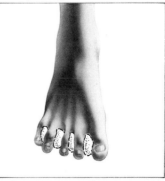

7 Separate toes with cotton wool or tissue to stop polish smudging from one toe to the next. Damp cotton wool slightly to prevent fluff sticking to polish. Paint nails with base, varnish and sealer as for manicure. Clean up edges with remover on orange stick. Dry with cotton wool between toes and go barefoot for a while to give polish time to harden.

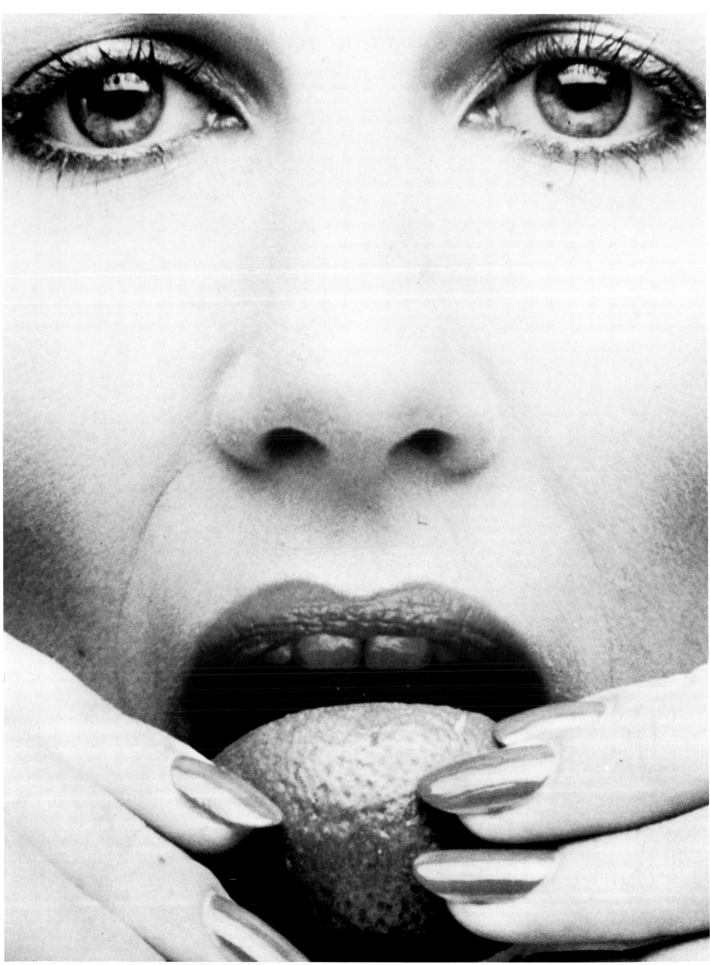

Eyes and Teeth

Good eyesight and a healthy set of teeth are invaluable assets to your general well-being. What is more, your looks benefit greatly from proper care and attention to them – the eyes and teeth are, after all, among your most noticeable features, and if they look unhealthy your appearance as a whole always suffers.
The person who has grown into full adulthood with perfect vision and without a single tooth filled is comparatively rare. But that doesn't necessarily mean that the rest of us must suffer for our imperfections. Improved dentistry and ophthalmic care must surely be counted among the areas in which scientific 'progress' *indisputably correlates with increased human happiness – how many people have been spared untold misery from near-blindness, or from all the pain and minor discomforts attendant on bad teeth, by treatment by the optician or dentist? Fortunately, too, medical care is able to take the appearance into account when putting right most of the common vision and dental defects – you have only to think of the invention of contact lenses and the crowning of teeth to realize this. These treatments are not cheap. But if they make your body more efficient, and boost your confidence by making a lasting improvement to your looks, they are worth it.*

EYES

Our eyes are in effect our windows on the world – it is through these complex sensory organs that the brain receives much of its information about the outside environment. It is worth detailing the constituent parts, and their functions, to show how the eye works as a whole. Starting at the front, from the outside in, the parts are as follows.

The conjunctiva is the mucous membrane which covers the front of the eyeball, and then doubles back to line the inside of the eyelid. It thus attaches the eyeball to the lid while still allowing movement. It must always be kept moist, and is extremely sensitive.

The cornea is the transparent layer in front of the eye, over the pupil and iris, which lets in the light. Its continuation is the sclera – the white of the eye – which surrounds the rest of the eyeball, except where the optic nerve enters at the back.

The iris, inside the cornea, controls the amount of light entering the eye by contracting or expanding to enlarge or reduce the size of the pupil. One cell layer of the iris, the stroma, contains pigment cells which determine eye colour. Albino eyes are pink because they lack pigment; most white babies are born with blue eyes, a sign of little pigment, but as more is deposited the eye colour often changes.

The pupil is the tiny hole through which light enters the eye. It looks black because the light is not reflected back from the inside of the eye.

Behind the cornea lies the anterior chamber, filled with a clear liquid, the aqueous humour, and behind this is the lens which, by being made less or more convex, focuses light rays on the back of the eyeball. The lens is held in place by the suspensory ligaments. These are attached in turn to the ciliary body, the muscles of which control the shape of the lens, stretching and elongating it when they contract, to adapt for long-distance focusing, and making it rounder and fatter when they relax, for short-distance focusing. This 'accommodation' to different focusing lengths occurs involuntarily, being controlled by the autonomic nervous system.

The rest of the eye behind the lens is filled with the vitreous body, a transparent jelly which keeps the eye's shape. The black spots that you sometimes see when looking at a pale surface are caused by specks floating in the vitreous body.

The choroid tissue lies inside the sclera round the back of the eye. It contains blood vessels, and its brown or black colour absorbs excess light inside the eyeball.

The innermost lining of the back of the eye is the retina, the complex nervous structure which contains the photosensitive cells, the rods and cones. These cells are densest at the fovea centralis, a small pit or depression in the retina where light has almost unrestricted passage to them; this is the area where vision is most accurate.

The optic nerve, which enters the eyeball at the rear, is a direct extension of the brain. The point at which it enters the eye is called the blind spot, since it has no light-sensitive cells.

Eye movement is controlled by six muscles attached to the sclera: four recti muscles, which run from front to back behind the eye, and two oblique muscles, running round the eye. Eyestrain is caused by the contraction of these muscles.

Protection from injury

Being ultra-sensitive, the eyes are protected from injury in several different ways:
1   The bony sockets of the skull frame and enclose them.
2   The eyebrows collect moisture from the brow and stop it from running into the eyes.
3   The eyelids keep the conjunctiva moist by blinking, thus sweeping fluid over the surface at regular intervals, every two to ten seconds, and during sleep they cover the eyes to prevent evaporation. The lids also prevent injury from foreign bodies by the automatic blink reflex.
4   The eyelashes catch particles of dust and grit, and may set off the protective blink reflex.
5   The lacrimal glands,* above and towards the outside of the eyes, produce tears – the salty fluid that cleans and lubricates the eye surface.
6   The lacrimal ducts drain the fluid into lacrimal sacs, leading into the nasal passage.

EYE CARE

The brain is a hard taskmaster to the eyes, constantly requiring them to pass on the maximum amount of information. If your eyes cannot function properly – either because they have an inherent focusing defect or because they are working in adverse conditions – they compensate by working extra hard, and this is where eyestrain occurs. Because the body's complex nervous system is heavily dependent on the eyes, eyestrain can give rise to fatigue, irritability and nervousness, which in turn are reflected back in the eyes, making them look dull and the surrounding skin lined.

Eyestrain commonly occurs after you have worked too long in a bad light, as a result of tension arising from bad posture, or when the eyes are trying to make up for a vision defect, as in the short-sighted child trying to see the blackboard from the back of the class. Reading or other close work need not necessarily strain the eyes, so long as it is done in the right conditions. The Association of Optical Practitioners in Britain stresses the importance of correct lighting: ideal conditions are 'a good *general* level of illumination with good *local* or possibly directional lighting' – in other words, a reasonable amount of overhead light supplemented by a table or desk light for close work like reading or sewing. *Don't* watch television in a dark room. The television screen is being bombarded with light from behind, and is glowing brightly; a light elsewhere in the room softens the glare without spoiling the image. This is quite different from cinema viewing when the picture is being projected from behind the audience on to the screen, and would disappear if the lights were on.

Ophthalmic opticians may tell you that since you are exercising your eyes ceaselessly throughout your waking hours, specific eye exercises are unnecessary except to treat particular muscular defects and after certain types of eye surgery. However, it is a good idea to give your eyes a break every now and then. Rest them by (a) blinking rapidly; (b) closing your eyes and covering them with the palms of your hands for a few minutes, while leaning your elbows on a table or desk so that your body is comfortable; and (c) bathing the eyes with cold water or covering them with a flannel soaked in cold water for a few minutes when they feel tired.

Diet is important for healthy, attractive eyes. You should be eating plenty of food rich in Vitamin A, lack of which causes night blindness (see below), and in the Vitamin B group. See page 40 for the best foods to eat to obtain these vitamins.

If you damage your eyes in any way, you should seek medical attention. It is usually possible to remove small 'foreign bodies' in your eye by pulling the upper lid out and down over the lower lid, or with the corner of a handkerchief. But if it refuses to budge, and your eye continues to be sore, have it attended to in case of infection. For information on conjunctivitis, styes, and other eye problems, see page 212.

You should see an ophthalmic optician if you experience any of the following: constant blinking, frowning, squinting, headaches, dizziness, blurred vision or blotches before the eye. He will be able to prescribe glasses for ordinary vision defects or refer you to a specialist in the case of eye disease.

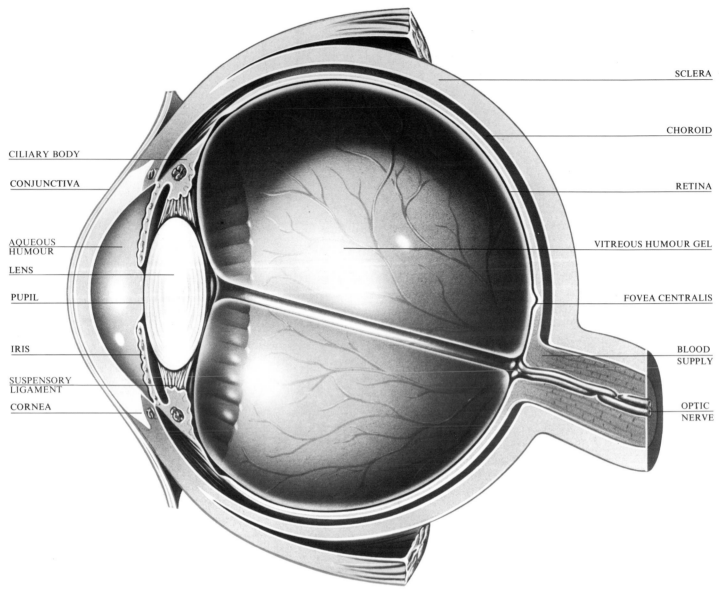

CILIARY BODY

CONJUNCTIVA

AQUEOUS
HUMOUR

LENS

PUPIL

IRIS

SUSPENSORY
LIGAMENT

CORNEA

SCLERA

CHOROID

RETINA

VITREOUS HUMOUR GEL

FOVEA CENTRALIS

BLOOD
SUPPLY

OPTIC
NERVE

CROSS-SECTION OF EYE

DEFECTS IN VISION

In normal sight, light rays passing into the eye are focused exactly on the retina, giving a small, sharp image, which is upside down and is reversed by the brain. It is amazing that emmetropia or normal sight *is* normal, given that $\frac{1}{25}$ in (1 mm) variation is enough to distort the image. However, the common forms of defective vision can usually be rectified by glasses or contact lenses.

Healthy young eyes have a tremendous focusing range, from long distance down to a few inches. This focusing range alters and reduces with age, and the change is particularly noticeable after the age of about forty. Don't worry about this, it is absolutely normal, so much so that if change of focus does not occur within a few years of the expected time you should have your eyes tested. Some people actually find that the change in focusing noticeably improves their sight.

Myopia or short sight occurs when the lens is too rounded and thick, or the eyeball is too long from front to back. The light rays are then refracted in front of the retina, making the image blurred. Glasses or contact lenses must be concave to correct the focus.

Hypermetropia or long sight occurs when the lens is too long and thin, or the eyeball is too short from front to back, so that the focus falls behind the retina again making a blurred image. Many people become mildly long-sighted as they get older. Convex lenses correct the focus for reading or close work.

Astigmatism occurs when the cornea is unevenly curved, so that the refractive power of the eye varies, and it cannot focus on vertical and horizontal objects at the same time – for example, in letters such as E, F or T. Corrective lenses compensate by affecting the light rays on only one plane.

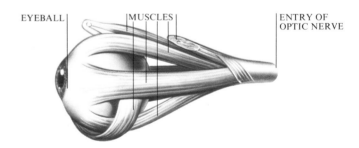

EYEBALL

MUSCLES

ENTRY OF
OPTIC NERVE

MUSCLES RESPONSIBLE FOR EYE MOVEMENT

Strabismus or squint occurs when the eye muscles fail to hold the eye in place – hence the term 'lazy eye'. It is a common condition in children, who often outgrow it. Most people who have a 'cross eye' know that it becomes more pronounced when they are tired. Conventional treatment is to build up the eye muscles by covering the strong eye with a patch and making the weak one do the work. Acute cases can be corrected by surgery.

Night blindness – when the eye fails to focus in semi-darkness – is often due to a dietary deficiency in Vitamin A, and commonly improves with the regular intake of foods containing this vitamin, such as eggs, milk, carrots, liver and kidneys.

Colour blindness, as it is commonly called, though it is really colour-defective vision, occurs in approximately 8 per cent of men and in less than 1 per cent of women, though some surveys have shown a slight increase in colour blindness among women who take the Pill. Total colour blindness or mono-chromatic vision, when only shades of black and white can be seen, is extremely rare. The most common form of colour-defective vision is the failure to distinguish between red and green.

EYE AIDS

Glasses and contact lenses are both used to correct the focusing defects of long and short sight and astigmatism. The advantages of contact lenses, tiny plastic discs which rest directly on the eye surface, are that they often give better vision than glasses and the cosmetic consideration that they do not alter the appearance. On the other hand, they tend to cost more than glasses, especially some types of soft lenses, are more fragile and subject to loss and wear and tear, and may not be acceptable to some eyes. Glasses genuinely suit many people, and are probably the best solution for those with only a minor vision defect who don't have to wear glasses all the time. But for others who have suffered through childhood with thick, heavy glasses, wearing contact lenses can seem like a miraculous release.

Hard lenses
Hard lenses can be 'scleral' lenses, covering all the visible part of the eye, or, very much more commonly now, 'corneal' lenses, covering only the pupil and iris. Some eyes simply cannot become accustomed to hard lenses, and a sizeable number of would-be wearers have to resign themselves to buying soft lenses or glasses, or to wearing hard ones for only part of the day. It takes about three months for eyes which do tolerate them to work up to all-day wear. But most people whose eyes have accepted hard lenses find them highly satisfactory. In general, the British Association of Optical Practitioners' advice in choosing between hard and soft lenses is to stick to hard ones if you can wear them, since they are cheaper, more durable, and give consistently good vision.

Care of hard lenses. Even after cleaning with the recommended fluids, hard lenses sometimes become coated with a greasy substance secreted by the eyelids, which blurs vision and makes the lens surface resist its normal coating of fluid. Some specialists suggest cleaning lenses periodically with washing-up liquid or methylated spirits. But make *absolutely* sure you thoroughly rinse and dry the lenses afterwards. As plastic scratches easily, lenses should ideally be sent back to the manufacturers to be given an annual polishing.

Soft lenses
Soft lenses are made from flexible, water-absorbent plastics. Their great advantage is that the more water they contain, the easier it is for them to adapt to the shape of the cornea and the more comfortable they are for the wearer. Unfortunately, the higher water content also means a more fragile lens. Experiments and research are still being done to produce a lens which is soft, tough and resistant to contamination. Unlike hard lenses, soft ones do not have to be specially shaped for the individual eye, but are ready-made in various curvatures which quickly adapt to the eye. Expert fitting is essential, for while a badly-fitting soft lens may be perfectly comfortable it will cause imperfect vision. Soft lenses can't always help some forms of astigmatism because, by following the shape of the eye, they simply repeat the distortion.

Care of soft lenses. Storing, wetting and sterilizing instructions vary according to the material that soft lenses are made of. But always make sure your finger nails are smooth, since the smallest nick on the edge of the lens can cause a tear, and never let the lenses dry out. Care of soft lenses is more complicated than for hard ones, but most wearers do not find this a problem once it has become routine. What they *do* find is that soft lenses are amazingly comfortable, particularly if they have already tried and failed with hard ones, and take only a week or two for the eyes to tolerate them all day. They are much more expensive than hard lenses and you should consider insuring them, though premiums covering loss or damage can also be high.

Sunglasses
Nowadays sunglasses are more often bought for purely cosmetic reasons, as a fashion accessory, than for their original purpose of sheltering the eyes from bright light. There is a massive range of shapes and shades available, and a corresponding range in quality.

The lenses of some sun-glasses simply consist of tinted glass or plastic. A medium-depth brown or greenish-brown tint is usually the most restful in temperate climates; some blue and pink tints will only alter every colour you see through them. Cheap mass-manufactured sun-glasses may cause eyestrain if the lenses distort your vision. When buying a pair, test the glasses by holding them at arm's length and looking through them at any straight edge, such as a window frame. Then rotate the glasses. If at any angle the straight edge looks wavy, choose another pair.

Some sunglasses have polarized lenses, which filter out glare from horizontal light waves

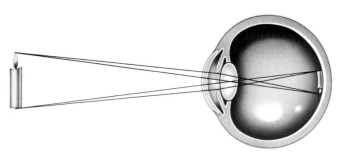

NORMAL SIGHT

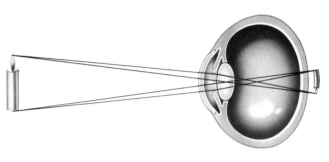

LONG SIGHT

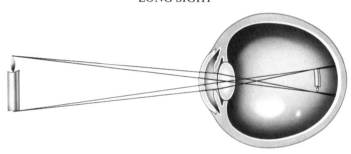

SHORT SIGHT

When eyeball is correct shape, lens focuses light exactly on retina. Long sight (hypermetropia) occurs when eyeball is too short from front to back. Light entering eye is focused by lens at a point behind retina, resulting in blurred image of objects close to eye. Distant vision is not affected. Short sight (myopia) occurs when eyeball is too long from front to back. Light entering eye is focused at a point in front of retina. Image becomes blurred as light rays disperse again before reaching retina. Objects close to eye are usually in focus.

by an ingenious filter in the glass which works rather like a venetian blind, but running from top to bottom rather than from side to side. Most 'dazzle' which causes discomfort to our eyes comes from reflected rather than direct light, and as most reflected light is polarized on a horizontal plane, it is effectively screened by the 'shutters' in the lens.

Photochromic sunglasses are a relatively new invention. Photo-chromic glass contains crystals which make the lens sensitive to ultra-violet light, so that they darken when exposed to bright light, fade to a pale tint on a dull day and go light when indoors. However, even at their palest they still retain some tint, and like other sunglasses can cause the eyes to become over-sensitive to light if worn all the time. Bear in mind, too, that the lenses take anything from half a minute to half an hour to adjust to light changes; if you consider how

quickly you pass from light to shade while driving, you'll realize that they cannot keep up with the changes under these conditions and can therefore be dangerous.

It is possible to have your normal prescription glasses made up with a tint in them. But do remember that sunglasses are rarely actually essential, and if worn constantly can make the eyes unable to cope with ordinary light.

Eye drops
Models sometimes use vegetable dyes with their contact lenses to change the eye colour temporarily. The dyes, supplied by opticians, last a few hours and are harmless to the eyes. But specialists do *not* recommend the blue eye drops currently being marketed, which are intended to whiten the sclera or whites of the eyes and thus enhance the contrast with the iris. These eye drops cause the blood vessels in the sclera to contract, thus draining the area of blood, which could be harmful.

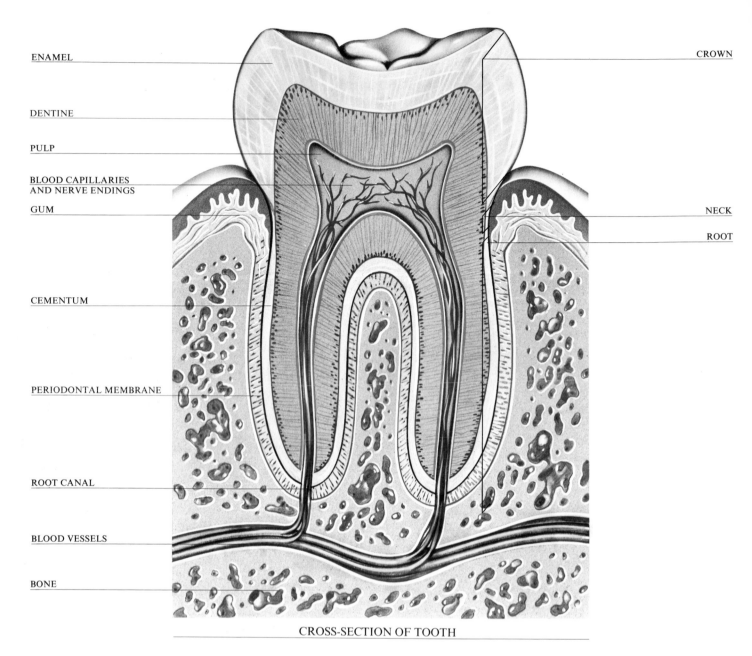

ENAMEL

DENTINE

PULP

BLOOD CAPILLARIES
AND NERVE ENDINGS

GUM

CEMENTUM

PERIODONTAL MEMBRANE

ROOT CANAL

BLOOD VESSELS

BONE

CROWN

NECK

ROOT

CROSS-SECTION OF TOOTH

TEETH

Teeth, like most other parts of
our bodies, are purpose built.
Their prime function is to help us
to bite and chew the food we need
to eat to survive. In addition, they
help us to articulate when we
speak. Human beings have two
successive sets of teeth. The
first set, often called 'milk' teeth,
start to appear when a baby is
about six months old; all twenty
have usually arrived by the time
the child reaches two-and-a-half
years. Around six years the milk
teeth begin to come out and are
replaced by a second set, which
we have to make last for the rest
of our lives. The growth rate varies
from one child to another.

The fact that a third of the
British population over the age of
sixteen have lost all their natural
teeth shows how dismally many of
us fail to give our teeth the full
attention they require.

An adult with a full com-
plement possesses thirty-two teeth,
though in cases where the wisdom
teeth do not appear or are
malpositioned, which is not at all
uncommon these days, he or she
will have only twenty-eight
functional teeth. We have three
basic types of teeth: incisors, at
the front, sharp-edged teeth which
we use for cutting; canines, next
to them, long, pointed teeth for
gripping and tearing; and
premolars and molars, at the
sides and back of the mouth,
square teeth for grinding. Each
tooth is made up of enamel, the
hardest tissue in the human body,
which coats and protects the
outer surface of the crown of the
tooth; dentine, which forms the
bulk of the tooth; cementum, a
thin, hard layer which covers the
root of the tooth; and pulp, the
soft tissue inside the dentine
containing the nerves and blood

vessels which enter the root of
the tooth by a small canal. The
root of the tooth, which con-
stitutes about two-thirds of the
structure, is embedded in the bone
of the jaw and the crown, the
visible part of the tooth, projects
above the gum line. The point at
which the root and crown meet
is called the neck of the tooth.

Building healthy teeth

The buds of a baby's first teeth
are formed in the mother's womb
as early as the sixth to ninth week
of pregnancy. At birth, part of the
crowns are already formed and
the crowns of the second teeth are
starting to grow. It is vital,
therefore, for the health of her
child's teeth, and also her own,
that a woman pays particular
attention to her diet from the
moment she knows she is pregnant.
The size and shape of a child's
teeth are inherited from the
parents, but the structural quality

will be determined by the health
and diet of the mother while the
teeth are being formed.

Diet. To build strong teeth
and healthy gums you need a
well-balanced diet which contains
sufficient proteins, vitamins and
minerals (see page 35). The
minerals which play the most
important part in tooth formation
are calcium and phosphorus; the
essential vitamins are A, C and D.
Without Vitamin D the body
cannot make proper use of the
calcium and phosphorus.
Normally the body makes enough
Vitamin D naturally in response
to the action of sunlight on the
skin, but it can be deficient in
young children and pregnant
women. Eating eggs and oily fish
will ensure that sufficient of the
vitamin is obtained. In a properly
balanced diet there should be no
lack of calcium and supplements
in the form of tablets are not

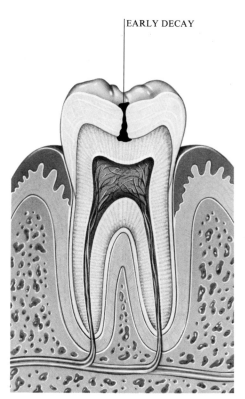

EARLY DECAY

Bacterial activity of plaque and sugar causes acids which eat into enamel of crown of tooth.

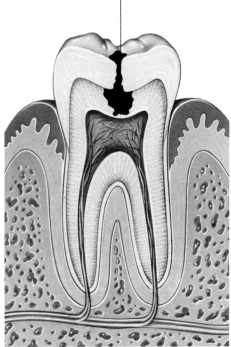

DECAY
REACHES DENTINE

Enamel is destroyed and area beneath affected. Decay spreads rapidly through softer dentine.

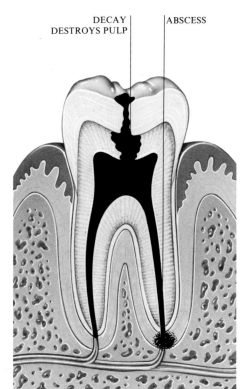

DECAY
DESTROYS PULP | ABSCESS

Decay progresses through pulp of tooth causing severe pain. Abscess develops around root.

necessary. However, children should be encouraged to drink plenty of milk to make sure they have sufficient calcium while their bones and teeth are growing.

Fluoride. Much controversy has surrounded the fluoridation of water supplies. Fluorine is a tasteless, colourless, odourless mineral. Many exaggerated claims have been made for its beneficial properties and just as many scare stories have been published of possible side-effects. The facts are that research showed that in areas where water was naturally fluorinated there was better dental health among the residents. This discovery led to government legislation in Britain and the United States enabling local authorities to add fluoride, a compound of fluorine, to water supplies. By simply adding one part of fluoride to one million parts of water a drop in tooth decay in children in these areas by as much as 60 per cent was achieved. Excessive fluoride can cause mottling of the teeth, but in the recommended quantities there are no hazards. Fluoride has been well proven to help build and maintain strong teeth, especially in children under the age of fourteen. Most dentists believe that the topical application of fluoride in the form of toothpaste or gel treatments is also very effective and in areas where the water is fluorine deficient the mineral may be given in tablet form to children from the age of weaning to the end of adolescence.

	GROWTH BEGINS 6-8 YEARS
CENTRAL INCISOR	
LATERAL INCISOR	7–9 YEARS
CANINE	9–12 YEARS
PREMOLAR	10–12 YEARS
PREMOLAR	10–12 YEARS
MOLAR	6–7 YEARS
MOLAR	11–13 YEARS
WISDOM TOOTH (MOLAR)	17–21 YEARS

PALATE

Permanent teeth start appearing at six years. The full adult set of thirty-two teeth is usually complete by the age of twenty-one.

TOOTH DECAY

Sugar is the greatest single enemy of teeth, along with all the sugar-based sweets, puddings, biscuits and drinks which have become part of the daily diet of most adults and children in the Western world. Nutritionists consistently tell us that we do not need sugar other than that which occurs naturally in fruit and vegetables, that sugar is harmful in our diet not only as a cause of tooth decay but also for exacerbating weight problems and coronary conditions. However,

children are still rewarded with bars of chocolate and given chewing gum or bags of toffees to keep them quiet on a journey. Little wonder then that few survive to the age of five with even their milk teeth intact.

Even if we keep sugar to a minimum in our diet, our teeth need to be freed of the deposits which all food leaves behind and of the layer of bacteria, saliva and food debris known as plaque which, if not removed, coats our teeth. Plaque combined with sugar produces acid which attacks the

enamel, eventually causing dental decay. If plaque is left to build up it will damage the gums as well. It is a good idea to finish each meal with a glass of water and something raw and crunchy such as a carrot, apple or stick of celery, which encourages the flow of saliva to help clean the mouth, but the only way to remove food deposits and plaque completely is by regular, careful and thorough tooth-cleaning.

How to clean your teeth Ideally teeth and gums and the upper surface of the tongue should be brushed after every meal, but a really thorough cleaning after breakfast and before going to bed is better than half-a-dozen token efforts during the day. Cleaning your teeth and gums properly should take at least two-and-a-half minutes – the average dash of forty seconds is completely insufficient to do a good job. The object of tooth-cleaning is not just to have a fresh mouth and sweet breath, but also to remove completely the particles of food which coat surfaces and lodge between the teeth and to remove plaque. Fierce scrubbing is not essential to do this, in fact it may even be damaging to the enamel and neck of the tooth; gentle, thorough brushing is necessary.

Your toothbrush. Choose a brush which has fine, tightly-packed filaments, all of the same length and with rounded ends to prevent scratching. Bristle brushes tend to harbour germs; they also take longer to dry, which

CLEANING YOUR TEETH

The only way to remove the sticky plaque deposits which cause tooth decay is by really thorough brushing. This does not entail violent action, which can damage teeth and gums, but a gentle, careful brushing of every single surface of the teeth. This should take at least two minutes. If you cannot brush your teeth after a meal, try to finish with a glass of water, or a raw fruit or vegetable to make saliva flow over teeth. A good toothbrush should have a small head, to get into every corner of the mouth, and lots of fine, tightly-packed, flexible filaments to enter all the crevices where food deposits may linger.

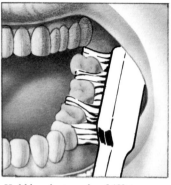

Hold brush at angle of 45° to outside of teeth, tufts half on gum, half on teeth. Make short vibratory movements to clear debris under gums. Brush from gum to tip.

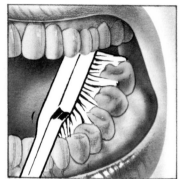

For inside of teeth, use brush in same manner as for outside. Clear deposits under gums and between teeth and brush with sweeping motion from gum to tip.

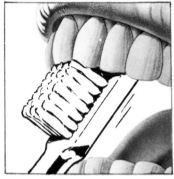

To clean inside of top and bottom front teeth, hold brush vertically with tufts still at an angle of 45° to teeth. Brush up and down, gum to tip, with short strokes.

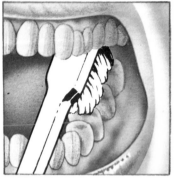

Finish off by brushing biting surfaces. Apply tufts straight on to surface and brush backwards and forwards with short, scrubbing strokes. Do not brush too harshly.

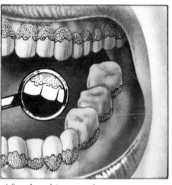

After brushing, teeth may appear clean but often have plaque still adhering to surface. Special disclosing tablets stain plaque pink and make it easy to see and remove.

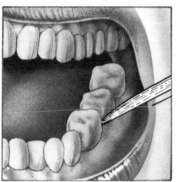

Softwood sticks are designed to remove plaque from small spaces between teeth. Pass stick gently backwards and forwards, taking care not to damage gum.

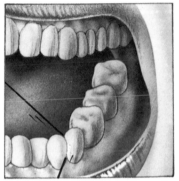

Dental floss is strong nylon thread for cleaning narrow gaps between teeth. Wrap floss around each middle finger and with thumb and forefinger work gently to and fro.

causes the bristle to rot, so synthetic fibre brushes are usually better – but it is wise to ask your dentist to recommend a brush that would be suitable for your particular teeth. Your toothbrush should be strong and flexible, but the texture must never be too hard or the filaments will scratch the enamel of your teeth, and you should have a new one at least once every three months. Electric brushes look tremendously efficient, but they may provide an excuse for skimpy brushing and the batteries run down surprisingly quickly. As a novelty they can be helpful in encouraging children to clean their teeth regularly, but they are no better than a properly used manual brush.

It is not easy to make a good job of cleaning your teeth. Plaque is a sticky substance and taking a brush to it could be likened to trying to sweep up treacle with a broom. In the future someone will invent a more efficient tool for cleaning teeth, possibly one which works more by rubbing than brushing. Some dentists already recommend using a cloth rather than a brush for cleaning, but the brush has the advantage of the many single filaments to get into slight crevices.

How to brush. When brushing your teeth remember that each tooth is like a cube, with one of its six sides embedded in the gum. Good cleaning means including all five other surfaces, each surface requiring a different brushing action. You should use a side to side motion only on the biting surfaces and on the backs of the front teeth; for the rest, working always from root to tip, including gums, and always beginning with the brush fibres resting on the gum, brush with firm sweeping movements along the tooth towards the biting surfaces. Thus each jaw is cleaned by making brushing movements towards the opposite jaw, dealing in turn with the inner and outer surfaces of all the teeth.

Cleaning aids. A brush, however well used, cannot penetrate all the little corners of teeth and gums, nor can it get between the teeth. For these areas it is a good idea to get into the habit of using dental floss. Ask your dentist to show you how to use floss properly, as care needs to be taken not to cut or scrape the gums. Ideally you should floss every night before you brush, then use the brush to clean away loosened debris. Well-made tooth picks are also useful, particularly after meals when it is impossible to brush your teeth, but again it is important not to damage teeth or

gums in the process by prodding carelessly or too enthusiastically. Some patients are advised by their dentists to massage gums with special softwood tooth picks to toughen the gums. Just because your teeth look and feel clean, it is no guarantee that they are. The only way you can be absolutely sure that you have brushed correctly and removed all the plaque is by using a disclosing tablet or solution which stains the plaque pink. The disclosing agent can be used before you clean your teeth to identify the affected areas, or afterwards as a check to see that you have succeeded in removing the plaque. Try using it a few times to give yourself some idea of just what degree of brushing is called for, and then occasionally as a spot check to make sure your teeth are still plaque free.

It is wrong to confuse white teeth with clean teeth. In fact, the healthiest teeth are often not white but yellowish, since hard enamel is thin and translucent and reveals the yellow tinged dentine beneath. Very white teeth often have soft, porous enamel and may need special attention.

Toothpaste. A good toothpaste should contain three basic ingredients: detergent, polishing agent and fluoride. The detergent

should foam well to lift out food particles. A polishing agent does what the name suggests, but should not employ rough abrasives to do the job as these damage the enamel. Special toothpastes or powders for smokers are rarely recommended, as most contain harsh abrasive agents. Fluoride will help to strengthen enamel against decay. When you have finished brushing your teeth and rinsing your mouth, there should be no hint of the toothpaste flavouring; the taste is not just to make your breath smell fresh, but serves as a reminder that toothpaste is simply a cleansing agent. If you can still taste the flavouring rinse until it has completely gone, then you will be sure that you have flushed out all the detergent and the food debris it may hold. Although some people find it harsh and unpleasant to taste, salt is quite effective as a tooth-cleaning agent; it is also good for the gums and is cheap and easy to obtain.

YOU AND YOUR DENTIST

Most people look on the dentist as a repair man to be visited only when pain drives them to his door. It would be far better for us if we made use of his specialized skills to prevent dental disease from occurring in the first place. If he

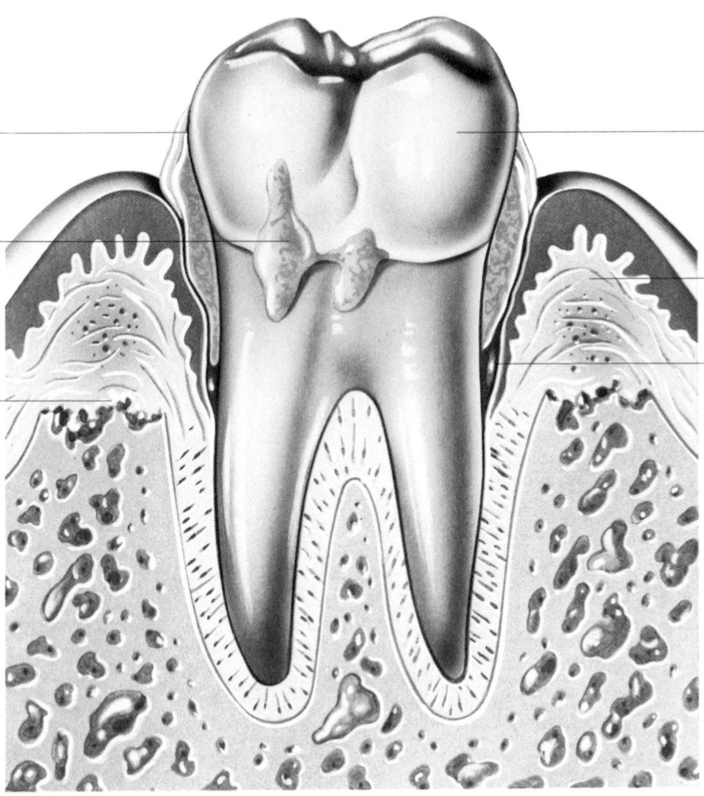

MINERALIZED PLAQUE (CALCULUS)

MINERALIZED PLAQUE (CALCULUS)

BONE DESTRUCTION

PLAQUE

GUM INFLAMMATION

CREVICE POCKET

Gum disease is the main cause of tooth loss in adults. An accumulation of plaque is mineralized into calculus around neck of teeth which separate from gums, forming pockets that fill with bacteria. In early stages of infection gums are inflamed and may bleed. If unchecked, bone supporting teeth is attacked and even healthy teeth may become loose.

is visited only when you need a filling, his role is inevitably limited to repair work; if on the other hand you visit him regularly every six months, preventive dentistry will mean that corrective treatment is minimal, and you stand a far better chance of keeping your teeth for life.

Preventive treatments
Scaling. Your dentist can help to prevent the trouble caused by a build-up of plaque or tartar on the teeth by scaling. This is a thorough cleaning, scaling and polishing treatment which removes all the deposits on the teeth, leaving them feeling and looking clean. Even if you are not a sweet-eater your teeth still need regular cleaning of this sort, as all food leaves a deposit. Tea and coffee if drunk in abundance and regular cigarette smoking will stain your teeth and scaling will remove this, too. Gum diseases which lead to loosening of teeth are also minimized by scaling.

Fluoride. For children and adolescents, fluoride applications at regular intervals will help to protect and strengthen teeth against decay. Fluoride is applied in a gel or fluid form to the surfaces of the teeth, left for several minutes and then rinsed off thoroughly. This should be repeated every six months.

Balancing the 'bite'. Your dentist will check to make sure that your teeth bite together evenly, and will adjust surfaces which are functioning incorrectly. An uneven bite produces unbalanced and destructive pressures on the bone holding the teeth, eventually causing them to loosen in their sockets.

Repairs to teeth
Tooth decay starts when the enamel, the first line of defence, perishes under the attack of the acid produced by plaque. What begins as a tiny spot on the enamel of the crown can enlarge through the dentine and eventually reach the pulp and cause an abscess.* You will usually experience some pain when the decay has progressed to the dentine; if left, it will progress into the pulp and you will certainly have toothache. Obviously it is better to detect decay in its very early stages and for this reason your six-monthly check-up at the dentist is vital. The longer a tooth is left to decay, the more complicated the repair becomes and the greater the likelihood that you will lose your tooth altogether. The treatment used to fill or restore your tooth will depend on the severity of the decay, but even if there is only a small part of the tooth left healthy, possibly only the root, a

good dentist will do all he can to preserve and build on it. Removing teeth and replacing them with artificial ones is always less satisfactory. When teeth are removed the jaw-bone shrinks and the mouth and face begin to lose their shape. Provided treatment is given in time and the cavity is small, teeth can be filled using amalgam, gold or one of the white filling materials; where decay is severe the entire crown of the tooth may have to be replaced by gold or porcelain in order to make it healthy, strong and functional.

Today the dentist has at his finger tips a range of high-speed drills and local anaesthetics which usually make a visit to his surgery a painless experience. However, if your tooth problem is severe and treatment likely to be uncomfortable even with these aids, or if you are particularly nervous, some dentists will use intravenous injections of sedatives which have the effect of relaxing the body and depressing the central nervous system to abolish anxiety as well as pain. If the work to be done is very extensive, or will take a particularly long time, a general anaesthetic may be given.

Gum disease
Gum disease is more common than tooth decay, and beyond a certain stage is more difficult to

put right. Gum disease usually begins when hardened plaque or tartar attacks the gums. There may initially be no sign that anything is wrong or there may be inflammation, soreness and bad breath. At this stage, gingivitis is the general term for the condition and professional cleaning around the neck of the teeth may be all that is required for the gums to right themselves. If gingivitis progresses there may be puffiness and bleeding and the gums will detach from the teeth, leaving hollow pockets where bacteria and food particles can collect. This condition, perio-dontitis, is much more serious. The dentist may have to cut away areas of the gum to get rid of the pockets. If gum disease is allowed to go further still, the bone itself may become so damaged that the teeth become irretrievably loose. The irony is that the individual teeth may be healthy but the bone attachment has become hopelessly inadequate.

Pregnant women frequently suffer from a hormonally induced form of gingivitis which inflames the gum margins. The effects can be minimized by meticulous oral hygiene and the condition corrects itself after the birth of the child.

For information on mouth ulcers, see page 216.

ORTHODONTICS

This is a specialist branch of dentistry which is concerned with correcting developmental problems of teeth and jaw, the work usually being undertaken when the patient is about twelve years old when teeth will move along the jaw quite easily. By taking steps to correct faults at this age future cosmetic and functional problems can be avoided and a lot of embarrassment and misery spared. Treatment varies according to the fault. For example, teeth can be overcrowded or too spaced out, perhaps because the patient has inherited the jaw of one parent and the teeth of the other. If the jaws themselves are dispropor-

tionate the child may have buck teeth or a protruding lower jaw; in either case the teeth fail to meet properly, eating is difficult and the condition unsightly. The successfully-treated teeth not only look better but are obviously easier to clean and thus better proof against decay. Orthodontic work is usually achieved by using appliances which correct the positioning of the teeth while they are growing. Correcting adult or fully-grown teeth involves the use of porcelain crowns and white fillings which enhance the colour, position and shape of the teeth. This work is usually referred to as cosmetic dentistry.

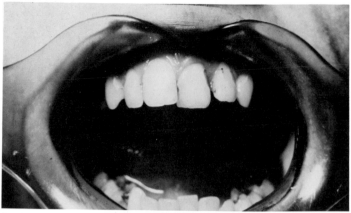

1   Seriously filled and crooked teeth. Inner structure was sound, correction of shape and position reasonable, so jacket crowns could be used.

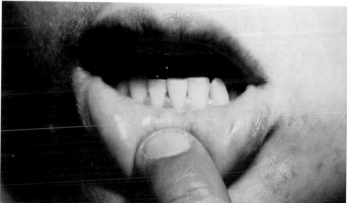

Childhood habits can damage teeth. Thumb-sucking forces teeth out of position. Constant pressure of nail-biting can cause pulp abscesses.

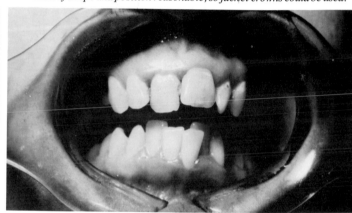

1   A combination of stained and crooked teeth, so malpositioned that to grind down enough to make corrections nerve tissues would be damaged.

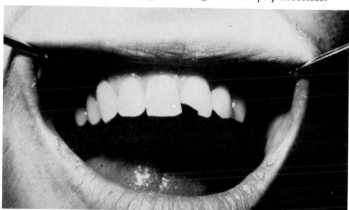

1   A corner broken off a tooth is unsightly and vulnerable to decay. An ordinary filling would be too weak and noticeable in this position.

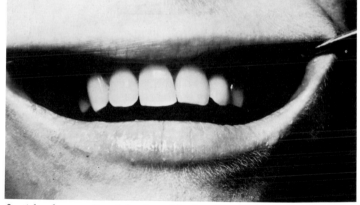

2   A hard composite of plastic and finely pulverized glass, fixed by both acid etching and micro screws, makes the repair strong and invisible.

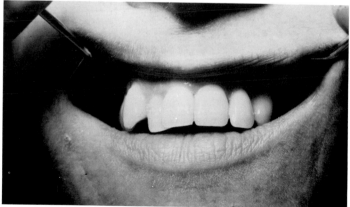

1   Extremely crooked teeth which could have been straightened easily in childhood with an orthodontic appliance. Jacket crowns are now required.

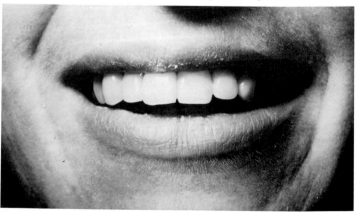

2   Porcelain crowns are fixed. Plastic crowns are inadvisable as flexible plastic gives under constant impact; bacteria may penetrate causing decay.

204

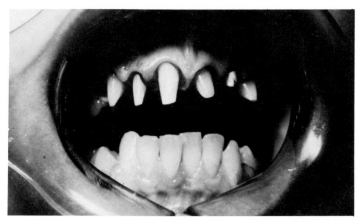

2 Cores of teeth after stripping off outer enamel casing, leaving narrow ledge just below gum. Enamel casing was used as a model for crowns.

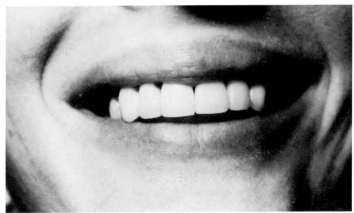

3 Porcelain crowns, bonded on to platinum for strength, are cemented into position. Properly fitted these should last as long as natural teeth.

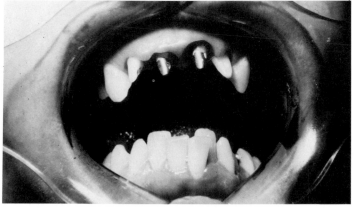

2 Nerves are removed and teeth ground to below gum level. Central teeth needed root filling. Angled stainless-steel posts are fitted into roots.

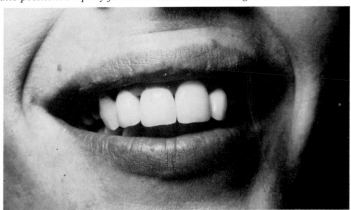

3 New porcelain crowns are bonded on to metal posts. Post crowns are made when corrections required are too extensive to apply jacket crowns.

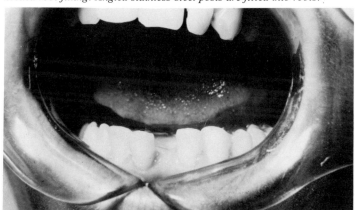

1 This patient had an incisor missing in the centre of her lower jaw. She had always worn a removable denture, but a permanent bridge was made.

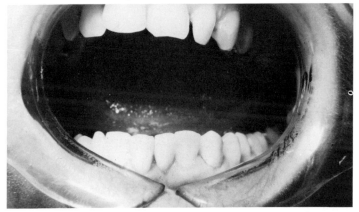

2 Fixed bridge is attached to the nearest adequately strong tooth – second to left of space. Bridge does not show and need not be removed.

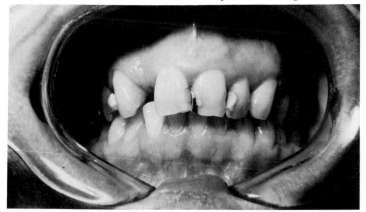

1 New crowns and fixed bridges were made to improve this mouth full of stained ugly teeth with extensive and deteriorating fillings and gaps.

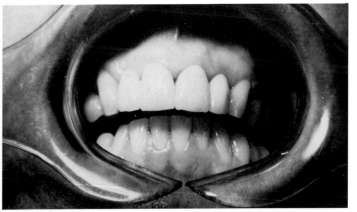

2 Inverted, bone structure of face beneath horizontal line across pupils gives shape for upper central incisor. Crowns may be made to this model.

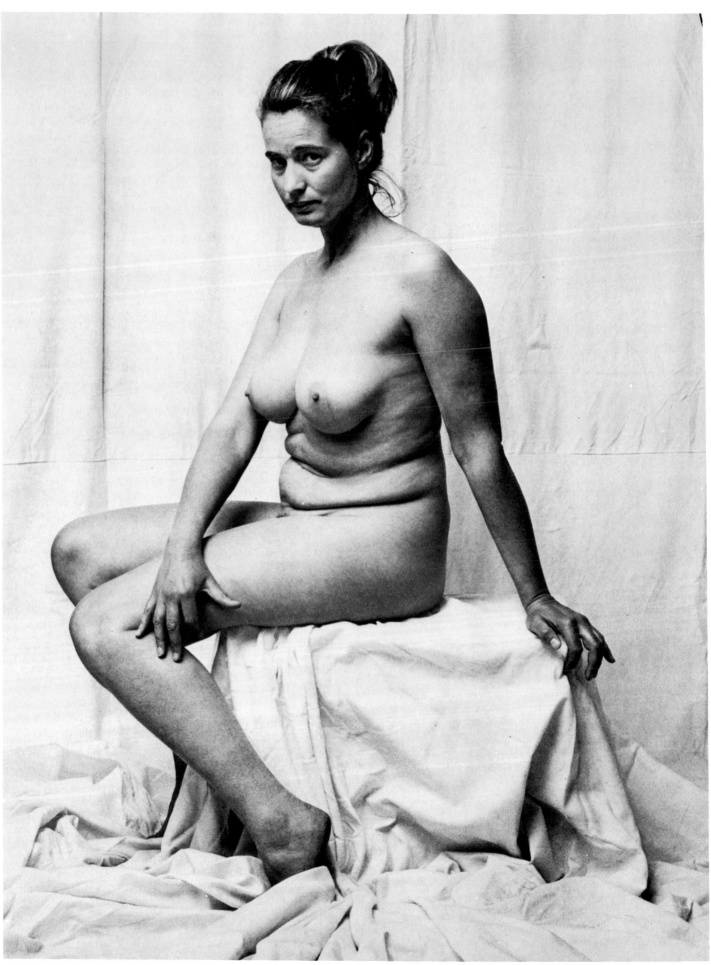

Plastic Surgery

The woman who ardently desires major plastic surgery may feel at first that no one understands the problem. 'No one I knew seemed to recognize my desperation,' said a girl with an overlarge bosom who wanted it reduced. She described how one doctor to whom she spoke simply smiled and said, 'I wouldn't worry about it. You're just very well developed.' This girl was very young, only sixteen, and British surgeons in particular are conservative about operating on teenagers – often justifiably, since at this age physical development is not complete and the figure has not yet 'settled'. Nor have the emotions. An aspect of the appearance which seems hideous and embarrassing in early years may simply become a fact of life, or even an asset, later on.

Arranging an operation will often take a great deal of determination if you are seeking the services of a reputable cosmetic surgeon. Over-worked family doctors can be unhelpful and unsympathetic about referring you for operations which they feel spring from vanity rather than medical need. Good cosmetic surgeons are also careful about whom they take on as patients. 'It is very important to examine the motives of a patient,' says one top Harley Street doctor, 'to be assured that her expectations of what the operation will do for her are reasonable. I am always wary of someone seeking cosmetic surgery at a crisis point in their life.'

What are reasonable expectations from cosmetic surgery? They are, broadly, that the operation will make you look better and thus make you feel better psychologically. In the most positive cases, cosmetic surgery simply makes you happier about certain exterior aspects of yourself. A woman who had had a big nose said: 'Having my nose altered just means that I don't have to worry permanently about whether I'm sitting in profile to a man I like.'

However, expecting an operation to change your life or your personality fundamentally is not 'reasonable'. People often expect a change in looks to change their identity in some way, but of course the personality remains the same. 'If an actress comes to me and says she wants her nose bobbed because she thinks it would make her a bit more photogenic, I think she has a reasonable attitude,' says a psychiatrist who works with plastic surgery cases. 'But if an actress says she wants her nose bobbed because the nose she has is the only thing standing between her and instant stardom, I know she is in for a disappointment. Her expectations are unreasonable. She is imagining that the shape of her nose is determining everything, and when her nose is altered and she is not a famous star overnight she will be bitterly disappointed.'

Doctors cannot always judge who will benefit from cosmetic surgery, but they can sometimes judge who will suffer – psychologically, that is. These include people with over-inflated expectations of how it will change their lives. Fading beauties with insecure marriages are, alas, a rich area of exploitation in the plastic surgery business, but they are often doomed to disappointment. 'It is much harder to adjust to the idea of ageing if you have been a great beauty,' says the psychiatrist quoted above, 'and it is much harder if you have made your living out of your looks in some way. Consequently, for some once-beautiful women, all their emotional investment is in their looks which they cannot accept *must* change with age. There is nothing wrong in itself with having a face-lift or a bottom-lift or a bosom-lift; it is just false to imagine that that *in itself* will win back the love of a straying husband, or make you once more the talk of the town. A face-lift is something that can help you to look better, but it does not restore youth. Paradoxically, to benefit most from this kind of surgery, you should be the sort of person who accepts the fact that ageing is inevitable.'

Sometimes, too, a person seeking cosmetic surgery may be in a state of deep self-rejection which really needs psychiatric care: for example, a black person who wants a 'white' type of nose may be seeking not simply a new profile, but a different racial identity. And surgeons have also to watch out for a rare mental condition called dysmorphophobia – the overwhelming feeling of deformity unaccompanied by any objective evidence.

The people who often derive the most from cosmetic surgery are those who have their shapes altered for purely professional reasons and approach it in a practical, almost casual, manner. People who have had the misfortune to be in motor accidents, fires or other kinds of mishap, and need major skin grafts and cosmetic surgery, are also usually positively and reasonably motivated. And women who have had a breast or part of a breast removed have every right to expect a good remodelling job, depending on how radical the mastectomy (page 100) has been.

FINDING A PLASTIC SURGEON

In Great Britain your general practitioner should refer you to a plastic surgeon, whether the operation is to be done on the National Health or privately. Because of the stringent regulations concerning advertising by doctors, there is no list of plastic surgeons available to the public. However, GPs usually know the specialists practising in their area, and if not they can refer to the British Association of Plastic Surgeons for information. If your doctor considers your physical and mental well-being warrants it, you may have plastic surgery paid for by the National Health Service.

Reputable plastic surgeons warn: 'Never go to a clinic that advertises.' The best plastic surgeons never take anyone 'off the street', they always seek a referral, usually from the patient's GP. In America much cosmetic surgery is accomplished through the grapevine – women like to recommend their friends to a certain doctor or clinic. Of course, a recommendation through a general practitioner is also the correct way of finding a plastic surgeon in the United States. Again, *don't* go to clinics that advertise, unless you have a recommendation from someone who has already had a successful operation there.

British doctors have a highly conservative reputation when it comes to plastic surgery. They are often over-cautious and over-burdened with fancy psychological theories. They are not at all like the Americans, who take a positive view of 'image-enhancing'.

It must be said, however, that the American system can lead to great abuses. An investigation into plastic surgery in California, published in an American magazine, estimated that 25 per cent of the doctors practising plastic surgery there are completely unqualified for it. Moreover, the injunction against advertising is so widely flouted that the convention has now established its acceptability. There is a huge demand for plastic surgery, in California especially, and wherever there is a wide demand for a commodity the quality varies. After five botched breast operations to enlarge her bosom, one woman wound up having radical mastectomies because the breasts had become diseased from being messed about. This is the result of too lax an attitude. Plastic surgery is an area which needs controls.

Even in conservative Britain things can go wrong, for the simple reason that all surgery inevitably involves a risk. In 1978, the case was reported of a fat man who had a number of stomach-reducing operations and finally died in the operating theatre; and a thirteen-year-old girl suffered severe brain damage when a simple operation to pin back her ears went wrong.

If you have been treated by a reputable surgeon, the chances of post-operative complications should be small. Having an operation on your breasts, for instance, should not interfere with the functioning of your breasts and you should be able to breast-feed afterwards in the normal way. But, as you grow older, the effect of breast enlargement may wear off, and you may need another implant. Some women also complain of scars: the two marks under the breasts where the cuts have been made show on some people more than others.

A face-lift averages a ten-year innings; after that you may have to have it repeated. The most common operation, nose alteration, is also the most noticeable; one 'nose-job' can nearly always spot another. Sometimes there is a diminution of the sense of smell, and some people complain of more congestion when they have a head cold.

However, caution is always justified where cosmetic surgery is concerned. This attitude can be frustrating for the person who knows that she is willing to take the risk of an operation, but the too-suggestible have to be protected. For the truth is that almost no woman is entirely happy with her appearance, but turning to surgery to change it must still be considered a last resort.

NOSE
Shortening, straightening or building up of nose. In reduction excess bone, cartilage and tissue are removed. To enlarge a small nose silicone and cartilage are implanted. The short operation is performed from the inside so there is no scarring. The nose is in a plaster cast for a week and, although face is heavily bruised at first, recovery is quick and the effects are permanent. A few people complain of a diminution of the sense of smell and increased congestion with a cold, but the operation is recommended when the shape of the nose is a professional drawback or causes psychological problems. It can be performed once features have settled after adolescence.

CHIN
Chin remodelling. Corrects a receding or prominent chin by adding or removing bone or cartilage; sometimes a silicone implant is inserted. An incision is made in the mouth for the operation and, depending on the extent of the surgery, two to twelve weeks are spent recuperating. The operation is often done in conjunction with orthodontic work. A simple double chin, however, may be corrected as part of a face-lift or by a shorter operation in which a Z-shaped incision is made under chin and excess fat and tissue are removed. The effects of a chin operation usually last for ever and often rebalance a profile in such a way as to make other surgery unnecessary. Remodelling should not be done until features have settled.

BREASTS
Breast reduction or augmentation. To reduce breasts or lift drooping ones is a complex operation involving three incisions: under breast; down from nipple; and round nipple. Excess fat and skin are removed and usually repositioned. Scars fade in a few months but seldom disappear altogether and function of nipple may be impeded. Post-operative care is strict and complete recovery takes up to a year. The effects last for ten years or more and the operation can be performed on mature women from seventeen onwards. The breast augmentation operation stretches the skin so that it will cover inserted implants (prostheses), which are filled with either gel or saline. These are inserted through incisions, made either under breast or at the side near armpit, and then stitched to wall of chest. The augmentation operation is most helpful in cases of non-radical mastectomies or if breasts are of very different sizes. It should not be considered until child-bearing years are over.

EYES
Removal of 'hoods' or sagging excess skin round eyes. An incision is made either below lower lashes or in hollow under brow bone and a section of skin and fat is removed. Scarring is rare as tissue round eye is particularly resilient, but swelling is unpleasant at first. This simple operation can be performed any time after adolescence, as eye problems are sometimes inherited rather than caused by age. You should never have all eye wrinkles removed as this creates an unnatural look, but the successful operation is remarkably effective and should be considered before a full face-lift. It lasts up to ten years.

EARS
Repositioning or 'pinning' of ears. To correct fly-away ears a tiny incision is made behind each ear and excess cartilage is removed. The skin is then tightened and stitched up and each ear is bandaged flat against head and left to heal for two weeks. The effect of the operation is permanent and side-effects are extremely rare. It can be performed at any age after four.

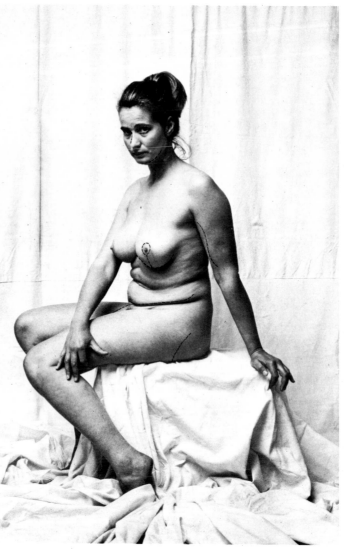

STOMACH
Stomach reduction. A very delicate operation removing excess skin (often the result of pregnancy stretching the skin and abdominal muscles). An incision is made low in stomach along groin crease and up over hips; the slack skin is drawn down and removed and muscles are tightened. The lower scar is hidden by pubic hair but hip scars rarely disappear completely. The operation is effective for up to ten years but should not be performed until you have decided not to have any more children, nor in cases where over-weight is the real problem. However, excessive slack caused by drastic weight-loss can be treated.

INNER THIGHS
Inner-thigh lift. Removes unsightly bulges and controls fat as far down as knee. An incision is made in groin on inside of thigh and excess fat and tissue are removed. Often a second incision running vertically down thigh is necessary, and of course this will leave a scar. The operation takes up to four hours and again is only performed in cases where strict dieting and exercise have failed. It should not be contemplated after middle age.

FACE-LIFT
Full face-lift. Surgery here rectifies the sagging that occurs in three facial areas: drooping eyebrows, crow's feet and frown lines; slack cheeks and nose-to-mouth lines; loose chin and neck. The three-to-four-hour operation involves working on underlying muscles as well as simply removing excess skin. For a full face-lift the skin is lifted in three parts and incisions are made in hair line above temples, in fold in front of ear, and under lobes. The only scar which really shows is that in front of ear; it should fade in a couple of months. Some surgeons prefer to take this incision behind ear. Recovery depends on individual skin chemistry but puffiness may be prolonged and loss of facial expression can result, causing a bland look. The effects of the operation last from five to ten years. It is not recommended for women under forty and it is often a good idea to try a simpler operation round eyes first. Beware of a 'mini face-lift' which simply treats the skin at temples – it will not last.

UPPER ARM
Removal of excess skin and fat from upper arm. The incision 'lifting' upper arm is hidden beneath limb, and a long incision running down inside of arm takes care of the rest. This is usually S-shaped, following the skin's natural relaxation lines. However, the scars are difficult to conceal. This is not a very common operation and is only performed if you have already had other body surgery.

BUTTOCKS & THIGHS
Correction of fat buttocks and outer thighs. Lifting a dropped bottom and reducing outer-thigh bulges. This long and complicated operation involves cutting away crescent-shaped sections of skin and fatty tissue from the area where thigh and bottom join. Scars do not fade completely and recovery is slow and uncomfortable. The operation should only be contemplated by young and middle-aged people and most surgeons will only perform it when persistent dieting and exercise have failed.

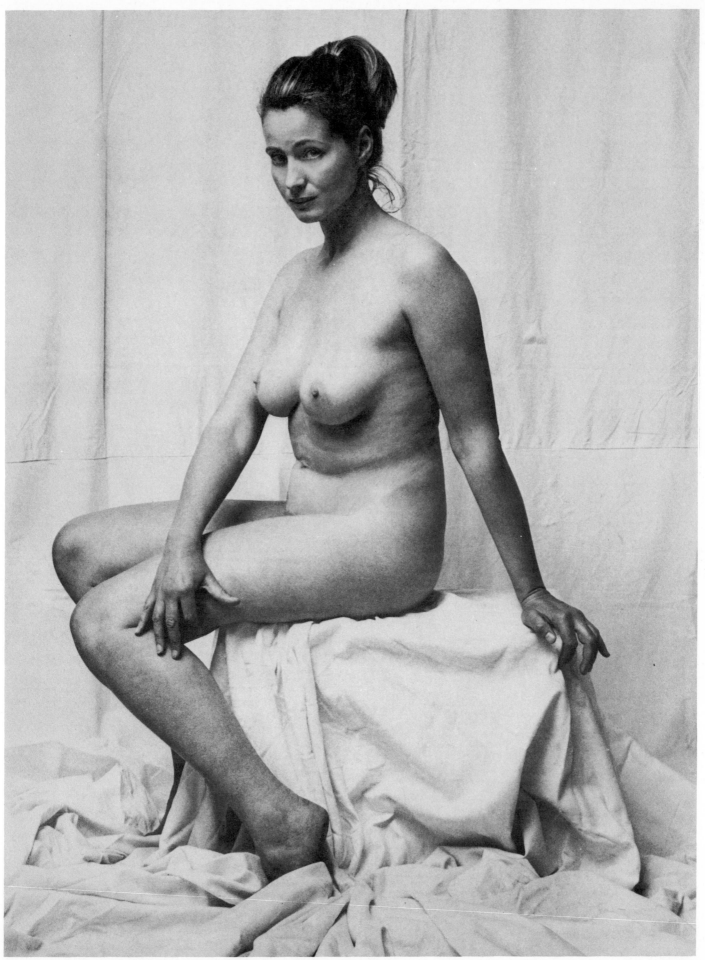

A

Abscess An abscess may appear anywhere on the body, but the most common are tooth abscesses or gumboils. These occur when pus formed by bacteria from an infected tooth collects in a cavity, often at the root of a tooth. Treatment is generally effective once the cause has been isolated and remedied. A doctor will usually prescribe oral antibiotics and will sometimes lance the abscess, so that the poison can drain away and relieve pressure.

Adrenal Glands See Glands.

Agoraphobia Agoraphobia means literally a morbid or irrational dislike of open places. A person suffering from this will find it difficult, often impossible, to go out, and the prospect of having to do so can make him or her physically ill. The distress caused can manifest itself in the form of vomiting, palpitations, raised temperature or migraines. Like all phobias, agoraphobia is a kind of protective mechanism by which a person who is suffering from other deep-rooted psychological or emotional problems finds a means of expressing his or her fears. Agoraphobics are often unable to describe what or who it is that they fear 'outside', but the fear is totally real. There is no point in adopting a blunt 'pull yourself together' attitude with a genuine agoraphobic person. He or she needs sympathy and professional help to get to the root of the underlying emotional disturbance. Agoraphobic associations have been formed which enable victims to talk to experts and fellow sufferers.

Allergic Conjunctivitis See Allergies.

ALLERGIES An allergy is the altered susceptibility of a body produced by a sensitizing dosage of or exposure to some foreign material. The term is most frequently used to describe an abnormal sensitivity to the action of a particular foreign material or allergen, such as a food, a chemical substance or pollen. Substances that cause allergic reactions can be roughly grouped into four categories: inhalants (such as pollen, grasses, scents); ingestants (food and drinks); injectants (stings, bites, certain injected medicines); contactants (chemicals, fabrics, cosmetics). There is evidence that a tendency to allergy is inherited, though the form may vary. Men are more prone to the disease than women, as are people of a highly-strung or nervous disposition.

Allergic conjunctivitis This is an allergy, usually to something in the air such as dust or pollen, which manifests itself in the form of conjunctivitis, i.e. inflammation of the mucous membrane that lines the inner surface of the eyelids and is reflected over the eyeball. If you suffer from conjunctivitis, see your doctor. If symptoms persist, he will probably refer you to a specialist for treatment to alleviate the condition.

Asthma This is a respiratory disorder characterized by paroxysms or attacks of difficult breathing, wheezing and gasping for breath. During an attack, spasmodic contraction of the smaller bronchial tubes and swelling of the tube lining cause the difficulty in breathing. In many cases the cause is an allergic reaction, often to pollen, some item of food, animal or bird hair, or even ordinary house dust. Many asthmatics also suffer from other allergic reactions, such as nettle rash or hay fever. Asthma tends to start in childhood (though in certain cases it does not manifest itself until middle age), is more common among men than women, and is frequently associated with and precipitated by stress for reasons which are still not totally clear. The taking of antihistamines, either orally or by injection, can help to ward off an asthmatic attack once the allergen or allergens have been isolated, but this may take a long time as there are such a vast number. Inhalants which reduce the swelling of the bronchial linings may also help. Antibiotics may be used if the lungs are so congested that a bacterial infection develops.

Cosmetic allergy This is best prevented by using products, usually called hypo-allergenic, from which any known allergens have been screened, although even these products may produce an allergic reaction in a few people. Occasionally, a person who suffers an allergic reaction to a cosmetic may feel like taking action against the producer, retailer or, in the case of a hairdresser, the salon itself, because she feels that the allergic reaction should not have occurred. In such a case, the potential litigant should bear in mind that in Britain all cosmetics now carry labels listing the known allergens included in the product, and in the United States *all* the ingredients are printed on the label in descending order of priority. Also, the manufacturer of any cosmetic product is required to use only those substances and colouring agents allowed by the government and to carry out sufficient tests to guarantee the safety of the product. Medicated cosmetics must comply with additional regulations, since they are strictly speaking medicinal products. In short, there are laws governing the production, distribution, sale and use of cosmetics, and though an allergic reaction may prove to be idiosyncratic and not the fault of manufacturer or user, if you feel you have a case, take legal or medical advice. For instance, if a hair dye causes an allergic reaction and the mandatory test was not carried out on a patch of skin beforehand, you may be able to sue successfully the hairdresser responsible. If, on the other hand, you use a product without performing an allergic reaction test yourself, when this was prescribed on the label, you have only yourself to blame.

Dermatitis See Skin Problems.

Eczema See Skin Problems.

Hay fever (rhinitis) This is an allergic disease which generally 'attacks' its victims in the spring and summer, when the pollen from various plants and grasses irritates the mucous membranes of the eyes, nose and throat. The symptoms are similar to those of a severe cold or flu: violent sneezing, inflammation and swelling of nose and eyelids, watery discharge from nose and eyes, itching of eyes, a dry cough and sometimes asthmatic paroxysms. The reaction can be caused by allergens other than pollen, such as household dust, animal hair or feather pillows, but if the attacks occur regularly in summer the cause is almost certainly pollen. Ideally a person allergic to pollen should avoid it, but this is obviously almost impossible in normal life, although precautions can be taken if weather forecasters predict a particularly high pollen count. Injections of vaccine prepared from pollen can be given in the winter months or antihistamine preparations in tablet or injection form can be taken throughout the season. These are generally effective, though they can produce side-effects, including drowsiness in some people, so care is necessary when driving or operating machinery.

Hives (urticaria) See Skin Problems.

Rhinitis See Hay fever above.

Amniocentesis Amniocentesis is the removal from the uterus, through the abdominal wall, of a small amount of amniotic fluid, about ¼ fl oz (10 ml), for analysis. Ultrasound should first be employed to tell the doctor where the placenta lies in the uterus so that it can be avoided when the needle used to draw out the fluid is inserted. The procedure is usually carried out between the twelfth and sixteenth weeks of pregnancy and is done under a local anaesthetic. The cells in the amniotic fluid can carry indications

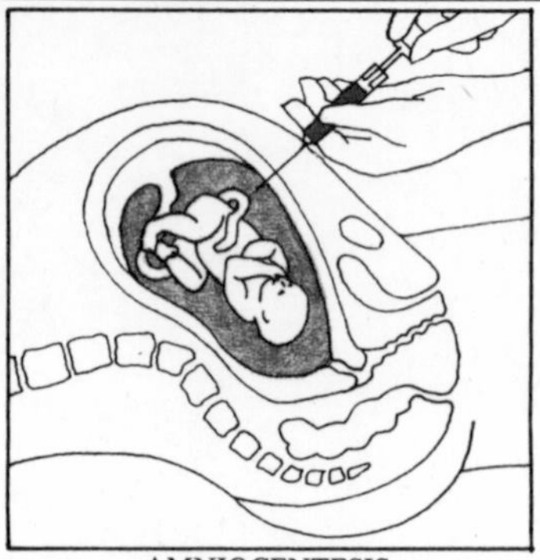

AMNIOCENTESIS

of abnormalities in the foetus such as mongolism and Rhesus incompatibility. As a by-product of amniocentesis the cells also indicate the baby's sex, but as amniocentesis carries a 1 per cent risk of spontaneous abortion it would never be carried out for this reason alone. It is usually recommended for women over the age of thirty-five, who have a one in three hundred chance of bearing a mongol child, and for a woman who has already borne a defective child or knows that she carries a serious hereditary disorder. If the results of amniocentesis show that abnormalities are present in the foetus, a therapeutic abortion can be carried out if the parents wish.

Amniotic Fluid Within the uterus the foetus is cushioned inside a bag of membranes filled with watery amniotic fluid. The 'breaking of the waters', or leakage of this fluid through spontaneous rupture of the membranes, heralds the onset of labour in some cases. The amniotic fluid provides a sterile environment of constant temperature in which the baby can grow and move freely. It also acts as a shock absorber as the mother moves about. The average quantity of amniotic fluid is about 2 pt (1.2 litres).

Anaemia Anaemia means literally lack of blood, but in fact it is the medical term used for a shortage of haemoglobin, the oxygen-carrying compound of protein and iron in the red blood cells. It may be caused by an abnormal loss of haemoglobin due to bleeding or excessive destruction of red cells, or to defective production due to iron deficiency, vitamin deficiency, chronic infection or certain poisons. The simple kind of anaemia which affects many people is iron deficiency, caused by a lack of iron in the diet, and is easily corrected. The causes other than iron deficiency are likely to be more serious, such as bleeding ulcers or inefficient bone marrow. The symptoms are vague unless the anaemia is severe and may include feelings of weariness and inefficiency, pallor, headaches, slight fever and physical weakness. Sometimes the heartbeat accelerates to keep the available haemoglobin circulating more quickly, so compensating to some extent for the deficiency, but in time this can over-tax the heart. Anaemia is not a disease in itself, but is a symptom of an underlying disorder. It is generally more common in women than in men, one-sixth of adult women in Britain are anaemic, as there is a special risk of iron deficiency at certain times in their life. At puberty, for instance, if no reserves of iron have been built up during childhood, a girl may become anaemic when she starts menstruating. Also, during pregnancy, a woman has to provide for her baby's needs from her own iron stores, although the fact that she is not menstruating accounts to some extent for this loss. There is no iron in breast milk; the baby has enough iron stored in its liver for the first six months, after which mixed feeding should begin. Treatments for anaemia vary, but try to avoid the problem by following a good mixed diet which is adequate in vitamins and minerals, especially iron.

Androgen See Hormones.

Anorexia Anorexia means literally want of appetite. Today the term is usually used in conjunction with the word 'nervosa', to denote a self-induced, wilful starvation, not at all the same thing as lack of appetite. The anorectic in most cases does have an appetite, but suppresses it. The disease is most common in teenage girls and, while the exact causes are not known, there is general agreement that they become anorectics as a result of emotional or psychological stress. Most anorectics have low self-esteem and often resent one or both parents strongly; becoming anorectic makes them the centre of attention and is a gesture of defiance, rebellion and independence. Far from being the weak creatures they appear to be, most anorectics are extremely strong-willed. The first symptoms of anorexia can be confused with a 'normal' teenage girl's fear of becoming or being plump as she enters adolescence, becoming choosy about meals, especially those that are associated with getting fat. A mother's instinct may be to chastise her daughter for not eating properly, but if she is wise she will collaborate with her as far as possible, offering non-fattening foods, possibly eating these herself, and reassuring her daughter that she looks good and is not fat. If a refusal to eat persists and the girl starts to balk at all food, picks at and finds 'disgusting' what is on her plate and others, and gradually loses weight, her mother should seek professional help. Once anorexia gains a firm hold it is hard to break. Persistent weight-loss affects the body in many ways: skin and hair lose lustre and elasticity, hair on the head may fall out while more body hair is produced, skin becomes sallow or discoloured, and menstruation will probably cease. Confirmed anorectics have a greatly diminished chance of bearing children. In their desire to be slim—anorectics often consider they are over-weight even when they are grotesquely thin—they will lie, hide food that they are supposed to have eaten, or gorge quantities of food and then force themselves to be sick. If anorexia has reached this stage, short of a miracle only highly-skilled professional help can remedy the situation. Even so, deaths as a result of anorexia continue. Treatment can be through drug therapy and bed rest in a hospital or nursing home. This can be combined with 'behaviour modification techniques', whereby the patient is presented with a system of rewards as weight is gained. Increasingly treatment involves psychotherapy, either with the patient alone or preferably with her parents and siblings as well. Discovering and attempting to cure the root causes of the stress situation which led to anorexia in the first place, though difficult, represent the best long-term solution.

Anovulatory Cycle See Ovulation.

Antihistamines See Tranquillizers.

Apocrine Sweat Glands See Glands.

Asthma See Allergies.

Athlete's Foot See Foot Problems.

B

Barbituric Acid See Tranquillizers.

Bartholin's Glands See Glands.

Benzodiazepines See Tranquillizers.

BIRTHMARKS Birthmarks are skin blemishes which are present at birth. The most common are strawberry or raspberry marks, port-wine stains and liver spots, which have all been so named because of their resemblance to these objects.

Liver spots These are dark bluish or brownish areas of skin which look like very large freckles. Like freckles, they are cellular concentrations of the pigment melanin. They can be disguised by cosmetics, but are often not really unsightly enough to do more than leave them alone.

Port-wine stains (a form of haemangioma) These are areas of skin which, like strawberry marks, contain enlarged blood vessels. Unlike the latter, however, they are flat, purplish-red in colour, and tend to cover a larger area. If port-wine stains cover part of the face and neck they can cause great distress. It is possible to have the marks removed surgically, especially where only a small area of skin is affected, but removal on a large scale can result in severe scarring. Research is still continuing into other ways of removing these birthmarks. If you or your child has them, consult a good dermatologist to see what can be done. Special cosmetics are available which help to disguise the condition.

Strawberry and raspberry marks (haemangioma) These are raised red areas of skin, slightly sponge-like in appearance and texture because of the enlarged blood vessels which they contain. The marks often grow rapidly in the first few months of the baby's life, but the majority, about 75 per cent, usually disappear of their own accord before the child reaches the age of seven. If the marks do not go, and are causing anxiety, they can be made smaller or removed altogether by by surgical means.

Blushing Blushing usually occurs as a reflex action to an 'exciting' stimulus, be it embarrassment, guilt or desire. The face, neck and sometimes other parts of the body become pink as blood capillaries in the skin dilate and blood 'rushes' to the surface. Many young girls and some older women are prone to blushing, and whilst to the observer the result may be attractive, it rarely is to the sufferer. Very little can be done about blushing; as the person matures, and becomes more confident, the problem may disappear, though many women continue to blush when in a state of high sexual arousal. *Hot flushes* are involuntary blushes, sometimes suffusing the entire body and accompanied by sweating, a feeling of prickly heat and giddiness. Flushes, or flashes, occur frequently at the onset of and during menopause and can be very discomforting for the woman suffering, both physically and because they may appear to be an emblem of the fact that she is undergoing the change of life. The flushes happen as a result of the hormonal changes taking place in the body. Hormone replacement therapy (HRT) seems to help reduce the incidence and severity of hot flushes in some women, as well as alleviating other symptoms of menopause. If you are troubled by frequent hot flushes during menopause, consult your doctor or gynaecologist, who may be able to prescribe hormone or other drugs which will help.

Boils These are hard, inflamed suppurations which contain a core of dead skin tissue surrounded by pus. They occur as the result of infection in or around a cut, an abrasion, a sweat gland or, most often, a hair follicle, usually at a point where there is friction or pressure such as round the collar or on the buttocks. Boils can be very painful, but they are best left alone and covered with a simple dressing. Squeezing must be avoided, as this can spread the bacteria and infect the surrounding area and bacteria may enter the bloodstream. Boils will often disappear by themselves once the core has been released. If you notice that the skin around the boil is becoming increasingly inflamed, see your doctor. He will probably prescribe antibiotics, or he may lance the boil so that the infected matter can be released. Boils are often a sign that a person is not in good general health. They can be caused by malnutrition or a lack of certain vitamins, or may occasionally be symptomatic of something more serious such as diabetes or anaemia. If they persist, or are very painful, medical advice should always be sought.

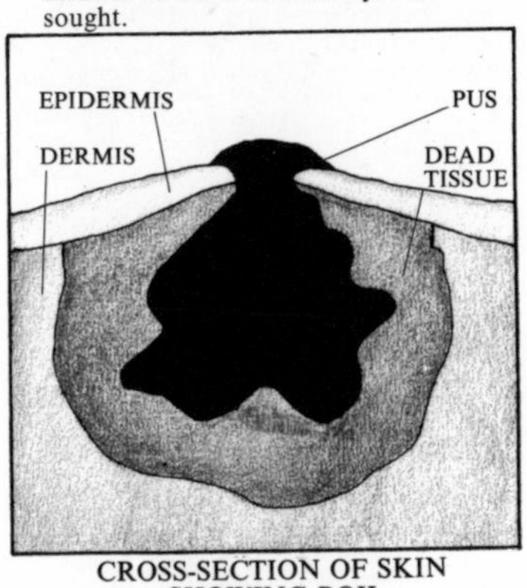

CROSS-SECTION OF SKIN SHOWING BOIL

Breast Cysts See Cysts.
Breast Self-Examination See Well Woman Check-Up.
Brittle Nails See Nail Problems.
Broken Veins See Veins.
Bruises See Skin Problems.
Bunions See Foot Problems.

C

Caesarian Section This is an operation performed on a pregnant woman to deliver her baby through the abdominal wall, when delivery is not possible through the vagina. Reasons for a Caesarian section include foetal distress, a low-lying placenta, a very small pelvis, obstructive fibroids, a transverse foetal position and previous uterine injury. A general anaesthetic is usually given before the operation, although Caesarians are now sometimes performed under epidural anaesthesia. A cut is then made below the navel into the abdomen and uterus. The baby is lifted out and the layers of the incision are stitched. A woman whose first baby is delivered by Caesarian section has a fifty-fifty chance of delivering her next baby vaginally. There is no limit to the number of Caesarian sections that can be performed on one woman, although the risk to mother and baby increases slightly with each one. Caesarians now account for 10 per cent of all deliveries in the United States, where they are often used in preference to difficult forceps deliveries. In Great Britain and Australia, the incidence of Caesarians is 4 to 8 per cent.

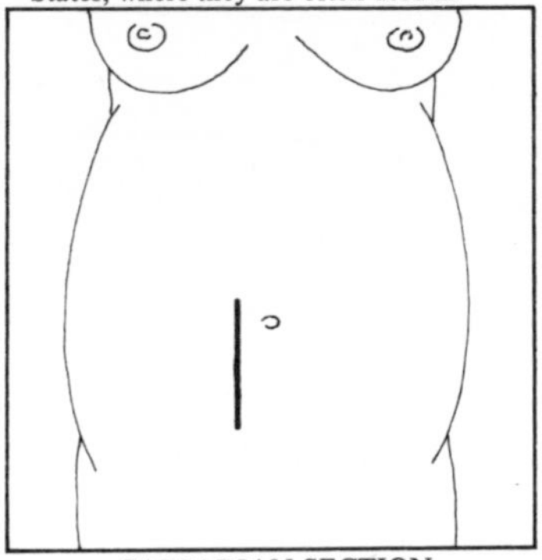

CAESARIAN SECTION CLASSICAL

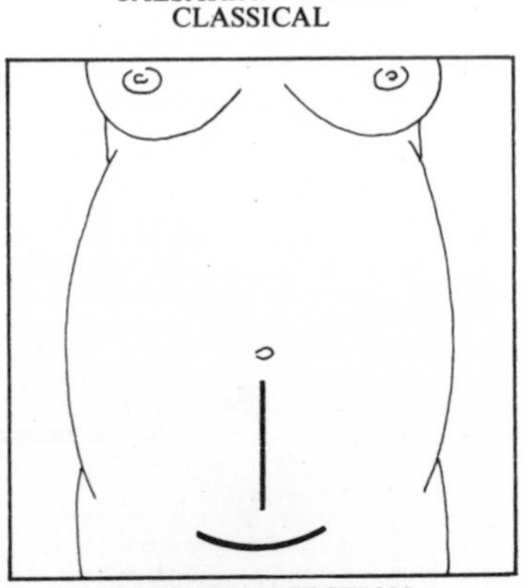

CAESARIAN SECTION LOWER SEGMENT

Callouses and Hard Skin See Foot Problems.
Candidiasis ('Thrush') See Vaginal Infections.
Cataract See Eye Problems.
Cervical Erosion See Uterine Disorders.
Cervical Smear See Well Woman Check-Up.
Chapped Skin See Skin Problems.

Chilblains (Erythema Pernio) A chilblain is an inflamed condition of the hands, feet, ears or nose which is nearly always the result of defective circulation. General ill-health, a poor diet and inadequate clothing or protective covering can all contribute to chilblains. They develop in three stages: first, the skin becomes purple and itchy; second, blisters form on the affected area; third, the blisters break, leaving an ulcerated surface which may not heal easily. The best way to prevent chilblains is to keep to a good diet, exercise regularly to ensure good circulation, and avoid extremes of cold, particularly to hands and feet. Constricting shoes or socks should never be worn. Hands and feet which have become very cold should be warmed gently, rubbing is a good method, and never subjected to intense heat such as a fire or hot-water bottle. In the second or third stages of a chilblain, relief can be obtained from the application of boracic ointment and the chilblain may be covered with a simple dressing.

Chromosomes Chromosomes are minute rod-like structures containing the genes which are found in the nucleus of every human cell. Each ovum and each sperm has twenty-three chromosomes, containing all the genes which provide the blueprint for the future human being. When the ovum has been fertilized by the sperm, it contains twenty-three pairs of chromosomes. In women each pair matches exactly, but in men the sex chromosomes are different and this pair alone holds all the information necessary to make the difference between male and female. The normal female cell contains a pair of X chromosomes. The male cell contains one Y and one X chromosome. If the ovum is fertilized by a sperm containing an X chromosome, the baby will be a girl. If the fertilizing sperm contains a Y chromosome, the baby will be a boy. The determination of the baby's sex is therefore a male responsibility.

Conjunctivitis See Eye Problems.
Corns See Foot Problems.
Cosmetic Allergy See Allergies.

Cuticles The word cuticle derives from the Greek words for small and skin (cutis). The cuticle is composed of layers of the outer, epidermal skin. Its function is to protect the nail matrix where the nail is formed and emerges from beneath the skin. Cuticles should therefore be looked after, not damaged by rough treatment, biting or cutting. If they are kept soft and supple by regularly massaging in cuticle cream or lanolin and gently pushing back with a towel after the bath to keep them separate from the nail itself, they will protect more efficiently.

Cystitis Cystitis is inflammation of the bladder. Symptoms include pain in the bladder or small of the back, pain during intercourse, and frequent passing or wanting to pass water, occasionally associated with pain and cloudy, strong-smelling urine. In chronic cystitis, a typical factor is the very frequent passing of small quantities of urine, sometimes accompanied by incontinence. In acute attacks, the patient may also suffer from high temperatures and shivering, and the attacks may be recurrent. Causes are usually associated with bacterial infection, either in the bladder itself or as a result of infection from the anal area, neighbouring organs such as the vagina in the case of gonorrhoeal infection, or from sexual activity if male hygiene is at fault. Any blockage, such as a stone, or constriction of the urethra, possibly due to changes which take place during the menopause, which might prevent the free flow of urine can also cause cystitis. Prolapse of the womb is frequently associated with the condition, too. Treatment usually involves taking drugs, either sulphonamides or antibiotics, to destroy the bacteria causing the infection. Where a stone or stones are present in the bladder, their surgical removal may be necessary. Palliative treatment during an attack of cystitis includes rest in bed, a bland diet, plenty of fluid such as water or barley water (not alcohol, tea or coffee, which will only aggravate the condition), and heat applied to areas of pain such as the abdomen or small of the back. If you suspect you have cystitis, consult your doctor immediately so that the cause can be isolated and the complaint treated.

CYSTS Cysts are abnormal swellings containing fluid. They are usually benign (non-cancerous) and often do not cause any discomfort. Some cysts, however, may become malignant or interfere with normal body functions, perhaps by pressing on a neighbouring organ, so it is wise to consult a doctor.

Breast cysts These are most common in women between the ages of thirty-five and forty-five. They are usually harmless, but may swell until pressure on the nerves or neighbouring tissues causes pain and their removal becomes necessary. About 75 per cent of breast lumps are non-malignant, but any lump or pain in your breast should be reported to your doctor. For breast self-examination, see page 222.

Ovarian cysts Small cysts in the ovaries either disappear of their own accord or grow larger and sometimes cause pain, which may be mistaken for appendicitis. Most do not require treatment, but large and troublesome cysts, which may cause haemorrhage, are generally removed by surgery. About a third of gynaecological operations are for ovarian cysts and their removal may enhance the possibility of pregnancy.

D

D and C See Dilatation and Curettage.
Demeral See Pethidine.
Dermatitis See Skin Problems.

Dermatologist A dermatologist is a doctor who specializes in the study of the skin and the diagnosis and treatment of skin complaints and diseases. Many skin problems which cause the sufferer great distress may seem trivial or a problem of vanity to a doctor in a general practice, who has patients who are seriously ill. If you have a skin problem and find that you are getting little response from your doctor, ask him to refer you to a dermatologist.

Diabetes This is a disorder in which the body is unable to control the use of sugars as a source of energy. Symptoms include passing large quantities of urine, constant thirst, weight-loss and lack of energy. Women may also suffer from irritation in the genital area. Antenatal checks will reveal diabetes if it has not already been detected. Diagnosis is made by finding sugar in the urine and high levels of glucose in the blood. The patient eats sugar in the form of glucose and about every half an hour the urine and blood are examined to discover the amount of sugar present. Proper control of diabetes can only be obtained by regular blood tests for sugar as the amount of insulin (a hormone normally produced by the pancreas) that a diabetic requires during pregnancy fluctuates. Regular antenatal visits at short intervals are therefore essential. It is usual for a woman with diabetes to be admitted to hospital in about the thirty-second week of pregnancy. As the foetuses of diabetic women tend to be puffy and fat, and thus difficult to deliver, they usually require induction by the thirty-eighth week, but each case needs individual attention.

Dilatation and Curettage This is a fairly common operation, performed while the woman is under anaesthetic, which involves enlargement of the cervical opening using dilators and gentle scraping of the uterine wall with a metal curette, a surgical scoop or ring. It may be performed for any one of the following reasons: to diagnose cancer, pregnancy outside the uterus, or causes of abnormal bleeding or discharge; to clear waste after miscarriage or abortion; to cause abortion; to help cure infertility; to curtail profuse and irregular bleeding; to remove cysts, polyps and other growths; and sometimes as a routine preparation for gynaecological surgery. Recovery from the operation may take anything from six hours to two days.

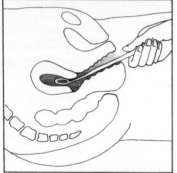

CURETTAGE

Down's Syndrome See Mongolism.
Dreams Everybody dreams, even those who claim they never do because they have no memory of it. Dreams are vital to our health in several ways: they allow the brain to sort and catalogue overflow information acquired during waking hours; they allow expression for desires and urges which are either suppressed or unformulated during the day; and they act as 'bridges' between sleep and wakefulness (for example, hunger experienced while we are asleep may prompt dreams of food or dreaming of someone whispering to us may actually reflect that someone is trying to wake us in this way). The evidence suggests that we dream for a number of periods, of up to twenty minutes each on average, every night. We dream mostly during what is known as 'paradoxical' sleep, when the body is deeply relaxed but the mind alert. This phase is characterized in man by irregular breathing and rapid eye movements beneath the lid. Deprived of paradoxical sleep, and hence the ability to dream, for any length of time we suffer from acute irritability, stress and eventually breakdown. It is as though dreaming is a vital part of the brain computer: failure to allow the dream programme to operate can result in the malfunction or total collapse of the machine.

E

Ear-piercing Ear-piercing is a simple, painless process provided it is done under sterile conditions, preferably by a doctor or reputable beauty salon. Usually a local anaesthetic is applied and the ear lobe is pierced either by diathermy or using a special 'gun'. A gold stud or ring or a silk thread is then inserted into the hole. It is very important to follow instructions carefully regarding bathing and turning the insertion, to avoid infection or the hole sealing. After two to three months, you should be able to wear the ear-rings of your choice. However, it is wise to avoid any made in metals which contain nickel, as this frequently causes an allergic response.
Eccrine Sweat Glands See Glands.
Ectopic Pregnancy This is a pregnancy in which the embryo does not develop

in the uterus. In most cases the fertilized egg becomes lodged in the Fallopian tube, although it may also develop on the ovary itself, within the abdomen attached to some organ like the large intestine, or at the bottom end of the uterus (very rare). The symptoms show in the second or third month of pregnancy, as the embryo grows, and may include acute pain on one side of the abdomen, slight swelling and vaginal bleeding. Any of these symptoms should be reported to your doctor immediately. It is usually necessary to remove the Fallopian tube and embryo by surgery, but recovery from the operation is quick and as a woman has two Fallopian tubes it is still possible for her to conceive and have further pregnancies. About one pregnancy in three hundred is ectopic and the problem is often due to prior inflammation of the Fallopian tube.
Eczema See Skin Problems.
Embryo This is the term used to describe the unborn infant from conception to the end of the second month of pregnancy. Thereafter the developing baby is known medically as the foetus. During the embryonic period all the main organs of the body are formed. Subsequent development, during the foetal period, consists of growth of the organs and sophistication of their function.
Endometrial Cancer See Uterine Disorders.
Endometriosis See Uterine Disorders.
Endometrium This is the mucous membrane which lines the body of the uterus. Once a month it undergoes various changes as part of the menstrual cycle and, if fertilization does not occur, is discarded as a period with blood and mucus.
Epidural Anaesthesia This is a local anaesthetic which deadens sensation below the waist. Its advantages during labour are that, while all the pain of labour is gone, the pregnant woman remains fully conscious and able to participate in the delivery. Also, although like all other forms of pain relief in labour the anaesthetic crosses the placenta, it has no systemic effect on the unborn baby. However, it does have disadvantages: it can only be used during the active stage of labour or contractions may cease; it doesn't work for every woman and can cause nausea, vomiting and a drop in blood-pressure; and the anaesthetic effect means that the urge to push is deadened so that the second stage of labour is often longer and the woman is more dependent on her attendants to control her labour. The rate of forceps delivery is markedly higher with epidural anaesthesia. It is administered via a very fine tube directly into the epidural space between the backbone and the spinal cord, from which the spinal nerves emerge. At present the technique is not universally available as it requires a skilled anaesthetist to carry it out.

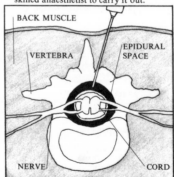

BACK MUSCLE

VERTEBRA

EPIDURAL SPACE

NERVE

CORD

EPIDURAL ANAESTHESIA

Episiotomy This is the medical term for a small incision made with scissors in the skin and superficial muscles of a woman's perineum, the region between the vagina and anus, during childbirth. It is performed under a local anaesthetic if there is a danger of the perineum being torn by the baby's

head. An episiotomy is easier to stitch than a jagged tear, is much less painful if stitched properly, and heals far better, although it may be slightly sore and uncomfortable for a couple of days. It is very important that the stitching of this delicate operation is not delegated to someone inexperienced, as problems can arise later if the job is not correctly done. An episiotomy is generally not necessary in an uncomplicated labour, but is common procedure during a forceps delivery.

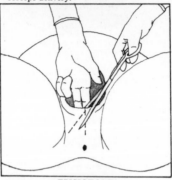

EPISIOTOMY

Ergometrine Originally made from a fungus which grows on rye, ergometrine is now made synthetically and is used during childbirth to make the uterus contract firmly to expel the placenta or 'afterbirth'. It is injected into the mother as the baby's head or shoulders emerge and is probably the best single method of checking bleeding after birth. In the United States, it is more commonly known as ergonovine.

EYE PROBLEMS

Cataract This is an opacity of the lens of the eye, or its capsule, caused by the lens becoming hard and thus opaque. Although cataracts may occur as the result of injury, excessive heat, radiation or electric shock, the most usual cause is age. The cataract can be surgically removed, usually under local anaesthetic, but the patient has to wait until the cataract has 'grown' fully, which may take some time. Strong glasses are prescribed afterwards to compensate for the loss of the lens.
Conjunctivitis This is the term used to describe inflammation of the conjunctiva, the mucous membrane that lines the inner surface of the eyelids and is reflected over the eyeball, joining this with the lids. A common cause of conjunctivitis is the presence of a 'foreign body', such as a speck of dirt, dandruff, a hair or an ingrown eyelash, which causes inflammation. Removal of the foreign body and soothing with warm water remedies the condition. If the inflammation is caused by infection, either from a virus or bacteria, antibiotic eyedrops are required so you should always consult your doctor. In itself conjunctivitis is not a serious condition, although occasionally it may lead to ulceration of the cornea. For advice on allergic conjunctivitis, see Allergies.
Stye A stye is caused by inflammation of the sebaceous gland surrounding an eyelash, usually a result of bacterial infection. Children are more prone to styes than adults, possibly because they rub their eyes, often with grubby hands, more frequently than adults. Treatment often involves removing the eyelash from the infected gland and bathing with warm, clean water. Doctors sometimes prescribe antibiotic ointments, but these should be used only under medical advice and supervision.

F

Fallopian Tubes The Fallopian tubes are the two ducts leading from the upper, outer corners of the uterus to the ovaries. Fertilization of the ovum by

the sperm takes place in one or other of the Fallopian tubes and after three or four days the fertilized ovum leaves the tube and enters the uterus. If it fails to do this, it will either die or form an ectopic pregnancy, which will have to be removed surgically. If the Fallopian tubes are blocked by mucus, fertility may be affected. The tubes can be tested for blockage by passing carbon dioxide along them (insufflation) or by injecting a radio-opaque dye into the uterus (hysterosalpingography) and along the tubes and examining them with the aid of X-rays.
Fibroids See Uterine Disorders.
Flaking Nails See Nail Problems.
Follicle Stimulating Hormone (FSH) See Hormones.

FOOT PROBLEMS

Athlete's foot This is a fungus, similar to that which causes ringworm, which grows between and under the toes. It thrives on warm, damp skin and is contagious. It makes the skin between the toes look soggy and white, and the skin itches, splits and peels. Powders and creams can be bought to cure the condition, but you can help yourself to avoid it by always being careful to dry between the toes and by washing and drying your feet carefully after a visit to a swimming pool or any other public place where people go barefoot. The infection may linger in socks and shoes for some time after the symptoms have disappeared from the feet. If possible, limit the shoes and socks you wear and discard them after the infection has cleared.
Bunions These are usually caused by wearing shoes that do not fit properly, causing the big toe to bend in. A bunion is the swelling and thickening of the main big toe joint in a bony outgrowth. Sometimes bunions become so severe that the whole foot looks deformed and a fluid-filled sac (bursa) may form on the joint. If you suspect that you may be developing a bunion, visit the chiropodist and ask his advice immediately. Prevention is better than cure. A bunion can be operated upon, but the recovery process is fairly painful and not always successful. It is far better to discard any shoes which cramp your feet, however much you like them.

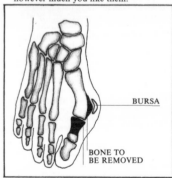

BURSA

BONE TO BE REMOVED

FOOT WITH BUNION

Callouses and hard skin Callouses can be uncomfortable and, if severe, can throw the foot off balance. They form across the ball of the foot or where shoes constantly rub or pinch. You can deal with mild callous formations yourself by rubbing with a pumice stone or special foot scraper after your bath. It is a good idea always to check your feet in the bath or when you give yourself a pedicure and to rub away dead skin to prevent callouses developing. If they become severe, you should go to a chiropodist to have them scraped or even cut away. If a callous keeps forming at a particular place on the foot, try to find out which pair of shoes is causing the rubbing or whether you are walking incorrectly.
Corns A corn is a type of callous caused by pressure from shoes, often on the little toe if it is squeezed by shoes which are too tight. It is cone shaped, with the

point often going deep into the foot, and can be very painful. Corns are best removed by a chiropodist, although temporary relief can be found in little felt rings which surround the corn and prevent direct pressure on it.

Ingrowing toe nails These occur when the sides of the toe nail start to grow into the skin of the nail wall. It is extremely painful and hard to correct once firmly established. At the first sign of an ingrowing toe nail, go to a chiropodist. You can help to prevent them forming by making sure that your shoes are wide enough across the toes and by cutting your toe nails correctly. They should be cut straight across, never down into the corners, and not too short.

Onychomicosis This is a fungal infection that attacks the nails, usually those of the feet and more often than not the big-toe nails. Like many infectious fungi, it grows and spreads in warm, damp conditions and will flourish where feet are sweaty, shoes and socks tight or non-porous, and in hot weather. Onychomicosis manifests itself in excessive thickening of the nail and discoloration, but pain is not necessarily a factor. If the affected nail is pressing on another toe, sores or corns may appear on this, too. To treat onychomicosis effectively the fungus must be killed with applications of a fungicidal liquid. Although this is essentially easy to apply, the thickened nail must be pared away to provide access to the source of infection and treatment may extend over weeks or months, until the offending nail has completely grown out and been replaced by new, unaffected growth.

Verrucas (plantar warts) These are ingrowing warts which may grow singly or in groups on the feet. The warts are flattened and pushed inwards and can be very painful, especially as they generally occur on the parts of the foot that receive most pressure. They are the result of a virus infection, which is catching, and are easily picked up in swimming pools, school changing rooms and other places where people go barefoot. The sooner verrucas are identified, the easier and quicker they are to remove, so if you suspect you have one visit a chiropodist at once.

Forceps Forceps are a pair of curved steel blades, not unlike a pair of spoons, which are fitted over the baby's head to facilitate a quick delivery. The aim is to protect the baby's head from undue pressure from the pelvic bones. A baby is delivered with the aid of forceps in the following circumstances: when the baby's head ceases to descend once the cervix is fully dilated; when the baby is thought to be in distress, indicated by the slowing of its heart rate, so that it is safer to deliver the baby as quickly as possible; in certain cases of maternal distress. A local anaesthetic in the pelvic area is necessary for a forceps delivery, unless the mother has already had an epidural anaesthetic.

G

Gas and Oxygen Mixture One method of pain relief in labour is the inhalation of a mixture of gas and oxygen during contractions. The gas, nitrous oxide, is mixed with oxygen so that there is never less than 30 per cent of oxygen in the mixture. It is usually stored in a cylinder with a mask attached, which the woman herself holds over her face. The best way to take the mixture is to begin breathing it in deeply at the very start of the contraction, so that the strongest effects coincide with the strength of the contraction. You will be taught how to use the mask at antenatal classes.

Genital Warts See Warts.

GLANDS Glands are organs which secrete and release vital substances which keep the body working properly. There are two main types: exocrine glands, which carry secretions to the surface of the body or lining of a hollow organ (e.g. sweat glands, sebaceous glands), and endocrine glands, which secrete hormones that are carried in the bloodstream and regulate the vital processes of the body (e.g. adrenal glands, pituitary gland). See also Hormones.

Adrenal glands The two adrenal glands are situated at the back of the abdomen against the upper ends of the kidneys. The outer layer of the adrenal body, the cortex, is an endocrine gland which produces three different types of hormone: cortisol, aldosterone and sex hormones. Cortisol and aldosterone help the body to cope with stress and control the water balance and are essential to life. Sex hormones on the other hand, i.e. oestrogen and progesterone in women, are also secreted by the ovaries from puberty to menopause. The changes which take place in the body at menopause are the result of a drastic reduction in oestrogen, an absence of progesterone, and a rise in pituitary hormones. It was once believed that oestrogen ceased to be produced altogether after the menopause, but it is now known that a small amount continues to be secreted by the ovaries well into old age. This is supplemented by the oestrogen produced by the adrenal glands and one woman in two continues to secrete enough oestrogen after menopause for her body's needs. The inner zone of the adrenal body, the medulla, is stimulated by the nervous system and produces adrenalin (epinephrine). When the body undergoes the kind of stress produced by shock, anger or fear, the glands increase their secretions of adrenalin which passes into the bloodstream and thence to every part of the body, speeding up the heartbeat, causing an increase in blood-pressure, and enabling the muscles to work faster and longer than usual.

Apocrine sweat glands A sweat gland is a coiled tube made up of secretory cells which absorb fluid from the surrounding cells and capillaries and pass it through the tube to the surface of the skin. The apocrine sweat glands are concentrated in the armpits and groins, around the nipples and navel, and tend to respond more to emotional and nervous stress than to changes in temperature. The sweat they produce has a slightly 'earthy' smell.

Bartholin's glands These are two pea-sized glands on either side of the hymen. During sexual arousal they secrete fluid which moistens the entrance to the vagina, so that the man's penis may enter easily and without discomfort. Occasionally these glands may become infected.

Eccrine sweat glands The body possesses about two million sweat glands in all, both apocrine and eccrine. The eccrine glands cover the whole skin surface and are stimulated by an increase in temperature: the result of hot weather, eating spicy food, exercise or fever. The sweat they produce, which is 99 per cent water and 1 per cent waste salts, cools the body down again as it evaporates on the skin and acts as an efficient temperature control. In a temperate climate an average man loses about 1 pt (600 ml) of sweat a day. Both the liquid and the salt must be replaced; if water alone is taken the salt and water balance of the blood tissues will be upset and cramp may result.

Hypothalamus This is a part of the brain which is connected by nerve fibres to most other parts of the nervous system and attached by a thin stalk to the pituitary gland. The functions of the hypothalamus are numerous and include regulation of the autonomic nervous system, and so of the heart and abdominal organs; control over the emotions and mood; regulation of body temperature, appetite and thirst; increasing the flow of blood through the muscles during exercise; control over the water balance in the body by stimulation of the antidiuretic hormone (ADH) which is stored in the pituitary gland; stimulation of the production of oxytocin, which is also stored in the pituitary, to help the uterus to contract during childbirth and the muscles round the mammary glands to contract and eject milk; and control of the pituitary gland, which in turn regulates the output of other endocrine glands and the kidneys. The hypothalamus also, for reasons which are not quite clear, secretes substances called releasing factors which about four years before the onset of menstruation pass down the blood vessels connecting the hypothalamus with the pituitary and cause the release of hormones which trigger off the changes of puberty. The hypothalamus works very closely with the pituitary gland to regulate the amount of each hormone in the blood and together they are the real controllers of the hormone system. See also Pituitary gland.

Lacrimal glands These are the glands where tears are formed, situated under the upper eyelids. The ducts secrete a solution of sodium chloride, sodium bicarbonate and a germicide which keeps the exposed surface of the conjunctiva and cornea moist, washes away dust and other particles, and combats infection. Tear fluid normally evaporates from the eye as fast as it is secreted, but some may drain into the nasal cavity through the lacrimal duct at the eye's inner corner.

Mammary glands These are found in the breast. They develop during pregnancy and are stimulated to produce milk after childbirth by the hormone prolactin, which is secreted by the pituitary gland. During pregnancy, the release of prolactin is prevented by the effects of high levels of oestrogen and progesterone produced by the placenta, which prepare the breasts for lactation by actions on the ducts and alveoli, the milk-producing areas. After the birth, the level of oestrogen and progesterone drops and the pituitary gland starts to make and release prolactin, which circulates in the bloodstream and is taken up by the milk-making cells in the breast. At first only thick colostrum is secreted, but within forty-eight hours of the birth milk usually starts to appear. The amount secreted is regulated by the baby's demand. The secreted milk will remain in and distend the mammary glands unless it is forced, by contractions of the minute muscles which surround the mammary glands, to travel along the milk ducts to the milk reservoirs. These contractions are caused by the hormone oxytocin, which is released by the pituitary gland in response to stimulation of the mother's nipple by the baby. If a mother does not wish to breast-feed, or stops after a couple of weeks, treatment must be given to prevent the breasts becoming heavy, tense, warm and painful. This is usually in the form of bromocriptine, which suppresses lactation by directly stopping the release of prolactin from the pituitary and stops the production of milk without any discomfort.

Ovaries Progesterone and oestrogen are secreted here. Progesterone controls the normal progress of pregnancy and interacts with follicle stimulating hormone (FSH), luteinizing hormone (LH) and oestrogen to control the menstrual cycle. Oestrogen controls the development of female features at puberty and interacts with FSH, LH and progesterone to control menstruation.

Pancreas Glands here produce insulin, which helps to control the use of sugar in the body. Failure to produce enough insulin leads to diabetes.

Parathyroid glands These are four small glands located within the thyroid. They secrete parathyroid hormone and calcitonin, which control the amount of calcium in the blood and bones.

Pituitary gland This is the most complex of the endocrine glands. It is situated in a small niche at about eye level in one of the bones near the centre of the skull and is attached by a thin stalk to the hypothalamus. The gland works very closely with the hypothalamus and secretes numerous hormones, most of which act upon and regulate the activities of other endocrine glands, to such an extent that the pituitary is sometimes called the 'master gland'. In women, the main secretions of the pituitary gland are growth hormones, which influence the growth of bone and other tissues; prolactin, which maintains milk production; luteinizing hormone (LH), which triggers off ovulation and helps to control the menstrual cycle; follicle stimulating hormone (FSH), which acts on the ovaries causing the follicles to develop and in turn secrete their own hormone, oestrogen, and helps to control the menstrual cycle; and trophic hormones, which stimulate other hormone-producing glands to release hormones. See also Hypothalamus.

Placenta During pregnancy the placenta secretes human chorionic gonadotrophin (HCG) and human chorionic somatotrophin (HCS), which help to control the normal progress of pregnancy, and oestrogen and progesterone which prepare the breasts for milk production.

Small intestine This secretes enterogasterone, which switches off acid production by the stomach, and secretin and CCK-PZ, which trigger the release of digestive enzymes from the pancreas.

Stomach wall The hormone gastrin is secreted here, which sets off acid production by the stomach.

Sebaceous glands These glands open into the hair follicles in the skin and produce an oily secretion known as sebum. This keeps the epidermis supple, as the oil inhibits the evaporation of moisture from the tissue, and gives hair water-repellent qualities. It is believed that the fatty acids in sebum help to prevent the breeding of harmful bacteria and fungi.

Thyroid gland This gland is situated in the neck, in front of the windpipe. It secretes thyroxine, which controls the rate of general body processes, heat production, energy production from food, and growth and development of the nervous system. Women are more prone to thyroid problems than men, particularly goitre, which is any enlargement of the thyroid. Simple goitre is the result of a lack of iodine in the diet, the gland's most important raw material. Deprived of this, the thyroid produces more thyroxine and responds by over-growing. Toxic goitre is over-activity of the thyroid. The swelling itself may be hardly noticeable, but the patient becomes irritable and restless, loses weight, and suffers from an over-active heart. The surest form of treatment for this complaint is removal of the gland. Too little thyroxine on the other hand, often a problem for women in middle age, tends to lead to over-weight, loss of energy, low body temperature, dry and puffy skin, and a dulled mind.

Gonorrhoea See Venereal Diseases.

H

Haemoglobin Haemoglobin is the compound of protein and iron in the red cells of the blood. It is the means of transporting oxygen from the lungs to the rest of the body. Its task in pregnancy is to transfer oxygen via the placenta to the foetus. A fall in the haemoglobin level, which in a normal woman is 82–100 per cent, indicates a general fall in the efficiency of the blood and can be a sign of anaemia, which can be corrected with iron pills. See also Anaemia.

Haemophilia This is an inherited disorder in which the blood clots very slowly. Any injury, however slight, is dangerous as there is generally prolonged bleeding. There is also a tendency to bleed internally for no obvious reason. Transfusions of healthy blood are used to control severe bleeding, and may even be needed in very minor operations such as the extraction of teeth. Haemophilia affects only men, but is carried by women. Children of female carriers have a fifty-fifty chance of inheriting the disorder—girls as carriers, boys as sufferers. If a male haemophiliac has children, all his daughters will be carriers but all his sons will be normal. If there is any haemophilia in your family, or your husband's, think carefully and take genetic counselling before starting a family.

Haemophilis Vaginalis See Vaginal Infections.

Haemorrhoids See Piles.

HAIRCUTTING AT HOME There is no substitute for a professional haircut, but if you are unable to visit your hairdresser regularly here are some tips for trimming at home. Hair should always be cut wet, since this will help you to achieve a more even cut, and scissors should be sharp. You will also need Scotch tape, a comb, clips to hold hair out of the way, a blow-dryer and two mirrors (so that you can check the back of your hair).

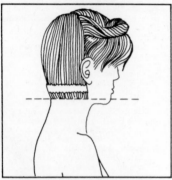

Bob If you have fine hair, simply tape it in place in the direction in which it was cut, just above the line you want, and trim. Thicker hair is slightly more difficult as you have to work in sections. Make a centre parting down the back of your head and clip hair out of the way. Then make a horizontal parting just above the nape, place a strip of tape around the back of your head above the line you want, and cut the hair little by little. When you have completed this section, make another horizontal parting above the first one, retape and cut again. Repeat the process until all the hair is cut, using two tapes as the hair gets thicker to hold it in place.

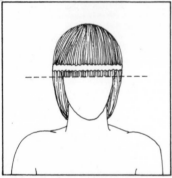

Fringe Comb your fringe down from a parting or the crown of your head, in the direction in which it was originally cut, and tape right round from one side to the other. Cut a small section in the front of the fringe above your nose, then cut towards the right and then the left. Leave the fringe a little bit longer than you want it, as the tape is pressing the hair flat against your forehead and it will look shorter when blown dry.

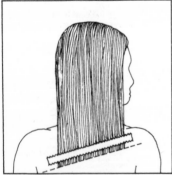

Long hair This is easy to trim yourself. Part your hair in the middle from the front to the nape, then comb it straight down and forwards from the back, slightly over the shoulder. Turn your head to one side, place the hair flat on your chest or neck depending on its length, and secure it firmly with tape. Make sure that this is perfectly positioned before you start, then cut right across using the tape as a guide.

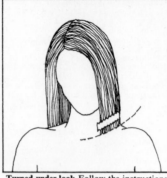

Turned-under look Follow the instructions for long hair, but tilt your head away from the cutting side when you tape and cut. This results in the top layer being longer than the bottom layer. Again, use the tape as a guide when cutting.

HAIRSTYLING EQUIPMENT Managing your own hairstyle may take some practice, but it is cheaper than a visit to the hairdresser and quite easy once you are used to it. Watch your stylist at work to learn how to create your personal look and try to avoid equipment which might damage your hair.
Brushes The best brush should glide through your hair like a comb. Expensive natural-bristle brushes, always thought to be the best, can in fact pull and damage some types of hair. Newer nylon brushes, if they are of good quality, have rounded tips and are set in a flexible rubber pad. Shun cheaper brushes with synthetic bristles and never use a brush on wet hair.
Bunches Never, *never* use elastic bands to hold hair in a pony tail or chignon. Tie your hair with silky-covered bands, ribbons or even pipe-cleaners.
Combs The best everyday comb is made of vulcanized rubber, hand-finished acetate or more expensively horn, and has a totally smooth surface which won't snag. Cheap plastic combs have spiky ends and unfinished rough edges between the teeth. A good comb should have wide and narrow teeth, and should be used primarily to section and style wet hair. The widely-spaced teeth of 'Afro' combs are excellent for combing through and fluffing up curly hairstyles.
Curling tongs These are useful for putting finishing touches to dry hair, such as turning under, flicking up, or adding curling tendrils around the face or at the nape of the neck. They are also good for straightening, temporarily, very curly hair and for ironing out fringes. The latest steamer tongs are especially good, since they moisten hair to inhibit dryness and make for a stronger curl because the hair is slightly damp as the curling process begins. Care is needed when handling curling tongs as butterfingers can burn the skin.
Hair-dryers Many hand dryers come with extra attachments such as hot combs, brushes and snap-on nozzles to concentrate and speed the air flow. Be wary of extra-fast dryers, as they can be hard on dry hair. Light dryers are easiest to handle, as arm ache can set in after minutes. Hair does not take a style until it is three-quarters dry, so save time and arms by drying naturally at first. Then part the hair into sections, pinning away top layers. Start at the back, holding hair in the required position. The hair-dryer should always be a good handspan away. Lift hair away from the scalp at the root to give height and movement. Hairdressers will blow-dry by holding the hair with a brush as they style; home hairstylists might find hands easier, and the use of the hand prevents hair from becoming too hot and dry. Salon-type driers are good for those who like free hands and a style set with rollers. They are expensive, but a good investment if you want a salon style at home. The rigid type with a stand are by far the best.
Hair grips Known as kirby grips, these should be chosen in colours nearest your hair colour and should be plastic tipped so as not to scratch. Grips can secure pin

curls when dry setting and will fasten wigs and hairpieces securely.
Hairpins Choose those with plastic-coated tips to avoid scratching. Large hairpins should be used to secure rollers; two in each roller is best, slipped sideways in opposite directions near the scalp. Hairpins can set short hair at the nape and cheek curls and are better than hair grips for setting.
Hair rollers Foam rubber or smooth mesh-covered rollers are the gentlest. Brush rollers, which have small hairy brushes inside to grip hair, are easier to use but can tear the hair. Plastic rollers with pronged teeth can also be damaging. The diameter of the rollers determines the size of the curl: small rollers give a tight, very curly style; large rollers are for long hair or a smooth style.
Heated rollers These are wax-filled plastic rollers which are heated on hot rods for about ten minutes and then wound into hair. The rollers will not burn your hands or head, but the rods will. A set of twenty gives enough for a whole head and will work quickly: a strong curl emerges after a few minutes and gradually drops out over a day or an evening. Use heated rollers sparingly, three times a week maximum, as they are very drying even if rollers dispense a conditioner. They are ideal for setting wigs and hairpieces, but should not be used on wet hair.
Wigs and hairpieces A whole-head wig is easier to handle than a hairpiece. Both can be made from real or synthetic hair; a real hair wig looks better and lasts longer, but a cheaper hairpiece can add body for an elaborate hairstyle. Both should be cleaned at the hair salon or with a special wig cleanser—never washed. They can be easily set with heated rollers or with ordinary rollers if heat is applied—try the airing cupboard overnight.

Hang Nails See Nail Problems.
Hay Fever (Rhinitis) See Allergies.
Headaches The types and causes of headaches are innumerable, ranging from a simple ache over the brow, caused by eyestrain and remedied by correcting the faulty vision, to a full-blown migraine. In relatively few cases, a headache can be symptomatic of a serious disease or illness, but most have a simpler origin: an infected tooth, rheumatism, sinus infection, high blood-pressure, fever and sunstroke can all lead to headaches. So too can anxiety, stress, constipation, excessive smoking, lack of fresh air or oxygen, continuous noise and the contraceptive pill. Many headaches are due to dilatation of or pressure on the intracranial arteries. Dilatation may be the result of stimulation of another part of the body, or it may start in the back of the neck or on the scalp. Headaches due to lack of fresh air can be alleviated by deep breathing, preferably accompanied by moderate exercise such as walking out of doors. Another cause, constipation, can be cured by taking an effective laxative to empty the bowels and again some form of exercise. Headaches caused by muscle tension in the shoulders and neck can be noticeably reduced by massage and exercise. Learning how to relax properly will also be of benefit in coping with or reducing the severity of headaches. Analgesics such as aspirin or codeine-based drugs give temporary relief, but should never be a regular precautionary measure; it is far better to diagnose the cause of the pain and remedy that. Some women find that they get more frequent and intense headaches in the days preceding a period. Premenstrual tension causes a great deal of discomfort for many women and drugs can be prescribed to alleviate the problem which, it is thought, has much to do with hormonal imbalances at this time. Similarly, hormonal changes which occur as a result of taking the Pill can precipitate headaches in certain women. Remember that there are a number of different types of contraceptive pill on the market and, if necessary, experiment until you find one which suits you better. Your doctor or gynaecologist will help you to do this. It is worth bearing in mind that the healthier your way of life,

and consequently the fitter your body, the less likely you are to be troubled by headaches.
Head Lice These small, parasitic insects (pediculi) are becoming an increasingly common problem, with as many as one million people in Britain now affected. The condition is highly infectious. The lice, which prefer a clean, healthy head, lay their eggs on the hair and are usually first detected by an itchy scalp or by seeing the insects themselves, especially when hair is washed. They can be most easily found on the scalp around the ears and underneath hair growth at the back of the neck. Treatment is with an anti-parasitic lotion which can generally be obtained directly from your local health clinic or pharmacist—there is no need for a doctor's prescription. A mild case will clear in a couple of weeks with application of the two necessary killing agents, malathion and carbaryl. The old cure used to be a mixture of DDT and gamma benzene hexachloride, but lice have become immune to this. A combination of both the new agents is recommended because lice tend to become immune to one after a time. Use first one, then switch to the other. This will kill both the existing lice and the fertile eggs, known as nits. The hair must be washed every day with a special shampoo and the lotion combed through with a very fine comb. Strict cleanliness is the rule for all members of the household; towels and pillows must not be shared and brushes and combs should be treated to daily disinfectant.
Heartburn This has nothing to do with the heart, but is a type of indigestion which is fairly common in late pregnancy. It is caused by small quantities of stomach content entering the lower part of the oesophagus, the tube from the mouth to the stomach. Heartburn occurs in pregnancy because the enlarging uterus pushes against the stomach and the valve at the entrance to the stomach relaxes. The condition is often worse at night, when there can be an intense burning sensation in the upper abdomen. An expectant mother can relieve heartburn by eating frequently but in small quantities and by sipping milk when an attack occurs. Sleeping propped up on one or two extra pillows may also help at night. If heartburn persists tell your doctor, who may prescribe antacid tablets or liquids to alleviate the condition.
Herpes See Skin Problems.
Hives (Urticaria) See Skin Problems.

HORMONES Hormones are chemical messengers released into the bloodstream by the endocrine glands (see Glands). They cannot be consciously controlled and are released in short bursts which vary in quantity and frequency. They make up an extremely complex and delicately-balanced network which controls a wide variety of processes in the body, including digestion, heat production, energy production, water balance, growth and development of the nervous system, acid production, emergency reaction, development of sexual features at puberty, and in women the menstrual cycle, pregnancy, childbirth and the menopause. The main hormones involved in the transformation of a girl into a woman and control of the reproductive cycle are listed below.
Follicle stimulating hormone (FSH) Secreted by the pituitary gland, FSH stimulates the growth of follicles in a woman's ovaries and helps to control the menstrual cycle.
Human chorionic gonadotrophin (HCG) This hormone, secreted by the placenta, acts with *human chorionic somatotrophin (HCS)* to suppress the mother's menstrual cycle and control the normal progress of pregnancy.
Luteinizing hormone (LH) Secreted by the pituitary gland, LH triggers ovulation and helps to control the menstrual cycle.
Oestrogen This is a female sex hormone secreted by the ovaries at puberty; it controls the development of female features and interacts with follicle stimulating hormone, luteinizing hormone and progesterone to control the menstrual cycle. During pregnancy,

oestrogen is also secreted by the placenta and acts with progesterone to control the growth of the uterus and prepare the breasts for milk production. In middle age, diminished secretions of oestrogen lead to the menopause. Small doses of oestrogen may be prescribed in hormone replacement therapy if the symptoms of the menopause are severe.

Oxytocin Stored in the pituitary gland, oxytocin helps the uterus to contract during childbirth and stimulates contraction of the minute muscles around the mammary glands during milk production. Synthetic oxytocin is often used to induce labour.

Progesterone Like oestrogen, progesterone is an important female sex hormone which is first produced at puberty and helps to control development of female features and the menstrual cycle, interacting with follicle stimulating hormone, luteinizing hormone and oestrogen. It also prepares the uterus for pregnancy and, during pregnancy, acts with oestrogen to control the growth of the uterus and prepare the breasts for lactation. In middle age, production of progesterone by the ovaries terminates, leading to the menopause.

Androgens These are male sex hormones and the principal androgen, *testosterone*, is secreted by the cells in a man's testicles. Androgens are also produced in small quantities in the ovaries and adrenal glands of women. If the secretion is excessive, a woman may develop certain male characteristics, such as excessive hair on the face.

Hot Flushes See Blushing.

HOT OIL TREATMENT

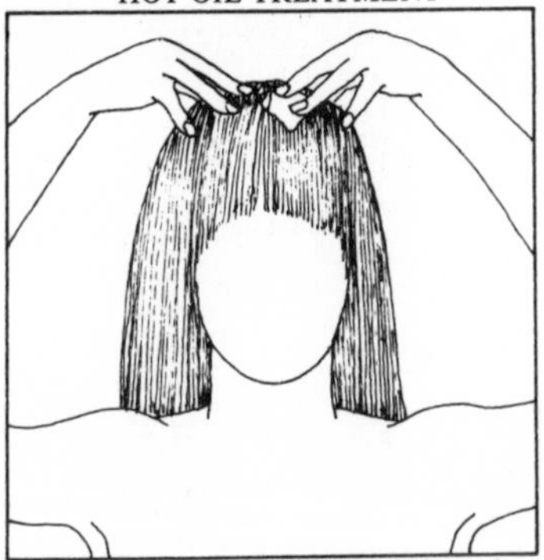

1 Section hair and apply warmed olive oil. Massage into scalp.

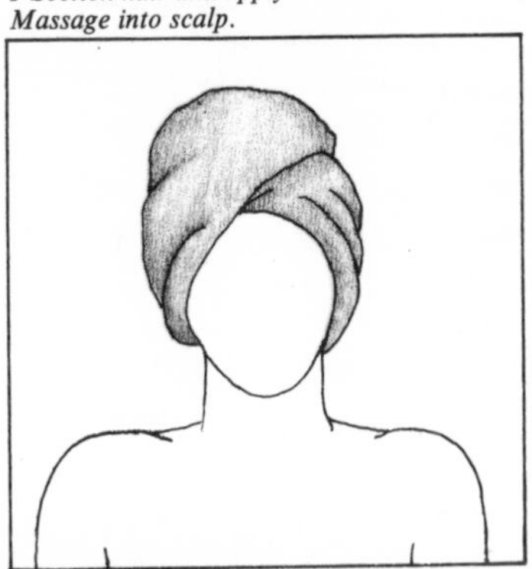

2 Wind hot towel round head. Leave for fifteen to thirty minutes.

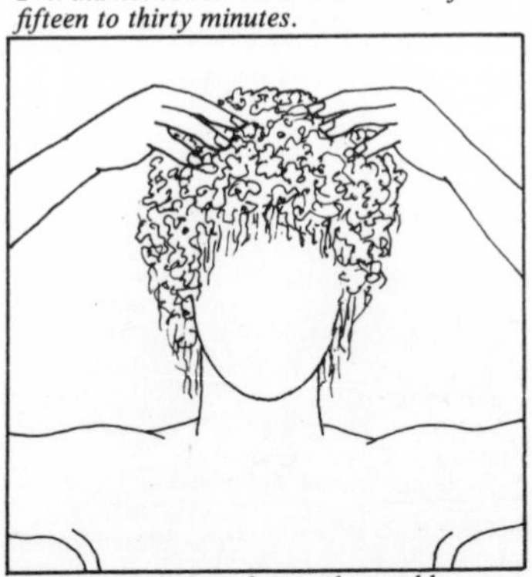

3 Shampoo hair and rinse thoroughly.

Hot Oil Treatment for Dry Hair Warm two tablespoons of olive oil and massage thoroughly into the scalp. Immerse a towel in hot water, then wring it out and wrap it round your head like a turban. When the towel cools, reheat and apply it in the same way as before. You may have to do this two or three times to achieve complete saturation. Then wash your hair with shampoo and rinse thoroughly.

Human Chorionic Gonadotrophin (HCG) See Hormones.

Human Chorionic Somatotrophin (HCS) See Hormones.

Hypo-allergenic Derived from the Greek word 'hypo', meaning less, and the word allergen, meaning something which causes an allergic response, hypo-allergenic is the term used to describe cosmetic products which have had all known allergens, such as perfume and certain chemicals, screened out of them. See also Allergies, Cosmetic allergy.

Hypothalamus See Glands.

Hysterectomy This is the surgical removal of the womb. It is total if the cervix is removed as well. The ovaries are removed only if they are abnormal, but a woman should always be asked for her prior consent to this as loss of the ovaries causes an immediate menopause and retention of even a small portion will avoid this. A hysterectomy is unavoidable if there is a malignancy or if some other condition such as fibroids, a prolapsed uterus or endometriosis becomes intolerable. It should not be offered as part of an abortion package (frequently done to poor women with large families) or as a routine procedure once child-bearing is over as a precaution against a future cancer. Surveys show that where hysterectomies have been performed unnecessarily they are more likely to be followed by depression and other problems. Where the woman is convinced that the operation was necessary, she is pleased to be rid of her troublesome condition and there are seldom any bad psychological after-effects.

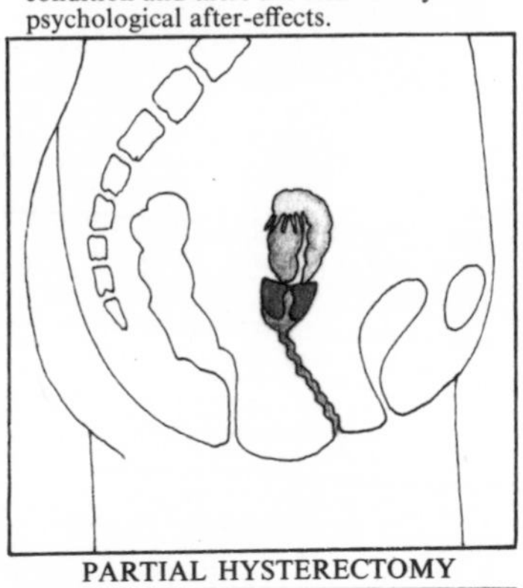

PARTIAL HYSTERECTOMY

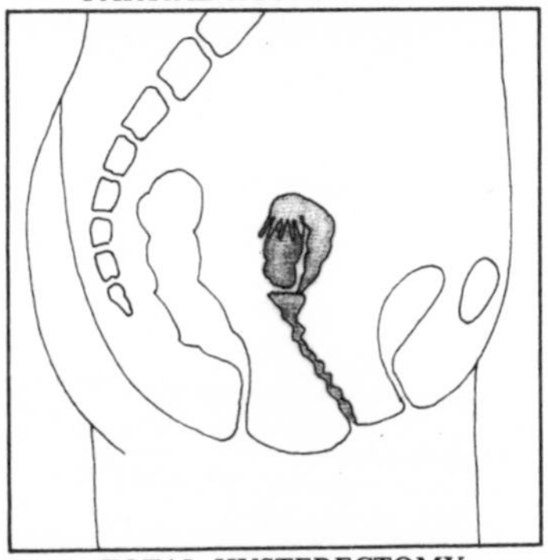

TOTAL HYSTERECTOMY

I

Incubator Premature and ill new-born babies will usually spend the first days of their life in an incubator. This provides them with a safe, warm, sterile environment, like an extension of the uterus, in which they can be cared for. Incubation of her baby is distressing for a mother, but there are ways in which she can be allowed to help and feed her baby even in the incubator.

Ingrowing Toe Nails See Foot Problems.

Insomnia Sleep is essential to our well-being, although we all need different amounts. A few people can survive happily on as little as four hours a night, whilst others need as much as eight or nine hours. The very young need a lot of sleep; conversely, as we get older we can generally manage with less. Deprived of sleep for more than a day or two, most humans will start to show signs of debilitation. They will function less efficiently and become irritable, and the effects of the deprivation will be reflected in their appearance. The reasons why people suffer from insomnia are numerous. There may be a temporary cause, or insomnia may have become a habit and, like all habits, prove hard to break. The first thing to do if you are having trouble sleeping is to try to establish the cause or causes. A simple check-list may help. Start by considering the following questions.

1 Is your bed comfortable, right for you? Some people like to sink into a deep sprung mattress, others prefer a hard bed; if you sleep with someone else there is no guarantee that you will both like the same kind of bed.

2 Are you ready for sleep? People's sleep needs and rhythms vary enormously and you may be trying to fit into someone else's pattern. There is a theory that you tend to wake and be at your most alert at around the time you were born which might, if true, explain why some people are up and raring to go at six in the morning whilst others only come into their own at midnight. The more usual explanation of these differences, however, is that our body rhythms vary and that we each have our individual peaks and lows during a twenty-four-hour period.

3 Are you too warm or too cold? Insomnia has been cured by something as simple as getting rid of nylon sheets or a duvet, or adding an extra blanket.

4 Is your bedroom conducive to sleep? Is it stuffy, too warm, too cold, too light? Not only sleep but also marriages can be disrupted if one of you likes to drop off at a steady temperature of 65°F (18°C) whilst the other prefers to sleep in a roaring gale.

5 Is your bed big enough? This is particularly relevant for couples. People differ enormously in the ways in which they sleep: there are snugglers, writhers, stretchers, grabbers of blankets, and if you differ in your habits what should be the quietest time of the day may turn into a battlefield. Separate beds may be the answer, or even separate rooms. This move doesn't have to signify that your relationship is cracking up, it could in fact be positively beneficial, particularly if we accept anthropologist Desmond Morris's theory that we all need territorial space and privacy when settling to sleep and waking up.

6 Are your eating, drinking and smoking habits inhibiting sleep? Eating late in the evening, particularly rich or spicy food, means a lot of work for your digestive system and can cause sleeplessness, as can too much alcohol or caffeine-based drinks such as tea and coffee, or too many cigarettes. If you are dieting or have been busy and skimped meals you may simply be hungry.

7 Is your mind over-stimulated? The old remedies for insomnia, a book at bedtime or a late-night movie, are only sleep inducing if they relax you. Anything that causes the adrenalin to surge round the body is not going to help you to relax and you can't expect to sleep if you have been working too late. If you have been cooped up indoors or in an office all day, you may simply not be tired because you have surplus physical energy; a walk last thing at night or a well-tried exercise routine may be all you need to tip you into the land of nod.

Perhaps the most common cause of insomnia is anxiety. If when you get into bed your brain starts wrestling with a particular problem, then obviously sleep will not come. The answer, of course, is to try to identify the cause of the problem and resolve it; this doesn't help much when you are tossing and turning, but it is worth remembering that nothing is ever as bad as it seems at four in the morning. If however hard you've tried you still cannot sleep, the sensible thing to do is to stop worrying about it; accept that you can't sleep and that you will not suffer irreparable damage because you have lost a few hours and get up. Risk waking your partner, who will almost certainly drop off again within seconds even if he does wake. Do something positive: iron some clothes, play a record, read a book, go for a walk, then you can try to sleep again. Lie down and practise the tense-relax technique (see page 59).

Internal Self-Examination See Well Woman Check-Up.

International Childbirth Education Association of America See National Childbirth Trust.

K

Keratin This is an organic, protein, horny substance (the word derives from the Greek word for horn). Hair is made up of dead keratinous scales and the nails on your hands and feet are outgrowings or extensions of layers of keratinous skin. It is the keratin in nails that makes them hard. The body normally manufactures sufficient of the essential constituents of nails—including keratin—to ensure strong, regular growth. The nails that you see are only the end growth of the original nail which is formed under the skin above the uppermost toe or finger joint. Good nail formation requires a diet rich in protein, calcium, iron, Vitamin B, iodine and potassium.

L

Lacrimal Glands See Glands.

Leboyer Method Frederick Leboyer is a French obstetrician who pioneered a method of delivery which concentrates on the baby's experience during birth. The Leboyer method tries to make the baby's entry into the world as unalarming and untraumatic as possible. Lights in the delivery room are kept very low, the attendants keep their voices down, and as soon as the baby is delivered, it is laid on the mother's stomach and gently massaged. Later it is placed in a bath of water at blood-heat temperature. Even though very few British hospitals practise the Leboyer method, many women and midwives find his ideas sympathetic, and his humanitarian and gentle approach to birth is having some influence on traditional thinking.

Lines or Ridges on Nails See Nail Problems.

Liver Spots See Birthmarks.

Luteinizing Hormone (LH) See Hormones.

Lymph Nodes The lymphatic system is a network of vessels in the body which collects fluids from the tissues and returns them to the blood through two veins at the base of the neck. The watery fluid which makes up lymph contains substances used by the body to fight germs. The lymph nodes or glands are swellings in the lymphatic system made up of small masses of spongy tissue and are particularly numerous in the neck, armpits and groins. Infection stimulates the lymph nodes to increase their activity and they may become swollen and painful. Cancer of the breast generally spreads through the lymphatic system, beginning with the lymph nodes in the armpit and sometimes those in the chest and spine as well. In cases of radical mastectomy some or all of the armpit lymph nodes are removed in an attempt to stop the spread of the cancer.

M

Mammary Glands See Glands.

Mastitis Mastitis is inflammation of the breast, caused either by infection or hormonal imbalance. *Puerperal mastitis* occurs after childbirth often as a result of poor breast hygiene. Infection usually enters lactating breasts through cracked nipples and they become hard, reddened, tender and painful. A doctor will usually prescribe antibiotics or sulphonamides to correct the condition, and a mother may have to stop nursing her baby. *Chronic cystic mastitis* occurs in women in their thirties and forties and is thought to be due to hormone imbalance. The breast can feel lumpy or rubbery, all over or in patches, and there may be some pain especially before menstruation or after lifting heavy objects. It is a normal bodily change for many women and may not need treatment, but check with a doctor.

Meditation Since the beginning of civilization, people have searched for ways to inner peace and serenity. In some respects, primitive peoples who acknowledge and have an institutionalized mechanism for dealing with 'the spirits' are more *advanced* today than we are when we try to lock the spirit away, or deny its existence, or have no ways of dealing with it. Yet inner peace and serenity can seldom be achieved without coming to terms with the spirit. Many people choose meditation as the means of doing this.

The techniques of meditation are curiously simple. The idea is to empty your mind completely of all everyday, transient worries, and then focus your concentration on one particular object. Think of flowers, for example: examine, in your mind's eye, what a flower is, its composition, the way it grows, blossoms, gives off pollen, and dies; how many kinds of flowers are there in the world, what colours, what sizes? Simply sit in a quiet room and compose yourself, and contemplate the wonder of flowers; after half an hour, you will feel pleasantly tranquil and relaxed.

If you don't feel too foolish about it, you can achieve a state of meditation by sitting alone in a room and repeating over and over again a word or a set of words: perhaps a key word like 'Me . . . me . . . me . . . me . . .' until you drift off into a type of trance. Repetition is used in prayer cycles in every religion; a Western form is the Litany, where the sing-song repetition of an invocation like 'Pray for us' after each supplication makes a rhythm whose cadences can lull and entrance.

Many Eastern philosophies help us towards inner serenity. Eastern mysticism emphasizes the power of non-doing, of *being* and of *essence*, and people are often attracted to it because it provides an antidote to the hectic, materialistic, aggressive element in Western society. The get-up-and-go aspect of the Protestant work ethic that has created the dynamism in Western civilization is noticeably lacking in tranquillity and spiritual succour. Zen, a Japanese form of Buddhism, is a religious manifestation of this emphasis on *being*, not doing. Yin and Yang, a Chinese philosophy of living in which everything rests on *balance*, is another way to reflective practice which has gained much acceptance in the West. But the most successful of all such philosophies is undoubtedly Yoga, which comes from Hindu thinking. Yoga is often regarded, and practised, as a physical exercise, but the aim in fact is to improve both physical and mental health to prepare the mind for higher consciousness. Beginning with the creation of physical well-being, Yoga then works on an upward spiral via the mental to the spiritual. It is, therefore, a physical expression of a spiritual exercise, in which the highest stage is union with God (the word yoga, from the ancient language of Sanskrit, actually means union or joining). This idea is common to almost all religions—that the body is the temple of the spirit, and the spirit is animated by the great life force, which should be sought in quiet ways.

Much meditation is accompanied by fasting, both in ancient religions and in contemporary health routines. When you withdraw substantial food, especially meat, from the system, you change the metabolic rate and thus the mental process. A one- or two-day liquid diet, in which you take nothing but fruit juices and water, can produce the effect of being 'high', with a strange and satisfying feeling of purity, cleanliness and innocence: renewal, in fact.

Melanoma See Moles.

Migraine This is the term used for an intensely painful form of headache, often recurring. The pain, frequently situated over one eye, is usually accompanied by blurred vision, 'seeing' bright, flickering lights, feelings of nausea and sometimes actual vomiting. Although research into the causes of migraine continues, there is as yet no proven cause, though there are a number of theories. One is that migraine may be due to a specific biochemical deficiency in the body, which means that the ingestion of certain foods —including chocolate, cheese and coffee —can trigger off the headache. Another is that a variety of circumstances—ranging from changes in the weather, physical or mental fatigue, alcohol and excessive smoking through to premenstrual tension and chemical changes during menopause—may individually or in combination produce a spasm or constriction of the blood vessels to the brain, followed by dilatation of the veins and subsequent release of fluid into the surrounding tissues. Yet another theory holds that the fluid thus released contains substances which lower the individual's threshold of pain. Whatever the cause, or causes, migraine is particularly painful as any sufferer knows. Treatment involves taking precautions against any of the factors that might, or seem to, trigger off an attack. If a migraine threatens, lying down in a quiet atmosphere and sleeping if possible may be enough to ward it off. If a migraine develops fully, the patient must lie down in a room with all sources of noise and light removed, abstain from eating, and take plenty of fluid, preferably water. Analgesics may help, as may drugs prescribed by the doctor to dilate the blood vessels. Migraine sufferers can join associations through which they can make contact with fellow sufferers and medical experts, which helps to reassure the patient that he or she is not unique and provides a source of practical help as well.

Moles A mole is a mass of cells, usually but not always raised, which contain a high concentration of the pigment melanin. Most people are born with a mole or moles somewhere on their body, although they sometimes appear in later life. During pregnancy moles tend to increase in number or grow bigger. It is also quite common for moles to contain one or several hairs. Most moles are perfectly harmless and have often in the past been regarded as a mark of beauty. Occasionally, however, moles may become malignant when *melanoma* occurs. Also known as black cancer, this is a tumour of the pigment-producing cells of the skin. Fortunately it is rare, but if you notice any abnormal changes in a mole such as sudden enlargement, bleeding or ulceration, particularly in a flat mole, consult your doctor immediately. If you are worried by the appearance of a mole and would like it or the hair growing from it removed, you should also consult a doctor. Tampering with moles or plucking hairs from them can cause infection and prove dangerous.

Mongolism (Down's Syndrome) Down's syndrome, named after the man who carried out the first major study of 'mongol' babies, so called because of their rather oriental looks and slanting eyes, is the most common of all congenital defects due to chromosome abnormality. Children born with this defect are mentally subnormal and usually delicate in health, although affectionate and often much loved. Down's syndrome affects one baby in every 1,500 born of mothers under the age of thirty, but the figure goes up sharply over the age of thirty-five to possibly one in every three hundred births. It is therefore usually recommended that mothers of this age undergo amniocentesis at around the fifteenth week of pregnancy to check whether their baby is affected. A therapeutic abortion would then be possible if the parents desired it.

Mouth Ulcers Ulcers which occur in the mouth are inflamed sores situated in the mucous membrane. The most frequent cause of these is a scratch or abrasion of the membrane which may result in a small infection. The ulcers will usually disappear of their own accord if this is the cause, but care should be taken not to irritate them with hot liquids or spicy food. Gels can be bought to deaden any pain, but as they are constantly washed off by saliva they give only temporary relief. Occasionally ulcers are a sign of other disorders, such as a high blood sugar level. If ulcers persist, visit your doctor and/or dentist.

N

NAIL PROBLEMS

Brittle nails Nails which grow a little and then become brittle and snap off can be inherited, or they can indicate that you are trying to grow your nails longer than your particular nail plate can support. Other causes are putting hands into detergent without wearing rubber gloves and incorrect use of nail hardeners and strengtheners, which should always be used in conjunction with a cuticle cream so that the moisture does not dry out of the nail. Cuticle cream, lanolin or petroleum jelly regularly massaged into the cuticle will stimulate the nail cells and encourage the growth of the nail; more important, they will ensure that the new nail is growing with the right amount of moisture between the layers, which is vital for bonding them together and preventing the nails from breaking and splitting. Incorrect filing can be another cause of this condition. Always use an emery board, never a steel file as this will tear the delicate keratin layers. Check that your diet is high in protein, calcium, iron, potassium and Vitamin B (foods such as yoghurt, celery, carrots, soya, eggs and fish) and take a daily dose of gelatine in the form of jelly cubes which will strengthen your nails. A course of iodine tablets may also be helpful.

Flaking nails The three layers of cells which form the nail plate separate and peel off, which seriously weakens the nail tip. Flaking nails can be hereditary, or they may be the result of crash dieting, when your body has been deprived of vitamins and minerals essential to healthy nails. (This would show up long after you had finished dieting, as the damage would have been done to the nail in the growing stage in the matrix and it takes time for the effects to grow up to the tip.) Certain drugs or medicines could also be a cause, as could harsh nail-polish solvents, an allergy to nail polish or solvent, or simply putting your hands into detergents too often without rubber gloves. As with brittle nails, it is wise to check your diet to ensure that you are eating the right foods, and a regular dose of gelatine is a good idea to strengthen the growing nail. To preserve the flaking, damaged part of the nail, file carefully in one direction only with an emery board to smooth layers which might snag and tear. Either stop wearing polish for a while or change to better quality products, and never use neat acetone as a remover. Always apply a base coat to protect your nails. Use a mending patch to stop the polish peeling off the layered part of the nail; it will both protect the weakened nail and help polish to adhere.

Hang nails These occur when the cuticle is firmly stuck to a nail. As the nail grows, it pulls the cuticle and eventually tears it. Hang nails can become infected and are then extremely painful. Avoid this condition by manicuring the nails regularly, using cuticle cream and loosening the cuticle away from the nail plate by pushing back gently with a towel after your bath. Never cut into the cuticle—this can cause a serious infection. Dead skin can be clipped off (but do not on any account pull the skin) and antiseptic dabbed on. Otherwise leave hang nails alone. If they become inflamed, see the doctor.

Lines or ridges on nails Ridges across the nails are caused by something damaging the newly-forming nail in the matrix. It could simply be a knock or a bump, but it is often caused by pushing back the cuticles too ruthlessly, which can damage the soft, new nail being formed below. Ridges can also be caused by illness. Once ridges have formed they cannot be removed, but they will grow out eventually. Faint lines or ridges going the other way, from cuticle to nail tip, can be inherited or caused by excessive dryness or acidity. Never use harsh polish removers and massage cuticles nightly with cream, lanolin or petroleum jelly. Vitamin A, calcium and iodine in your diet will help this condition.

Stained nails This can be caused by smoking or by the pigment in nail polish staining the nails. Using a base coat before varnishing prevents the polish infiltrating the nail plate. Nicotine stains can be removed by rubbing the nail with hydrogen peroxide or lemon, both of which are very drying, so thoroughly rinse and cream the nail afterwards.

White marks on nails These are usually caused by damage to the matrix either by a knock or bump, by too ruthless probing at the cuticle, or by picking at nail polish at the root of the nail. The injury causes the layers of keratin which form the nail to separate, and when air circulates between the layers a white spot appears. Once white spots have formed, they must just be allowed to grow out naturally. Occasionally white spots may be caused by a fungal infection, which should be seen by a doctor.

National Childbirth Trust and International Childbirth Education Association of America These are independent organizations which interest themselves in every aspect of pregnancy and childbirth. They are invaluable sources of information and support for the pregnant women who attend their classes, buy their pamphlets or seek their advice by telephone. Each association has trained teachers and counsellors all over the country who hold classes and act as points of contact for pregnant women and young mothers. They also help with problems such as breast-feeding once pregnancy is over.

Natural Childbirth Natural childbirth is based on the belief that most of the pain and trauma traditionally associated with labour are caused by ignorance and fear. A woman who gives birth following the principles of natural childbirth will have prepared her mind with a full knowledge of what is happening to her body during pregnancy and what to expect during labour. She will also have prepared her body by learning simple relaxation techniques that will help her to stay in control during powerful labour contractions. Natural childbirth is not a guarantee of painless labour and those extreme supporters who claim that it is do more harm than good. A woman who has been led to believe that all labour is a joyful, painless affair can be badly let down when the real experience comes, and can be made to feel a failure. However, whatever kind of labour is in store, classes in natural childbirth can be invaluable in giving self-confidence, helping relaxation and abolishing ignorance.

Non-Barbiturate Hypno-Sedatives See Tranquillizers.

Non-Specific Urethritis See Venereal Diseases.

Non-Specific Vaginitis See Vaginal Infections.

Nymphomaniac This is the term used to describe a woman, or the behaviour of a woman, who has apparently uncontrollable sexual desires and appetites. Most psychiatric opinion concurs in the theory that nymphomania is just one of the many possible manifestations of a psychologically or emotionally disturbed state. Women who relentlessly pursue sexual gratification are often basically insecure, unable to form or maintain a satisfactory relationship. Sexual encounters may provide an escape from anxiety and feelings of inadequacy. There is also evidence to suggest that so-called frigidity, the inability to achieve orgasm, can lead a woman into nymphomaniacal behaviour in an attempt to find gratification. Nymphomania is a term also applied, wrongly, to women who enjoy sex with a variety of people, or whose libido (sexual drive) is strong. The condition can be helped by tranquillizers or psychotherapy. The male equivalent of nymphomania is called satyriasis.

O

Oedema This is an abnormal accumulation of fluid in the tissues of the body, producing swelling. It is not a disease in itself, but may be a symptom of disease. During pregnancy some swelling of the legs towards evening is quite common, but swelling of legs in the morning, or of hands or face at any time, is a warning sign that toxaemia may be developing. If you notice that your shoes or wedding ring are uncomfortably tight, you should see your doctor at once.

A mild degree of toxaemia is fairly common in one woman in ten in first pregnancies and one in twenty in later pregnancies, and it is more frequent in multiple than single pregnancies. Treatment generally includes bed rest, a restricted diet, and sometimes diuretic tablets to get rid of excess water and salt. In more severe cases hospitalization may be necessary. If toxaemia is detected early and treated properly, there is no danger to mother or child. Regular attendance at the antenatal clinic is therefore extremely important. If the condition is neglected, serious complications such as convulsions and death of the baby can result, but this condition, known as eclampsia, is happily very rare.

Oestrogen See Hormones.

Onychomicosis See Foot Problems.

Osteopath An osteopath is a person who practises osteopathy, a system of healing in which diseases are treated by the manipulation of bones and other parts of the body in order to restore functions which have become deranged or disordered. The theory on which osteopathy is based is that the deformation of the skeleton, and the consequent interference with the adjacent nerves and blood vessels, is the cause of most diseases. Osteopaths believe that when blood is circulating properly disease cannot develop; when it does, blockage in the spinal area is often held to be responsible. Osteopathy is still not recognized by orthodox practitioners of medicine. However, there is increasing evidence to support at least one central osteopathic tenet: that illness is often due to the condition of the whole body and not to one outbreak in a particular location. Believing that the body is incapable of functioning well unless it is structurally sound, osteopaths look for structural disturbances: malposition or misalignment of bones, dislocations, 'faulty' muscle function, lesions on the spinal column. Manipulation and massage of spinal lesions, soft tissue, muscles and ligaments, plus diagnosis of the blood and the lymphatic system, are offered to the patient to effect cures for a variety of illnesses and diseases. Many people claim to have been completely cured of an ailment by an osteopath, and if one follows the argument that the proof of the treatment is in the cure, osteopathy cannot be denigrated. Indeed, some medical practitioners will refer a patient whom they cannot themselves help to an osteopath, although this is not orthodox practice. Great care should be taken when deciding to visit an osteopath, as there is evidence that they have aggravated or worsened certain conditions. Consult your doctor if you are thinking of visiting one. If he is unsympathetic, but you still feel that you want an osteopath's opinion, make sure that the practitioner you choose is bona fide, well qualified in his field, has a good reputation, and has a good general medical background.

Osteoporosis This can be a serious condition involving general demineralization of the bones leading to increased brittleness and a tendency to fracture, and often accompanied by pain. The bones of the back are usually the first to be affected, causing severe backache and a decrease in height.

The cause of the condition is still unknown, though it has been associated with a reduction in the amount of oestrogen in the body after menopause. One woman in five over the age of sixty-five is disabled by the disease and it sometimes occurs in younger women who have had their ovaries surgically removed before the age of forty. Large doses of oestrogen with calcium will help a woman who has developed osteoporosis, but a good preventive measure is a diet high in calcium and plenty of exercise.

Ovarian Cysts See Cysts.

Ovulation The formation of a new human being starts with the fertilization of an ovum from the female by a sperm from the male. The female generally produces one mature ovum in the middle of each menstrual cycle and it is this process which is known as ovulation. The ovum comes from the part of the female reproductive system known as the ovaries and each girl baby is born with around 80,000 immature ova, of which 400 at the most will be released as mature eggs during her reproductive life. On ovulation, the ripe ovum is carried into the Fallopian tube where it is ready to be fertilized by the sperm. If it is not fertilized within twelve hours, it becomes reabsorbed into the tube lining and menstruation occurs. A cycle is called *anovulatory* if a woman, or more usually a young girl, has a monthly menstruation but fails to ovulate. *Spontaneous ovulation* is a rare occurrence in humans, although it is normal for rabbits. A woman can ovulate at intercourse out of her normal cycle under situations of great, good, emotional stress. Women became pregnant in this way, for example, during the Second World War when their husbands were on leave.

Oxytocin See Hormones.

Oxytocin Drip Oxytocin is a hormone produced by the pituitary gland which causes the uterus to contract during labour and plays a part in the release of milk during lactation. Synthetic oxytocin, given as an intravenous drip, is used to stimulate uterine contractions and induce labour. It can be used throughout labour, but should not be given for more than ten hours. Oxytocin may also be offered as tablets, which the woman puts in the pouch of her cheek and allows to dissolve. This is not quite such a satisfactory method as the drip, but over 95 per cent of women have delivered their babies within twenty-four hours of induction using oxytocin in some form.

P

Pap Test See Well Woman Check-Up.

Para Compound This is a rather loose expression, originally an abbreviation of para-phenylene diamine but now used generally to mean those dyestuff intermediates which are used in permanent hair tints.

Parathyroid Glands See Glands.

Pelvic Examinations See Well Woman Check-Up.

Pelvic Floor The muscles of the pelvic floor stretch across the lower part of the pelvis, supporting all the abdominal organs, including the pregnant uterus, and yet allowing urine and faeces to pass through their individual passages. For a baby to be born, the pelvic muscles must relax to their limit, but in order to stay taut and support the weight of the foetus they must be very strong. Every woman should be aware of her pelvic-floor muscles and keep them in good condition. The simplest way to feel the muscles working is to cut the stream of urine when you are passing water. The muscles that you squeeze to control urination are the pelvic-floor muscles. Do this simple, internal squeeze whenever you remember and you will not only be helping to avert future problems, such as prolapse of the uterus, but improving the quality of your sex life by keeping a taut, elastic vagina.

PERFUME

Choosing a perfume You choose to wear a particular perfume because it appeals to your sense of smell. Why you should love Je Reviens and detest a friend's Mitsouko can only be explained by saying that the sense of smell is entirely individual. Other people can and do give you their own ideas of what will suit you, because they think of you as an exuberant sporty type or a romantic, but this does not mean that you will necessarily like a single one of the range of green or floral perfumes, and there is no reason why you should.

There is great satisfaction in finding a perfume you like, whether you hit on it by admiring it on another woman and making discreet inquiries, or you are lucky enough just to try it by chance at a beauty counter. In the first case, be prepared to find that whereas it smelt marvellous on her, it may not combine well with your body chemistry. Your skin's acid balance (pH factor) does not alter the perfume technically, but it can detract from it and the end result may be a failure. On the plus side, the individual characteristics of your skin make a perfume smell unique and possibly even more attractive on you than on the other woman. A drastic diet can alter your skin balance, as can illness, so do not be surprised if you go off your favourite perfume in these circumstances.

If you set out to try perfume in a store, confine your testing to two or three samples: your nose cannot cope with any more. Do not buy then and there. A knowledgeable assistant will not pressure you, but will advise you to go away and let the perfume develop on your skin over several hours. You want to know how it smells when you are hot and cold, how long it stays, and whether it fades away pleasantly or has a nasty after-kick.

How to wear perfume When trying a perfume you will be lucky to get more than a dab on the wrist, but a spray, if it is offered, is a much better guide because spraying diffuses the fragrance best. If your chosen perfume essence does not come in a spray, invest in a spray bottle, and transfer small quantities as you need them.

In addition to the warm pulse spots—wrists, temples, behind ears and knees—try spraying lightly on hair and on the linings of clothes. Beware of spraying directly on to clothes as perfume may stain, and it can be very tenacious: you could regret branding your fur coat with your current favourite in years to come. Above all, go easy on perfume. Your nose grows accustomed to any smell after only a few minutes and cuts it out automatically. But whereas you may think that your scent has faded, anyone coming up to you will know it has not, so do not keep adding more.

There are women who believe that only the pedigree French classics such as Chanel No 5 or Je Reviens can be truly chic. Those who create perfumes will tell you that this is sheer snobbery. The sophisticated modern scents such as Charlie, Blasé or Rapport are every bit as technically complex and brilliant as the old classics. They cost less simply because they make use of synthetic ingredients, but even to the trained 'nose' these are indistinguishable from the real thing.

The advantages of the new crop of modern scents is that they allow women to experiment, precisely because they are not prohibitively expensive. They encourage us to *wear* perfume instead of keeping it in a drawer, to be used only for special occasions.

Perfume types Perfumes fall into five main groups, depending on their characteristic smell, which in turn is determined by the predominance of some ingredients over others. As the chart shows, these groups are: green, floral, aldehydic, chypre and oriental.

1 Green perfumes have a cool, biting edge to them. The wearer is often pictured by advertisers as the modern woman-about-town, sophisticated and independent. The perfume gets its green smell from a base of aromatic woods such as cedar and sandalwood, or grasses, ferns and mosses.

2 Floral perfumes can be young and 'innocent' like Blue Grass, or cool and pungent like Diorella, or maturely feminine like L'Air du Temps, but as the name suggests, the base is always a combination of flowers. The addition of spice, wood and musk makes the subtle differences.

3 Aldehydes are man-made chemicals, discovered in 1904. The term sounds unromantic, but some of the greatest and most popular perfumes are aldehydic because these chemicals add power and bite to flowers, fruit, incense or any other constituents with which they are combined. Aldehydes were first used to brilliant effect in the world-famous Chanel No 5, created in 1921 by Ernest Beaux for couturière Coco Chanel. It is still the world's top-selling scent.

4 Chypre perfumes derive their name from one original, Coty's Chypre, also a 1921 vintage. They are characteristically heavy and spicy, but have more bite than the similar group, the orientals.

5 The oriental perfumes often contain vanilla, which explains their heady, sweet smell. Other ingredients are exotic Eastern spices, woods and grasses. These are the evening perfumes, the seductive little-black-dress partners, best used in moderation as they can be overpowering.

PERFUME CHART

Type	*Perfumes*
Green	Y by Yves Saint Laurent Alliage by Estée Lauder Chanel No 19 Smitty by Coty Stevie B by Max Factor Blazer by Helena Rubinstein Vent Vert by Balmain
Floral	Joy by Patou Blue Grass by Elizabeth Arden L'Air du Temps by Nina Ricci Diorella by Dior, also Diorissimo and Dior-Dior Estée by Estée Lauder Rapport by Max Factor Jontue by Revlon Cabriole by Elizabeth Arden
Aldehydic	Chanel No 5 Je Reviens by Worth Arpège by Lanvin Caleche by Hermès Mme Rochas by Rochas Rive Gauche by Yves Saint Laurent Chamade by Guerlain Charlie by Revlon
Chypre	Chypre by Coty Mitsouko by Guerlain Ma Griffe by Carven Miss Dior by Dior Cabochard by Grès Intimate by Revlon Femme by Rochas
Oriental	Jicky by Guerlain Shalimar by Guerlain Youth Dew by Estée Lauder Bal à Versailles by Desprez Opium by Yves Saint Laurent Habanita by Molinard

Pethidine (Demeral) Pethidine is a pain-relieving drug used during labour and given by injection into the muscle of the upper arm or thigh once labour is established. An injection of pethidine lasts for about four hours and it may make you feel a bit intoxicated and drowsy as well as relaxing you and relieving pain. The injection may need to be repeated if its effects wear off before labour is completed.

Phenothiazines See Tranquillizers.

Piles (Haemorrhoids) These are varicose veins situated at the lower end of the bowel. They may be external, dark brown or purple in colour outside the bowel, or internal, bright red and covered with mucous membrane inside the anal opening, or a mixture of both. Whichever form they take, piles can be very painful. They often appear in women during pregnancy, largely due to pressure on the bowel by the enlarged uterus in the later stages. The more pregnancies a woman has had, the greater the risk of developing piles. Constipation and excessive straining to pass a motion is another frequent cause of piles. And people who lead sedentary lives are more likely to develop them than those who are active. Treatment involves avoiding constipation with a high roughage diet, drinking plenty of water and taking regular exercise. Cold water compresses applied gently to the anal area will temporarily relieve pain. There are also ointments which help to relieve pain and reduce swelling. If the piles are very painful, or if they bleed or protrude, you must consult your doctor. In severe cases, injections to shrink the piles or surgical removal may be advised.

Pituitary Gland See Glands.

Plantar Warts (Verrucas) See Foot Problems.

Polyps See Uterine Disorders.
Port-Wine Stains See Birthmarks.
Progesterone See Hormones.
Prolapse of the Uterus See Uterine Disorders.
Prostaglandins These are a group of substances in the body which have a variety of actions, including stimulating contractions of the uterine muscles. They are injected into the uterus to induce abortion and are safer and quicker to use than saline solution, although they may produce side-effects of nausea and fever. Some doctors also use prostaglandins to induce labour, instead of oxytocin, but there seems to be little advantage in this change. Experiments are being carried out with a view to using prostaglandins as a type of contraceptive for use *after* intercourse.
Psoriasis See Skin Problems.
Psychosomatic Derived from the Greek words for mind (psyche) and body (soma), this is used today mostly to describe diseases which are both physiological and psychological in origin. The inter-relationship of the mind and body in disease, both in causing and curing, is still not fully understood. Many disorders, such as heart palpitations, stomach ulcers, menstrual disorders and infertility, are held to be at least in part psychosomatic. Quite erroneously, the term psychosomatic is sometimes used in the pejorative sense, implying that someone suffering from a psychosomatic disease is in some way responsible for it or only imagines that they have it. The term really means that the emotions have caused the body to react in a certain way, for example to produce an excess of stomach acids, so causing the disease, which is very real indeed.
Pudendal Block This is an anaesthetic given to deaden pain in the pelvic region during a forceps delivery. The doctor gently puts his finger into the woman's vagina and injects a local anaesthetic around the triangular shaped bones on either side. This numbs the nerves which supply the vulva as they pass through the pelvis. Painful sensations in the vulva and lower vagina disappear quite quickly making the birth relatively painless, but contractions of the uterus are still felt.

R

Raspberry Marks See Birthmarks.

RECIPES FOR NATURAL SKIN CARE
Cosmetics are expensive and often, though not invariably, the best skin-care products are *very* expensive. This tends to make women regard them as luxury items, to be used sparingly. It is true that sometimes the instructions specify using a tiny amount of a cream or lotion, but on other occasions skimping lessens effectiveness, and may mean that the product lasts longer than was intended and so loses its potency.

The best way to save money on cosmetics is not to eke them out, or to buy cheaper brands, but to make your own. There is nothing difficult about it; all the ingredients are available from a chemist, drugstore or healthfood shop, although you may have to order some of them. The shelf-life of your home-made products will not be as long as the bought ones which have preservatives in them, but you can make up small quantities as you need them, or make up a larger quantity and store it in a refrigerator; most creams will last several months if you keep them in this way.

All the recipes that follow have been devised and tested by the beautician Clare Maxwell-Hudson, author of *The Natural Beauty Book*, who has whipped up her potions on television to demonstrate how quick and easy they are to make.

Equipment
Enamel or heat-proof bowls
Large frying pan or roasting tin
Metal measuring spoons
Set of measuring cups (optional, but an asset)
Electric beater (wooden spoons or glass rods will do, but are more work)
Liquidizer or strong metal sieve
Pipette or eyedropper for adding perfume
Jars and bottles
Labels
Roll of kitchen paper
Oleic acid (optional, for 'failures')

Method
Use the frying pan or roasting tin as a bain-marie (water-bath), in which you heat the separate bowls of oils or waxes and the water. Heating them slowly and gently in this way is important, as too intense a heat can spoil the cream. Keep the water in the bain-marie simmering, not boiling, until the oils or waxes have melted, then remove the bowls from the heat and combine together, stirring or beating on slow speed all the time. You *must* stir intermittently until the cream begins to thicken and cool, otherwise your cream may separate.

If the cream does separate, try beating it again slowly. If this fails, go back to the melting pot again. And if all else fails, a couple of drops of oleic acid will usually bind together any really obstinate cream.

Perfume is optional; it can irritate some sensitive skins, but if it suits you, add it as the cream begins to thicken and cool. Try a few drops of an essential oil such as lemon verbena, jasmine, orange, rose or herb. At the same time you can add a little colouring, such as cochineal, if you like.

If the cream should come out gritty it is probably because you didn't beat it enough, or the borax was not properly dissolved. As with that tricky item mayonnaise, practice makes perfect.

1 Cleansers
Ten-minute cleanser Ten minutes is the amount of time it should take to make, with a little practice.
½ tbsp beeswax
1 tbsp emulsifying wax
4 tbsp baby oil
2 tbsp coconut oil
2 tbsp water
¼ tsp borax
1 tbsp witch hazel
perfume (a few drops any essential oil—lemon verbena is lovely and fresh for a cleanser)
Measure the waxes and oils into a bowl and melt slowly standing in water. In a separate bowl heat the water and borax, adding the witch hazel when the borax is completely dissolved, but be careful not to heat the witch hazel for long or it will evaporate. When the waxes have melted, remove both bowls from the heat and beat or stir together. Keep stirring or beating frequently until the cream is beginning to cool. Add perfume. Continue beating until you have about half a cup of thick, light cream, which will suit all skins.
Rose cleansing cream This is based on a formula devised over 1,700 years ago by the Greek physician Galen.
1½ tbsp beeswax (or white paraffin wax)
1 tbsp emulsifying wax
4 tbsp baby oil
6 tbsp rosewater
½ tsp borax
perfume (rose oil)
Melt the waxes and oil together in one bowl and the rosewater and borax in another, making sure that the borax is completely dissolved. When the wax and oil have melted, remove both bowls from the heat and beat or stir together. As the white cream begins to cool, add a drop of rose oil. Keep on beating until the cream is really cool and you have about a cup of soft cleansing cream, to suit any skin.

2 Toners
Rosewater toner One of the oldest and best skin tonics, cheap enough to add to the bath or use as a final rinse for hair.
1 gal (4.5 litres) purified water
2 tbsp essence of roses
Simply mix together and shake thoroughly. Use the toner lavishly on any type of skin.
Vinegar toner Being acidic, this restores the skin's natural acid mantle.
1 part wine or cider vinegar
8 parts water
Keep a large bottle ready diluted in your bathroom for washing, rinsing hair and adding to the bath. It gets rid of the tight feeling you have after washing with soap, and it prevents itchiness.
Cucumber and mint toner A fresh, tingly and stimulating toner.
½ cucumber, peeled if you wish
4 tbsp mint
vodka (or pure alcohol) or witch hazel (optional)
green colouring (optional)
Blend the cucumber and mint in a liquidizer until the mint is very finely chopped, or chop both by hand and sieve. Add a drop of green colouring to the strained mixture and anything from a tablespoon to a wine-glass of vodka (astringent) or witch hazel (toner); either makes this toner cooler and longer-lasting. This makes a large bottle of refreshing skin toner.

3 Astringents
Hungary water astringent Used by Queen Elizabeth of Hungary in the thirteenth century.
2 tbsp rosemary
peel and pith of ¼ orange and ½ lemon
4 sprigs mint
¼ cup vodka (or pure alcohol) or witch hazel
½ cup rosewater
Mix together all the ingredients in a large bottle and let it stand for at least forty-eight hours, shaking frequently. Strain and bottle. Witch hazel will make it less astringent than alcohol.
Lemon and peppermint astringent
juice of 2 large lemons (4 tbsp) or bought lemon juice (not as good)
½ tsp peppermint extract
8 tbsp witch hazel
2 tbsp vodka (or pure alcohol)
Mix together all the ingredients in a large bottle and let it stand for a day. Strain, bottle and use. It makes ½ pt (300 ml) and is best for greasy skin.
Blue camphor astringent
½ cup rosewater
¼ cup witch hazel
¼ cup distilled water
1 tbsp camphor spirit
2 drops blue colouring (optional)
Mix together all the ingredients in a large bottle. This is quite a strong astringent, but you can tone it down by reducing the amount of camphor. It is good for tightening large pores, and for spotty or tired-looking skin. To make it *more* astringent, mix half a cup with a pinch of alum. Alum will make any of the above astringents more potent.

4 Skin foods and moisturizers
Sunflower moisture cream
4 tsp lanolin (anhydrous)
2 tsp emulsifying wax
2 tsp beeswax
5 tbsp sunflower oil
2 tsp glycerine
6 tbsp water
½ tsp borax
Melt the oils and waxes together in one bowl and the rest of the ingredients in another, making sure the borax is completely dissolved. While still on the heat, slowly add the water to the oils and stir well as you continue to heat for a couple of minutes. Remove from the heat and stir or beat. The cream will slowly whiten and thicken to give you about a cup of rich cream, which is instantly absorbed into the skin. It is good for any type of skin.
Jasmine moisture cream
2 tbsp emulsifying wax
2 tbsp almond or sunflower oil
1 tsp lanolin (anhydrous)
½ tsp borax
1½ tsp glycerine
8 tbsp water
1 tsp witch hazel
perfume (jasmine oil)
Melt the wax and oils together in one bowl and the borax, glycerine and water in another; when the borax has dissolved add the witch hazel. Remove from the heat and slowly mix the oils and water, stirring well until cool, then add a few drops of jasmine oil. This makes about three-quarters of a cup of cream.
As it is non-greasy, it is suitable for greasy and normal skins.
Wheatgerm nourishing cream
1 tsp beeswax
1 tsp emulsifying wax
5 tbsp lanolin (anhydrous)
3 tbsp sesame oil
2 tbsp wheatgerm oil
5 tbsp water
½ tsp borax
1 tbsp witch hazel
perfume oil
Melt the waxes and oils in one bowl and the water and borax in another, adding the witch hazel when the borax has completely dissolved. Remove from the heat and slowly mix together, stirring. Add perfume, then beat or stir until the cream is thick and glossy. This makes about a cup of very rich cream.
All-purpose honey cream Honey is a natural healer, attracts and conserves moisture, softens coarse and sensitive skin, and brings a glow to any skin. This recipe avoids the stickiness you would expect; it feels a bit tacky at first, but is soon absorbed by the skin.
3 tbsp lanolin (anhydrous)
½ tbsp liquid honey
1 tsp lecithin
4 tbsp warm water
perfume oil
Melt the oils and honey together and slowly add the water, beating fairly fast and continuously for the first minute then slowing down until it cools. Add perfume. This makes about a cup of pale-creamy-coloured firm cream which keeps well *out* of the refrigerator: if it gets too cold it separates.

5 Face masks
Nourishing egg yolk mask Egg yolk is full of lecithin and protein which is why it makes such a good skin food.
1 egg yolk
1 tsp almond oil
Mix together and leave on the face (or neglected feet, elbows and knees) for ten to thirty minutes. You can use the whole egg if you prefer.
Nourishing avocado mask Avocado is one of the most nutritious fruits, rich in vitamins, minerals and natural oils.
2 tbsp ripe avocado pear
1 tsp liquid honey
couple of drops lemon juice
Lemon juice stops the avocado going black; add it to the mashed and sieved avocado, then add the honey to make a paste. Leave on the skin as long as possible.
Apple mask The vinegar in this recipe restores the skin's acid mantle; the pectin in the apple is soothing and the other ingredients nourish.
½ apple, peeled and sliced
1 tbsp liquid honey
1 tsp ascorbic acid
1 egg yolk
1 tbsp cider vinegar
3 tbsp sunflower oil
Blend all the ingredients together in a liquidizer, or sieve until completely smooth. Leave on the skin for about fifteen minutes. This is good for all types of skin.

6 Hand creams
Almond hand cream
2 tsp lanolin (anhydrous)
1½ tsp cocoa butter
1 tbsp beeswax
5 tsp corn oil
1 tsp almond oil
2 tbsp water
¼ tsp borax
perfume (almond essence)
Melt together the oils and wax in one bowl and the water and borax in another. When the borax is completely dissolved, remove both bowls from the heat and stir together by hand; it sets very quickly to a pure white cream. Add a few drops of almond essence or, if you prefer, lavender oil, thyme or peach extract. This makes half a cup of cream, which is not at all greasy.
Satin hand cream
1 tbsp stearic acid
2 tsp almond oil
1 tsp emulsifying wax
6 tbsp water
1 tbsp glycerine
¼ tsp washing-up detergent
Melt the oil and wax in one bowl and the other ingredients in another. Remove from the heat and slowly add the water to the oils, beating or stirring all the time. This makes half a cup of white, satiny cream, which gives hands a pearly sheen. It is good to use as a body lotion, too.

7 Bath oil
Milk and honey dispersing bath oil
This oil does not rest on the surface of the water but sinks right in, turning the water milky, so your skin can absorb it all the time you are in the bath and not just as you get in and out. It is probably

the best bath oil you will ever use.
2 eggs
¼ cup almond oil
¼ cup sunflower or corn oil
½ cup safflower or olive oil
1 tbsp liquid honey
2 tsp washing-up detergent
¼ cup vodka or pure alcohol
½ cup milk
perfume oil (lemon verbena, pine or jasmine)

Using the low speed on your electric beater, completely blend the eggs and oils together, or do it the hard way by hand. Add the honey, then the detergent which makes it thick. Keep beating as you add the dispersant, the vodka or pure alcohol, then the milk which thins the mixture a little. Finally add the perfume. This quantity should last you a couple of weeks, but use it up fast as it does go off. *Warning*. Very hot water inactivates it (and you).

Retroverted Uterus See Uterine Disorders.

Rhesus Factor The so-called Rhesus factor is present in the red blood cells of 85 per cent of the population, whose blood group is thus denoted Rhesus positive. The Rhesus factor is a danger in pregnancy when the mother's blood is Rhesus negative. If the Rhesus negative woman marries a Rhesus positive man, their baby may also be Rhesus positive, and the foetal blood may therefore be incompatible with the maternal Rhesus negative blood. A first baby will be unaffected, but during the labour or birth it is quite likely that its Rhesus positive blood will be released into the mother's bloodstream and antibodies will be formed in the mother to counteract it. These antibodies may act adversely on the blood cells of a second baby, making it ill or even threatening its life. The blood test taken at the onset of pregnancy will establish whether or not a woman's blood is Rhesus negative, and later blood tests will discover the presence of Rhesus antibodies. The use of amniocentesis can detect the condition of the baby in the uterus and, if necessary, a severely affected baby can be given a blood transfusion in the uterus, although transfusions are usually given shortly after the birth to clear the baby's blood of dangerous antibodies. Regular antenatal care is therefore extremely important in this case. Rhesus incompatibility is also an indication for premature delivery by induction. Because medical intervention can help a baby in this situation, there is no longer any need for babies with Rhesus incompatibility to suffer as they once did.

Rhesus Incompatibility See Rhesus Factor.

Rhinitis (Hay Fever) See Allergies.

Ringworm This is a highly infectious fungus disease, in which the hairs are destroyed and break off leaving stubs of infected hair and inflamed or scaly patches on the scalp. The infection, which is allied to Athlete's foot, can spread to anyone in contact with the broken or loose hairs and can affect the skin, hair or nails. It needs immediate treatment by a doctor, but can be effectively cleared with a prescribed antibiotic. New anti-fungal creams can usually clear up ringworm of the skin in three to six weeks. If the nails are affected, it is likely to take a little while longer. Treatment must be continued until all traces of the infection have cleared.

Rodent Ulcer See Skin Problems.

Rosacea See Veins.

S

Salpingitis Salpingitis is inflammation of any tube in the body, but the term is usually used in connection with inflammation of the Fallopian tube caused by bacterial infection. This may be carried to the tube in the bloodstream or, more often, may spread from the vagina or uterus. Symptoms include severe pain in the lower abdomen. You should see your doctor immediately if you suspect salpingitis. In most cases the inflammation subsides promptly if treated with antibiotics. In severe cases abscesses may form and salpingectomy, the surgical removal or cutting of one or both Fallopian tubes, may be necessary.

Salt Bond This is a type of bonding within the hair structure which contributes to the strength of the hair.

Scars Scar is the word used to describe a healed wound, ulcer or breach of tissue. It consists of fibrous tissue which, in the case of superficial scars, is covered by an imperfect formation of epidermis—imperfect because the scar does not reproduce hair follicles, hairs or sweat glands. Scars are red and soft in the early stages because the fibrous tissue is full of blood vessels; as the scar heals the fibrous tissue contracts, loses its blood vessels and becomes denser, leaving a hard, white surface. The best scars, that is the finest and least noticeable, are the result of the fastest and most accurate joining of the skin edges after surgery or injury and the quickest healing time. Where the wound is allowed to gape, is badly joined, or there is infection and consequent inflammation, the scar is usually wider and thicker, with much puckering of the surrounding skin. Such scars are more prone to irritation and ulceration. Where a scar continues to give pain for a long time it is likely that a sensory nerve has been 'trapped' in the hard, contracting scar tissue. If scarring after surgery or an accident is bad and unsightly, it is possible to have some scar tissue removed using plastic surgery techniques.

Scorch Marks See Skin Problems.

Sebaceous Glands See Glands.

Self-Help Groups One of the most interesting social developments in recent years has been the formation and growth of self-help groups for all kinds of problems. Probably the first, and still the most effective, was Alcoholics Anonymous, which started in the 1930s. It is comprised of groups of people who have problems with their drinking habits and who meet to confess to each other, share their anguishes and find strength together.

There are now self-help groups for scores of personality problems. There is Weight Watchers for fat people and compulsive eaters; there are groups for smokers, for gamblers, for parents who fear they might batter their children, and for childless people who feel either upset by their infertility or unfairly pressurized by a child-orientated atmosphere. There are numerous self-help organizations for homosexuals; there is a society for phobics; there are groups for women who suffer from cystitis; there are associations for single parents and for parents with specific problems with their children—handicapped, specially gifted, autistic and so on. There are groups for dwarfs and widows, people with brittle bones and migraine sufferers, people who have had cancer and people with haemophilia, the blind, the deaf, prisoners, nursing mothers, back pain sufferers, spastics, people who have had colostomies, stammerers and paedophiles. There are also women's self-help groups which specialize in women's problems, both mental and physical. If you want counselling on abortion, to have menstrual extraction or learn how to do a full self-examination, try to find one of these groups which is active and well informed. If you have a problem, it is always worth trying to work it through with a group; if there is not a group for your problem, start one.

The best way to contact a self-help group is to look through specialist magazines and their small ads. Slimming publications, for example, usually have contact points for people who want to join or form a weight-watching circle. Gay newspapers and weeklies generally have small ads for people who want to talk over special problems about homosexuality. And progressive women's magazines, or even your local paper, will probably provide some information about women's self-help groups. If you don't have an organization in your area, think about forming one. The best way is to advertise, but if you don't feel confident enough for that, start by finding *one other person* with a similar problem.

Seminal Fluid The climax of sexual intercourse for the male is the ejaculation of seminal fluid from the penis. Seminal fluid is a sticky, whitish substance which contains the man's sperm. The average ejaculation produces $\frac{1}{12}$–$\frac{1}{8}$ fl oz (3–5 ml) of fluid, and each millilitre contains anything from fifty to two hundred million sperm. Only one of these is needed to reach and fertilize the ovum. When a man has a vasectomy, sperm are prevented from reaching the penis by cutting and tying the vas deferens, the tubes along which they travel. The aim of vasectomy is sperm-free seminal fluid.

Shingles (Herpes Zoster) See Skin Problems.

Skin Peeling See Skin Problems.

SKIN PROBLEMS

Broken veins See Veins.

Bruises A bruise or contusion is a minor injury where the skin becomes discoloured but not broken. A bruise occurs, usually as the result of a knock or blow, when tiny blood vessels under the skin break, releasing blood into the surrounding tissue. Bruises fade from blue-black to purple, green and yellow as the blood cells are gradually broken down and reabsorbed. A number of remedies for alleviating the pain or swelling of a bruise, such as cold compresses or the application of raw steak, are often advocated, but apart from cosmetic disguise there is nothing which will speed up a bruise's disappearance. If a bruise fails to fade and pain persists or the area becomes swollen, medical advice should be sought.

Chapped skin Chemicals such as those found in detergents and harsh weather conditions, particularly cold temperatures and wind, cause the skin to lose vital oils which normally keep the skin surface smooth and supple. Chapped skin occurs when the outer layer of skin, dehydrated due to this loss of protective oils, becomes rough, dry and flaky. As well as being sore and uncomfortable, there is a greater risk of infection through the cracked skin surface. The hands and face are particularly affected. The best way to guard against this is to protect your skin. Use rubber gloves or an efficient barrier cream when washing up or when the hands are constantly in water, dry carefully afterwards, and apply hand cream. Apply moisturizer and emollient (softening) creams to the face regularly, especially before and after going out in bad weather. Unless you have a skin particularly prone to easy tanning, usually dark and oily, do not allow your skin to dry by itself in windy conditions after swimming, even if the day is very warm and sunny. Pat yourself dry with a towel and apply more protective cream or lotion. While skin is chapped use a minimum of soap, add oil to your bath water, and use plenty of soothing cream.

Dermatitis Dermatitis means literally inflammation of the skin. It is not one skin disease, but a name covering the reaction of the skin to allergic or emotional disorders. Generally, the blood vessels in the skin become porous and the fluid from the cells collects so that blisters form. Eventually these erupt and the fluid forms a crust. The skin around the sore thickens and then flakes off in scales. Dermatitis is usually caused by the skin's reaction to certain substances, often chemical, such as those found in detergents, paints, insecticides and metals (often jewellery). Some people are allergic to more than one of these substances and are therefore particularly prone to dermatitis. For successful treatment, the cause or causes must be isolated and the allergen avoided. Wearing lined rubber gloves for housework will reduce the occurrence of dermatitis in most women. If the complaint is left untreated or if the skin becomes scratched or broken, infections can penetrate the skin and aggravate the condition.

Eczema A form of dermatitis, this is a non-contagious inflammation of the skin characterized by the presence of a red, itching rash and small blisters, which discharge a watery fluid that dries up and forms crusts. The condition often first appears in childhood and can recur throughout adult life. The itching may be severe and a vicious cycle of itch, scratch, break skin, crust can continue for weeks. The cause or causes of eczema have not been finally isolated. However, although repeated irritation by allergens such as detergents, rubber gloves, paint or even drugs may give rise to eczema, there is evidence to substantiate the theory that it occurs as a result of stress, and certainly that it happens when the skin temperature becomes raised, also symptomatic of stress situations or allergic reaction. Various medicaments are used to help alleviate the condition, but the doctor or dermatologist will need to trace the underlying cause before a real cure is possible.

Herpes This is the name given to a skin disease whose symptoms are patches of small blisters, often painful, which can affect almost any area of the skin, including the genital area. So far no effective cure for herpes has been found; it tends to disappear of its own accord. Some people are more prone than others to the two viruses which cause the different types of herpes, and once affected it is not uncommon for the disease to recur. *Herpes simplex*, the common cold sore, appears around the mouth or inside the nose usually as a result of a bad cold, throat or chest infection. The blisters are painful but become less so once they have erupted and a healing scab has formed. The sore will disappear in a matter of days. *Herpes zoster*, shingles, is a form of herpes where the blisters form along the course of a sensory nerve and may be accompanied by acute neuralgic pain. They usually appear on the abdomen, often encircling the body at the waist, the chest and occasionally the face. The latter can be serious if the eyes are infected. As the disease is caused by the same virus as chicken pox, any breaking or picking of the blisters can form crater-like scars which may take a long time to fade. Shingles generally lasts for two or three weeks.

Hives (urticaria) This is an eruption of the skin caused by an allergic reaction, usually to some form of food. The most common culprits are shellfish, chocolate-based food, soft fruit or citrus fruit. Some people also develop hives as a reaction to pollen, household dust, and even antibiotics. The skin of the affected person shows weals or raised red patches, which can be small or the size of saucers; in either case they itch and are painful. They occur because the food or material causing the allergy prompts the skin to release histamine, which in turn dilates the blood vessels and increases the flow of fluid to the skin surface. The condition usually disappears as soon as the substance responsible is out of the bloodstream. Soreness and itching can be relieved to some extent by soothing creams, lotions such as calamine, cold milk compresses, or pastes of bicarbonate of soda. Should the attack of hives affect the mouth and throat so that breathing or swallowing becomes difficult, a doctor should be seen immediately.

Psoriasis This is a chronic, but non-infectious, skin disease in which raised, rough patches of pimples covered with loose, silvery scales appear on the skin. Small bleeding points can often be seen under the edges of the scales. Psoriasis can appear anywhere on the body but is most common on elbows, knees, forearms, legs and scalp. The cause or causes of the disease, which results from an abnormal type and production of keratin, are still unknown, although stress, seasonal changes, gout and rheumatism have all been associated with psoriasis. There is probably a genetic connection, too. The condition may last for a short time or for many years; it may disappear as suddenly as it arrived and then recur. Although no permanent cure for psoriasis has been found, various treatments both internal and external can be prescribed by a doctor which will help to control and alleviate the condition.

Rodent ulcer This is the term used to describe a malignant ulcer which occurs most often in elderly people and is usually found on the face and nose. It increases in size very gradually but, although a cancer, does not spread to other parts of the body. It can be effectively treated by X-ray or may be removed surgically. It is important to consult a doctor immediately if you suspect you have developed such an ulcer.

Rosacea See Veins.

Scorch marks Scorch marks or superficial burns occur when the skin is exposed to intense heat, usually as a result of sitting too near a fire or in particularly hot sunshine. There is a burning sensation and discoloration, often showing a tracery of veins under the skin, especially on bony areas such as shins, chest or shoulders. The affected areas should be cooled as much as possible by cold compresses or by creams or lotions formulated to soothe burns and the sufferer must avoid extremes of temperature until the healing is complete. Discoloration of the veins may take many months to fade.

Skin peeling This involves the removal of the epidermis, the outer layer of skin, and sometimes the inner layer as well. There are two systems of skin peeling: deep peeling, or chemopeel, where chemicals are applied to burn off the outer and part of the inner layer, and dermabrasion, the less dramatic planing or removal of the outer layer of skin tissue by a rotating wire-brush-like instrument. Both methods must be carried out under medical supervision by fully qualified operators or the results of the treatment in the form of scarring can be worse than the original complaint. After peeling, the skin will look inflamed for anything up to six months. During this time it must be protected from the elements, particularly sunlight. Persistent cases of acne and other skin defects and blemishes may be helped by peeling or dermabrasion techniques, which may lessen pitting of the skin, but there could be pigmentation problems afterwards so treatment should not be undertaken lightly.

Spider veins See Veins.

Vitiligo This is a harmless skin disease which results in certain areas of the skin remaining white, rather like white freckles. There are drugs which help repigmentation to a certain degree, but the white marks are best ignored or camouflaged with cosmetics.

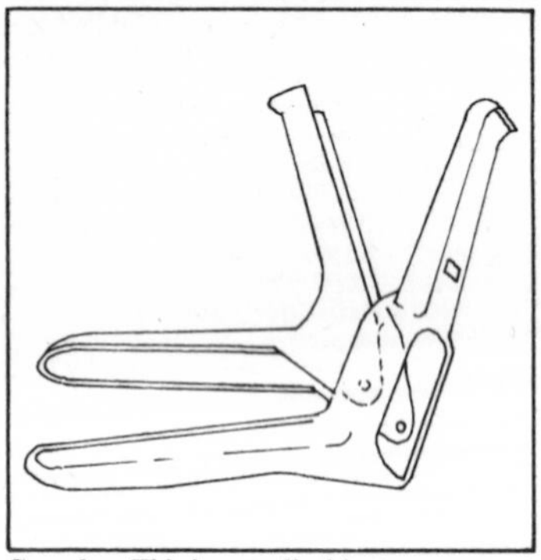

Speculum This is a medical instrument used to examine the female internal reproductive organs. It is made up of two rounded metal or perspex 'blades', which can be separated inside the vagina to give a clear view of the cervix and vaginal walls. See Well Woman Check-Up, page 222, for how to use a speculum for self-examination.

Sperm The human sperm is the reproductive cell produced by the male to fertilize the female ovum. Sperm are tiny tadpole-like organisms, $\frac{1}{600}$ in (0.04 mm) long, which find their way towards the ovum after they have been ejaculated into the vagina during intercourse. The average male ejaculation sends some four hundred million sperm into the passages of the female reproductive system, where one must survive to fertilize the ovum. The sperm carries the genetic contribution of the father to the child.

Spider Veins See Veins.

Spina Bifida Spina bifida is a congenital abnormality in which there is a gap in the baby's spine (vertebral column), leaving the spinal cord unprotected. There are many degrees of spina bifida, ranging from the very slight, in which the degree of physical handicap is minimal and mental handicap nil, to the very severe lesions where doctors have to decide whether or not to attempt any treatment at all. If they are not treated, many spina bifida babies die within the first few months of life. Even with treatment the prognosis is not good. Surgical techniques offer hope of a nearly normal life to the least affected, but certainly not to all spina bifida babies, and the decision to operate is not one to be taken lightly, although it is unfortunately one that must be made very soon after birth. Spina bifida is one of the conditions which can be identified in an unborn child by amniocentesis and Ultrasound techniques. Blood tests can also now be carried out at the seventeenth week of pregnancy to identify cases of spina bifida. The occurrence of the disorder varies from one country to another, from about ten in every thousand births to two in every thousand, the latter figure representing the proportion in Great Britain.

Spontaneous Ovulation See Ovulation.

Stained Nails See Nail Problems.

Strawberry Marks See Birthmarks.

Stye See Eye Problems.

Syphilis See Venereal Diseases.

T

Testosterone See Hormones.

Three Months Colic Colic is an attack of severe abdominal pain, which is common among babies in the first three months of life. The abdomen may be distended, the baby draws its legs up, cries from discomfort and releases wind. The basic cause is not really known, but there are many theories and research is continuing. The quality of milk does not seem to be the reason, although swallowing air during feeding may be a cause. To avoid this, wind the baby by putting it to your shoulder at intervals during and after the feed and rubbing or patting the back gently to release the air from the system. With some babies this may be a long process, but patience and persistence with winding will relieve the discomfort and thus the crying. Alternatively, allergy may be a factor in causing colic, as the baby may be sensitive to certain vitamins or milk, for example. If this is found to be the cause, your doctor may recommend a substitute. Fatigue may also play a part, and the baby is generally more comfortable lying on its stomach. There is no miracle cure for colic, but it will probably disappear by the time the baby is three months old, if not before. It will do the baby no permanent harm—indeed, the colicky baby prospers from the physical point of view, in spite of hours of crying, and will often gain more weight than average.

'Thrush' (Candidiasis) See Vaginal Infections.

Thyroid Gland See Glands.

TRANQUILLIZERS

Antihistamines Histamine is an organic substance released from the tissues during conditions of stress, inflammation and allergy. Antihistamine is thus the general name given to the group of synthetic drugs which counteract the effect of this substance. First used by the French in the late 1930s, some antihistamine drugs produce drowsiness as a side-effect. They may also be combined with a hypnotic drug to produce sleep, because antihistamines increase the effect of hypnotics. One of the most frequently prescribed has been Mandrax. In some such drugs, however, a high dose can produce the opposite of drowsiness and increase excitation and restlessness, possibly leading to hyper-activity or even convulsions.

Barbituric acid This was discovered in 1864 and has been used since the early twentieth century to produce sleep. Many known sleeping tablets, such as Nembutal and Seconal, have a barbiturate base. Barbiturates are powerful sedatives, but they are dangerous in overdose, cause drug dependence and can amplify tension and depression if taken over a long period of time. They can also disturb the body chemistry, since they interfere with certain enzymes in the liver.

Benzodiazepines The most widely prescribed benzodiazepine compounds are Librium, Valium, Tropium and many others of a similar type. They are principally considered as anti-anxiety drugs and produce four main effects: sedation, anti-anxiety, muscle relaxation and anti-convulsant. Although very valuable drugs on a short-term basis, they do have drawbacks. When taken on a long-term basis, they can make people confused. Side-effects include diminished ability to drive a car and use similar skills in operating machinery; drowsiness and lethargy; an impaired tolerance of alcohol; fall in blood-pressure; and sometimes excitement so that a person appears drunk rather than tranquillized. They can produce a form of physical dependence and, like all drugs, are subject to the law of diminishing returns. Benzodiazepine is also used as a sleeping draught. Two groups are used specifically for sleeping purposes: nitrazepam (Mogadon) and flurazepam (Dalmane).

Non-barbiturate hypno-sedatives These are used in the treatment of insomnia and include drugs such as Welldorm and Doriden. In this group, too, are old-fashioned sedatives such as bromide and chloral hydrate. Bromide potassium was much used in Victorian times to calm mental patients, but it can cause intoxication and can accumulate in the system to a poisonous level. Chloral hydrate is the oldest sleeping draught. However, it can irritate the stomach and acute poisoning may develop from a mixture of alcohol and chloral hydrate—this is known as a Mickey Finn.

Phenothiazines These are major tranquillizers, used to treat serious psychological disorders such as schizophrenia, paranoia, dementia and psychotic mania. Their most obvious effect is to sedate the patient; side-effects may include an impaired conditioned response, diminished attention and muscle rigidity.

Trichologist A trichologist is a specialist in hair and scalp disorders. They are not required by law to have training, but a qualified trichologist will be a member of a recognized institute of trichology.

Trichomoniasis See Vaginal Infections.

U

Ultrasound Ultrasound is a completely safe screening technique used very frequently in modern antenatal care. The pregnant woman lies on a couch and has her stomach rubbed with oil. The scanner is then moved slowly back and forth across the stomach, bouncing ultrasonic waves across the pregnant uterus. In this way a picture, rather like a radar, is built up on a screen. The picture produced by an ultrasonic scan gives the obstetrician a great deal of very valuable information. It tells him the size of the baby, so that he can see whether it tallies with the estimated dates, and shows him the position of the placenta in the uterus, which way the baby is lying, if there is an ectopic pregnancy, if the woman is carrying twins, and even the presence of abnormalities such as spina bifida or malformed limbs. Ultrasound is used with amniocentesis in the detection of mongolism and other conditions.

Urticaria (Hives) See Skin Problems.

UTERINE DISORDERS

Cervical erosion When the cells which line the cervical canal show as a reddened area at the head of the vagina the condition is known as cervical erosion. This happens naturally in puberty and during a first pregnancy and may also occur in women on the Pill or using IUDs. No treatment is needed unless the condition persists for over six months and leads to marked vaginal discharge, in which case a doctor will probably employ electric cauterization. This will produce a heavy, discoloured vaginal discharge which may last for four to six weeks, until healing is complete.

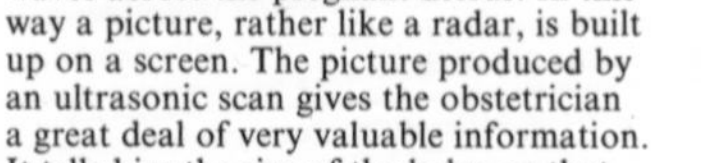

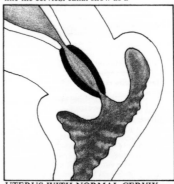

UTERUS WITH NORMAL CERVIX

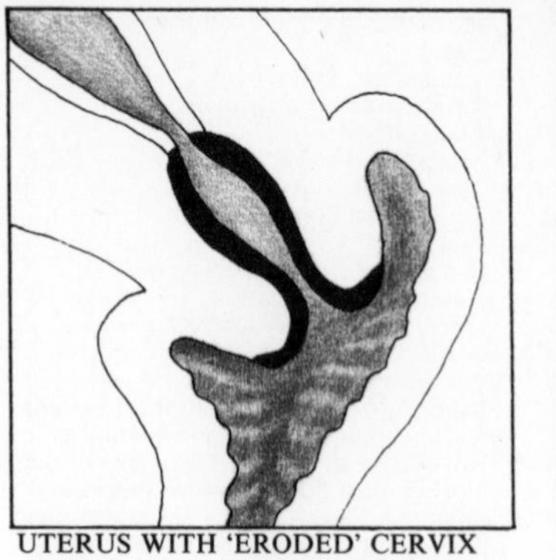

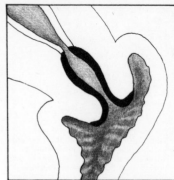

UTERUS WITH 'ERODED' CERVIX

Endometrial cancer Cancer of the endometrium, the lining of the uterus, occurs almost as often as cancer of the cervix but usually affects older women, between the ages of fifty and sixty. The obese and diabetics are also susceptible and it can run in families. A growth in the number of cases has been observed recently and there is some concern that this may be partly due to the increasing use of oestrogen over long periods, as in hormone replacement therapy. The disease is not easily detected by smear tests and doctors usually have to rely on symptoms. Any irregular bleeding after the age of thirty-five should be reported to your doctor at once. It is probably due to hormonal changes, but may be the first sign of cancer of the endometrium. Diagnosis is by scraping the lining of the uterus under anaesthetic and treatment involves hysterectomy and X-ray therapy. Endometrial cancer grows very slowly and is generally curable if treated promptly.

Endometriosis This condition occurs when cells like those lining the uterus (endometrial cells) grow in the wrong place, forming cysts in the muscle of the uterus, the ovaries, or other parts of the pelvis. It is most common in unmarried or infertile women in their thirties. The cells pass through the same monthly cycle as the endometrium: they swell before a period and then bleed, but as they have no outlet they cause severe pain in the lower abdomen for several days before menstruation. Depending on their position, the cysts may also cause pain during intercourse and, where they block the ovaries or Fallopian tubes, infertility will result. To discover the extent of the disease, a doctor may make a tiny incision beneath the umbilicus and insert an instrument rather like a periscope. This is a minor operation carried out under anaesthetic and is painless. Treatment is either by surgery or hormones, or sometimes by both.

Fibroids These are lumps of fibrous tissue growing in the muscle wall of the uterus, sometimes singly and sometimes in large groups. They are usually the size of a pea, but may grow as big as a tennis ball or even a grapefruit. The cause of fibroids is still not known, but there is reason to believe that it may be hormonal. They occur in about 20 per cent of women over the age of thirty, particularly the infertile, the sexually inactive and those who have children late in life. Doctors prefer to leave small fibroids alone if they cause no trouble, although they will want to check them from time to time. Large fibroids can cause pain, heavy and irregular periods, enlargement of the uterus which may interfere with urination and bowel action, and infertility through spontaneous abortion. They may have to be removed by surgery and in some cases, particularly in older women, it may be

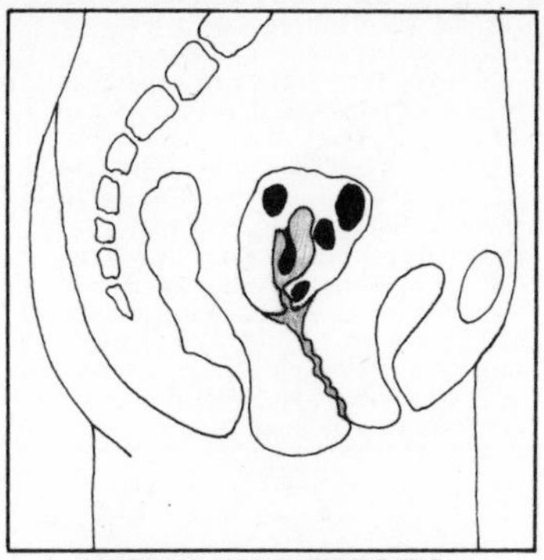

UTERUS WITH FIBROIDS

necessary to perform a hysterectomy.
Polyps Found in the uterus, as well as the bladder, nose and intestine, these are benign (non-cancerous) tumours which develop from mucous membranes and form dangling shapes. They are usually harmless, although they may cause an obstruction. In the uterus, polyps are generally removed by dilatation and curettage.

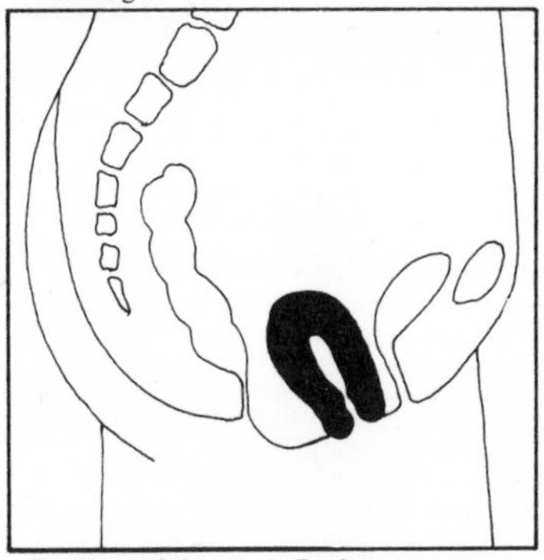

Prolapse of the uterus Prolapse means the displacement of an organ from its usual position and a prolapsed uterus will sag down into the vagina and perhaps even protrude between the legs. It is usually the result of an injury during childbirth, 99 per cent of women who suffer from prolapse of the uterus have given birth, but it may not become a problem until age further weakens the muscles and ligaments which support the uterus. Symptoms include frequent and difficult urination, incontinence, vaginal discharge, a feeling that something is coming out of the vagina, and above all the disappearance of all these symptoms on lying down. Mild cases require no treatment, but if the condition is troublesome a supportive pessary may be inserted by a doctor. In severe cases, the uterus may have to be corrected by surgery or even removed.

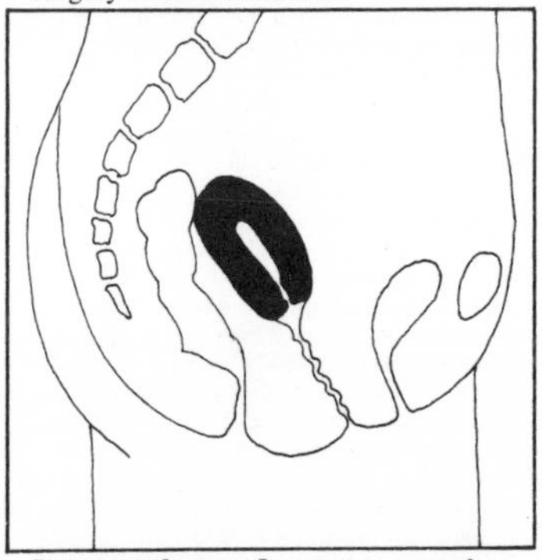

Retroverted uterus In most women, from puberty onwards, the uterus lies tilted forwards at an angle of 90° to the vagina, resting on the bladder, and moves backwards only as the bladder fills or when a woman lies on her back. In about 10 per cent of women the uterus is retroverted, i.e. it lies tilted backwards. Many ailments have been attributed to retroversion of the uterus in the past, including backache, sterility, vaginal discharge, pelvic pain, headaches, constipation, diminished sexual desire, frequency of urination and wind. It is now known, however, that it causes none of these symptoms and is usually troublesome only in pregnancy, when the enlarging uterus may fail to rise into the abdomen. Urine retention in the bladder results, but the problem can generally be corrected manually by a doctor. Retroversion can also happen after childbirth, or it may be caused by pelvic tumours, such as ovarian cysts, connective tissue joining to other structures, infection or endometriosis. In these cases, surgery may be necessary.

Uterus (Womb) This is a hollow muscular organ lying in the middle of the pelvis between the bladder in front and the bowel behind. It is pear-shaped and weighs only a few ounces. The upper part is broad and opens out at each side into the Fallopian tubes. The lower end narrows into the cervix, which leads into the vagina.

V

Vaginal Deodorants The purpose of a deodorant is, literally, to remove an odour. Deodorants which contain chemicals to destroy or neutralize smells arising from perspiration under the arms or on the feet have been in use for several decades and are safe for all but the most sensitive skins. Vaginal deodorants, on the other hand, are relatively new on the market and medical opinion that they may be harmful is increasing. Antiseptic deodorants used in the vaginal area can cause irritation to the delicate skin there and may interfere with the natural secretions of the vagina, some of which are 'natural' cleansers. The best way to cleanse the vaginal area is by regular washing with soap and water. Wear pants with cotton-lined gussets whenever possible and change them frequently.
If, in spite of regular cleansing, offensive odours persist, check with your doctor—particularly if you notice a discharge. The odour could be the warning sign of some vaginal disorder or infection and cure, as opposed to disguise, is called for.

VAGINAL INFECTIONS Many women experience some kind of vaginal infection during the course of their lives. Most of them are not dangerous, though they are troublesome and need to be cleared up as quickly as possible. Some vaginal discharge is natural, but the warning signs of an infection are unpleasant odour (check first that you have not left a tampon or contraceptive device, such as a Dutch cap, in situ), coloured or copious amount of discharge, soreness and/or redness of the vagina and labia, and irritation. If you use bath additives, particularly the foaming kind which contain some detergent, stop using them as a preliminary measure: they can cause irritation. If any or all of these symptoms persist for more than a day or two, visit your doctor. Never try to diagnose or treat yourself. See also Venereal Diseases.
Candidiasis ('thrush') Thrush is caused by a type of fungus, a yeast organism. It occurs naturally in the vagina, but is usually restrained by the acidic conditions. It can also be transmitted sexually, though men usually have no symptoms. Symptoms in women include itching and soreness of the vagina and vulva, getting worse at night or when the body becomes warm, usually accompanied by a thick, cheese-like, creamy discharge. Recurrent infection suggests possible lack of hygiene in both men and women. It may also result from taking certain antibiotics or oral contraceptives and, very occasionally, it may be the symptom of incipient diabetes. Treatment is usually by the insertion of nystatin pessaries high in the vagina.
Haemophilis vaginalis This is a bacterium which causes an infection whose symptoms are similar to those of trichomoniasis (see below). The differences are that the discharge is white or greyish and the odour produced is particularly unpleasant after intercourse. It is usually sexually transmitted and both partners should be treated.
Non-specific vaginitis The cause and nature of this infection are as yet unidentified. Symptoms include frequent or painful passing of water; white or yellowish discharge, sometimes streaked with blood; puffy vaginal walls, possibly with pus; pains in the lower back; and swollen glands in the abdomen and thighs. Treatment is usually effective through the application of sulphur creams or pessaries prescribed by your doctor.
Trichomoniasis This is the most common form of infectious vaginal discharge. It is caused by a single-cell parasite. Unless it is found in conjunction with other infections, the symptoms are a thin greenish-yellow or grey discharge, soreness and itching of vagina and vulva, and often clusters of red spots on the vagina and an unpleasant odour. Should the urinary tract become infected, cystitis may also occur. If, as occasionally happens, the Fallopian tubes become infected, sterility may result. It cannot be over-emphasized that vaginal infections must be diagnosed and treated as quickly as possible, since if the infection is trichomoniasis or gonorrhoea (the two sometimes occur together) a woman may become infertile. The infection is mostly transmitted sexually, and again men usually experience no symptoms, but very occasionally it can be passed on by wet or moist towels and flannels. Treatment involves both partners and, although vaginal pessaries may work for mild cases, oral antibiotics are usually required.

Varicose Veins See Veins.

VEINS
Broken veins Broken or enlarged blood vessels on the face may be caused by the skin disease rosacea (see below) or may be of the type known as telangiectases, where the capillaries have become permanently dilated. The reasons for this are not fully known, but as with broken or dilated veins on other parts of the body they may be the result of extreme heat or cold, too much spicy food or excessive sunshine. Heredity is almost certainly a factor, too, and liver damage can also be a cause. If the condition is mild, cosmetics will help to camouflage the redness; alternatively, your doctor or dermatologist may recommend the removal of the damaged veins by electrolysis (electrodesiccation) or cryosurgery (which involves freezing with dry ice).
Rosacea This is a skin disease where the face and nose become red and flushed because the blood vessels have become grossly enlarged. The skin is often oily with pimples in the same area, and the condition may affect the eyes. The cause of rosacea is not known, but it may be the result of an excessive intake of irritant foods and drinks, such as highly-spiced foods, tea, coffee and alcohol. Certainly, these seem to exacerbate the condition, as do extreme weather conditions and emotional problems. Treatment is by antibiotic drugs internally and soothing antiseptic lotions externally. A bland diet must also be followed. In some cases electrolysis may help to a certain extent, but this must be undertaken under the supervision of a dermatologist and results will depend on your age and the severity of the condition.
Spider veins The fine tracery of blue or purplish veins sometimes referred to as spider veins, because of a web-like formation, are usually found on the thighs, around the knees, and occasionally on the calves and feet. They are in fact blood-congested, dilated capillaries, particularly noticeable because they are very close to the skin. Pregnancy and hereditary factors play a part in their appearance, but the most common causes are constricting girdles or garters, excessive standing, and too much sitting with the legs crossed. Special leg make-up may be used to disguise the veins and in a few cases electrolysis can remove them. It is better, however, to avoid the predisposing factors mentioned above and to keep the body well toned and the circulation in good order.
Varicose veins These are veins which have become stretched and dilated out of proportion to the amount of blood they have to carry. The veins most likely to become varicose are the great saphenous veins, with branches on the inner side of the leg, knee and thigh, and the veins around the lower end of the bowel, which result in haemorrhoids or piles (see Piles). The veins of the legs are vulnerable because they have to defy gravity, pumping blood uphill back to the heart. If the valves which control the flow of blood become weakened, they allow blood to seep backwards. The early symptoms of varicose veins are aching and a feeling of weight in the limbs, sometimes accompanied by cramps, either at night or on getting up in the morning. Varicose veins are sometimes hidden, but they usually stand out above the surface of the skin. If they are not treated, they may become sore or inflamed and may ulcerate. There is also the danger that a blow may cause them to haemorrhage. Women who have had several children are vulnerable to varicose veins, as are those who are obese or spend long hours standing. Varicose veins which occur during pregnancy, due to foetal pressure, often disappear after the birth, but a few may remain and will become progressively worse with subsequent pregnancies. Where the condition is not severe, simple palliative treatment such as resting the legs and wearing supportive stockings or bandages may help. In more severe cases, injections may be used or the veins may be removed surgically.

VENEREAL DISEASES These are diseases which are nearly always passed on during sexual intercourse. The germs live and grow in the warm, moist linings of the sex organs and die almost immediately away from the heat of the body, so you cannot catch VD from lavatory seats, towels, bed-clothes, door handles or dirty cups. In the last twenty years, the number of cases of VD has multiplied three or four times in many countries. In Britain, one adult in every two hundred needs treatment and the frequency of gonorrhoea is second only to the common cold. The signs of VD are often difficult to spot, particularly in women, but if you know or suspect that you have had contact with an infected person, or if you notice any of the symptoms listed below, visit a doctor or clinic without delay. All the conditions are curable if treated early. See also Vaginal Infections.
Gonorrhoea This is the most common form of VD. In Britain, one thousand people catch it every week; in the United States, about five million people are infected every year; and worldwide there are about 150 million cases. The incubation period is longer in women than men and the eventual symptoms, if any, are less severe. They may include a burning sensation when urinating, frequent urination, whitish-yellow discharge with an unpleasant smell, fever, chill, abdominal pain and painful joints. However, over 70 per cent of women suffering from gonorrhoea experience no symptoms at all. Diagnosis is by laboratory analysis of any discharge or smear from the affected part; treatment is by antibiotics, which are generally effective if prescribed early, although alcohol may interfere with the cure. As not all gonorrhoea germs are exactly the same, some strains may initially resist treatment, so follow-up tests are necessary to make sure that cure is complete. If untreated, gonorrhoea has more serious consequences for women than for men. The disease may affect the glands at the entrance to the vagina, which can swell up as large as a golf ball; it may cause inflammation of the rectum, sometimes accompanied by discharge; it may spread to the bloodstream, cervix, uterus, ovaries and Fallopian tubes, sometimes leading to infertility; and it can infect the joints and cause arthritis. If it is undetected in a woman who becomes pregnant, gonorrhoea may result in an ectopic pregnancy, premature birth, umbilical cord inflammation, maternal fever or blindness in the child.
Non-specific urethritis Urethritis involves inflammation of the urethra, the tube leading from the bladder to outside. The cause of NSU has not yet been identified, but it does not always seem to require intercourse with an affected

person to develop. It is the most common of all sexual disorders in men, but in women the symptoms are often insignificant or hard to diagnose. They may include a burning pain on urination and discharge, which often contains blood or pus; untreated, the condition can lead to disease of the joints, eye disease and inflammation of the sex organs. NSU usually responds to antibiotics, but research is being carried out to find better methods of treatment and to discover more about the causes of the disease.

Syphilis This is the most serious venereal disease. Its prevalence varies: in Britain it is fairly rare; in the United States it is the third most common reportable disease; and worldwide there are about fifty million cases. The incubation period for syphilis is anything from nine days to three months, but symptoms usually appear three weeks or so after contact with an infected person. The first sign is a painless sore or ulcer (doctors call it a chancre), on or near the sex organs, which is round or oval, firm and just under ½ in (1.25 cm) across. It may ooze a colourless liquid and is full of syphilis germs, which can infect a minute crack in the skin of anyone coming into contact with them. The sore usually heals of its own accord in a few weeks and, as it is often inside the vagina or rectum, may pass unnoticed. Without treatment, the disease will now progress to the second stage and germs will spread through the bloodstream. A few weeks later there may be a general feeling of ill-health, sore throat, fever, headaches, swollen glands, loss of hair and skin rashes on the back of the legs and front of the arms, and perhaps on the body, face, hands and feet as well. These symptoms will also disappear eventually, even without treatment, lasting anything from three weeks to nine months. By this time the germs may have reached the brain, nervous system, eyes, liver and heart, where they can live for many years unnoticed but not inactive. They will slowly weaken, damage and cripple almost every organ and may cause paralysis, blindness, insanity and death.

Diagnosis of syphilis is by testing the sores for bacteria or the blood for antibodies; treatment is by antibiotics, which will cure the condition in most cases. Regular medical checks and blood tests are very important during and after recovery, often for more than two years, to make sure that cure is complete. If untreated, a woman who becomes pregnant can pass the germ into the bloodstream of her baby, which may be born dead or handicapped as a result. This is rare today as all mothers receiving antenatal care are given a blood test, known as the Wassermann test, to detect syphilis; if necessary, treatment can be given to cure both the mother and her unborn baby.

Verrucas (Plantar Warts) See Foot Problems.
Vitiligo See Skin Problems.

W

WARTS Warts are small, dry, tough outgrowths of the skin, formed usually in response to irritation of the skin by a virus. The growths are benign and are quite common in growing children and young people, especially on the hands. A wart may disappear of its own accord as suddenly as it arrived. If it persists it can be 'frozen' and cut off, burned off, or eroded by the application of certain chemicals. Warts should never be tampered with or removed except under medical supervision.

Genital warts Sometimes called moist warts, these are found in or around the genital area and anus. Although very infectious, they are rarely painful. The warts may take between one and six months to incubate and can be transmitted by sexual contact. A doctor may remove the wart by cauterizing it with an electric needle, freezing it or using chemicals, or he may prefer to remove it surgically.

Plantar warts (verrucas) These are warts which appear on the sole of the foot. For causes and treatment, see Foot Problems.

WELL WOMAN CHECK-UP

Every woman should know enough about her body to be able to recognize and understand the changes that occur. It is also vital for her health that she has a regular programme of check-ups and examinations, so that any problems can be dealt with before they become serious.

Breast Self-Examination

This is not difficult and should be done regularly once a month. The best time is after your menstrual period, when the breast is usually at its softest, or any day in the month if you have reached menopause so long as you make it a regular habit.

Choose a time when you will not be disturbed and then undress and sit or stand in front of a mirror with your arms hanging loosely at your sides. Study your reflection for any change in the size or appearance of your breasts, any irregularities in the outline, and any puckering or dimpling of the skin. Raising your arms above your head, turn a little from side to side and check your breasts from different angles. Then look down at your breasts, examining the nipples for any sign of bleeding or unusual discharge. For the second part of the examination lie down on your bed, with your head on a pillow, and make yourself comfortable. Put a folded towel or small pillow under your left shoulder to help spread the breast tissue and make examination easier. Put your left hand under your head and use your right hand to examine your left breast. Keep your fingers together and use the flat of the fingers, not the tips, feeling the breast gently but firmly. You will soon get to know what is normal for you, and must be on the lookout for any lump or thickening or anything unusual. Examine your breasts step by step, following the instructions set out below.

If you think you have found something in one breast, but are not sure, feel the same part in the other breast. If it feels similar, it is probably just the way your breasts are made. But if it feels different, and you think there may be something wrong, consult your doctor as soon as possible. Never neglect or ignore any change in your breasts.

Only one in five women who are referred by their doctors to a specialist because of these symptoms turn out to have breast cancer; the remainder have cysts, which can be cut out or aspirated (drawn out by suction), mastitis and other benign conditions. One in seventeen women do get breast cancer, but their chances of survival are enormously increased the earlier the cancer is detected and treated, so don't let your fear of surgery stop you going to the doctor. The most vulnerable women are those with a family history of breast cancer.

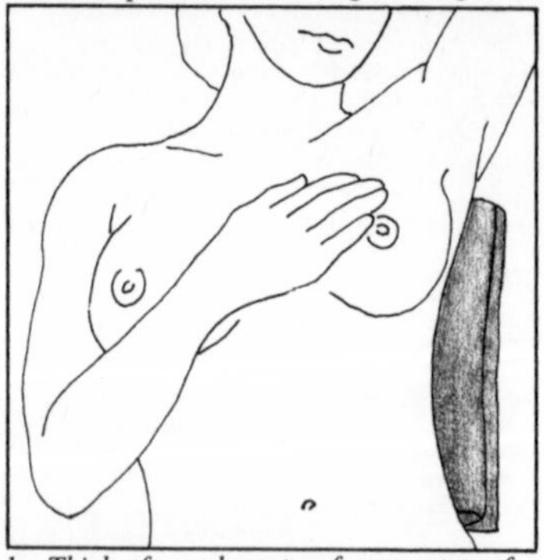

1 Think of your breast as four quarters of a circle. Begin by examining the inner, upper quarter. Start feeling well out from the breast and work your way carefully towards the nipple.

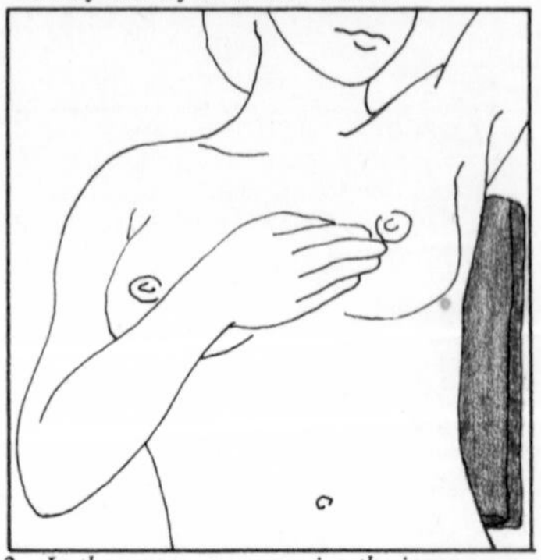

2 In the same way, examine the inner, lower quarter of your left breast, starting from the breast bone and from the ribs below the breast. Examine the area all round the nipple, too.

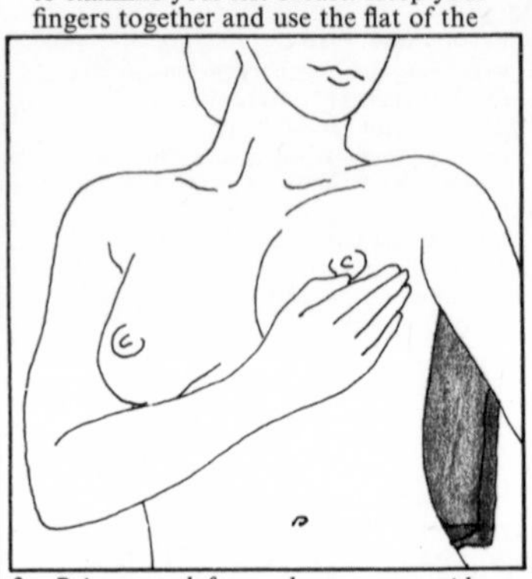

3 Bring your left arm down to your side and start to feel the outer, lower quarter. Again start well out from the ribs below and at the side of the breast and work in towards the nipple.

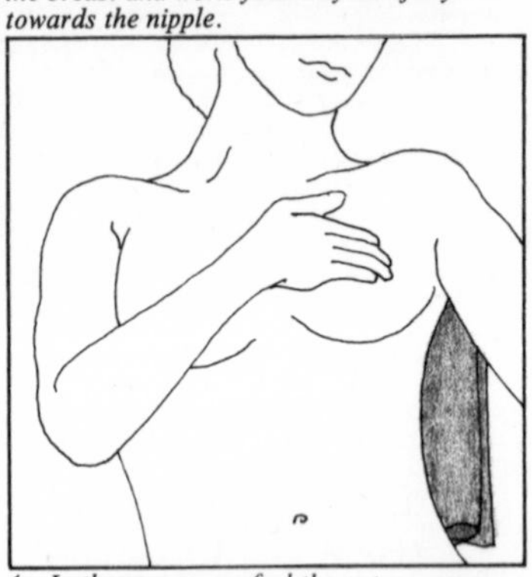

4 In the same way, feel the outer, upper quarter until you have come full circle. Then examine across the top of the breast again, feeling the extra section of breast tissue towards the armpit.

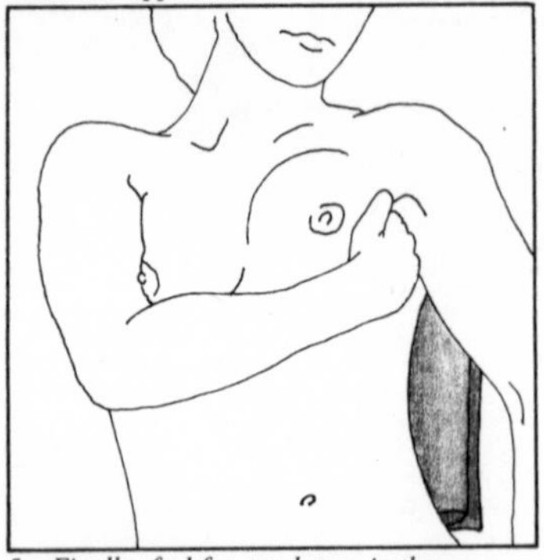

5 Finally, feel for any lumps in the armpit itself. Then, to examine your right breast, put the towel under your right shoulder, your right hand under your head, and follow the instructions as before.

Cervical Smear (Pap Test)

This test should be done every two years. Cervical cells obtained by gently scraping the cervix with a wooden spatula are analysed and if there are any suspicious cells a small operation can be done, called a cone biopsy, which removes the affected area entirely. The operation does not prevent a woman having children later. The test is free on the National Health Service to British women over the age of twenty-five.

Internal Self-Examination

Self-examination using a speculum is a very good way to get to know your body, particularly your reproductive organs, but it is not a substitute for a regular full pelvic examination by a doctor or clinic. A plastic speculum is easier to obtain than a metal one; try a good pharmacy which supplies the medical profession. Inserting it is painless if you are relaxed and self-examination is not difficult if you follow the instructions set out below.

1 Familiarize yourself with how the speculum works.
2 Sit or lie on your bed or a table with your knees bent and feet wide apart. Use a pillow to prop yourself up, if necessary.
3 Arrange a mirror beneath the vulva and direct a light against it so that the internal organs will be well lit up and clearly visible.
4 Rub the speculum with lubricating cream to facilitate insertion, if necessary.
5 Hold the speculum sideways with the blades closed and gently insert into the vagina in the same way as a tampon.
6 When it is all the way in, turn the speculum so that the handle points upwards.
7 Grasp the handle and firmly pull the

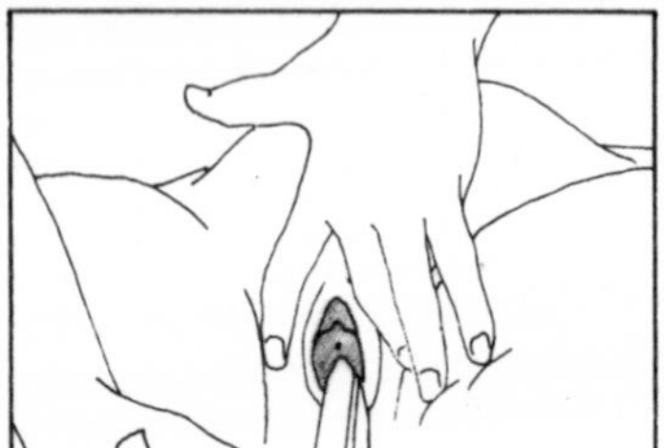

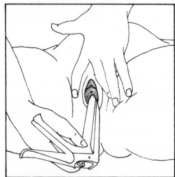

outside section towards you. This will open the blades of the speculum inside you.
8 Hold the part of the handle next to your pubic hair steady and push down the outside section until you hear a click. The speculum is now locked open.
9 With the light shining on the mirror, you should now be able to see clearly into the vagina. At the end you will notice a dome-like protrusion; this is the cervix. In the centre of the cervix is a small opening, the os, which leads to the uterus. The size and colour of the cervix depend on your age, the stage in your menstrual cycle, and whether you have had children. You may find that you have to move around or reinsert the speculum before the cervix comes into view. If you can't see it, gently draw the speculum out in the closed position and push down with your stomach muscles. Then reinsert the speculum in the same way as before.
10 Note the details of the cervix, os, vaginal walls and vaginal secretions. In this way you will learn what is normal for you and will be able to recognize any changes as they occur, and seek medical advice if necessary.
11 When you have finished your examination, remove the speculum with the blades in the closed position.
12 Wash the speculum with an antibiotic soap in warm water after each use.

Pelvic Examinations

These are carried out to confirm a woman's pregnancy and six weeks after childbirth. They are also done as part of a general gynaecological check-up, preferably once a year; when a woman needs advice about family planning; or whenever she reports a vaginal or pelvic abnormality. The following disorders should always be reported to your doctor.

1 Irregular or heavy bleeding, at any time before or after the menopause, which persists. Causes are many and various, most of them minor and easily cleared up, but they should be treated. Fibroids may be a cause, or polyps in the womb which can be removed by dilatation and curettage or shrunk with hormone treatment, but if they get very troublesome a hysterectomy may be advisable.

2 Sores, warts or any painful spots, boils or irritation in the genital area. They may be symptoms of sexually-transmitted diseases or caused by a virus.

3 Vaginal discharge which is abnormal in colour, smell, quantity, consistency or which causes itching. It may be caused by vaginal infections or VD.

Menstrual Problems

Troublesome or painful periods can be a constant drain on health and vitality. Too many women learn to 'live with' their menstrual problems and accept them as natural and inevitable. It is possible, however, to have treatment to help alleviate menstrual tension and pain. If you feel you need help, fill in the premenstrual tension chart below and take it to your doctor. It is also important to keep a regular check on the pattern of your periods, so that if changes in the cycle occur or there are any problems, such as heavy or irregular bleeding, you can take action. The menstrual chart below is of a woman with a five-day period on a thirty-day cycle. Make a similar chart for yourself to keep in touch with your own pattern.

Premenstrual Tension Chart

If you think that you are suffering from premenstrual tension and would benefit from treatment, record your symptoms on the chart below for at least one and preferably two menstrual cycles. Then show the chart to your family doctor. Once he agrees that your symptoms have a regular cyclical pattern, ask him either to treat them himself or to refer you to a specialist or clinic dealing with menstrual problems.

PREMENSTRUAL TENSION CHART

Symptom	Day of Cycle		Severity
	Start	End	* * * very troublesome * * unpleasant but not extreme * mild
Depression			
Irritability			
Anxiety			
Lethargy			
Lack of co-ordination (clumsiness, accidents, etc.)			
Breast tenderness			
Swollen abdomen			
Swollen ankles or fingers			
Headaches (not migraine)			
Loss of sex drive			
Other symptoms			
Date of last menstrual period			

MENSTRUAL CHART
showing regular cycle of thirty days and five days duration (p = period)

	Jan	Feb	Mar	Apr	May	Jun	Jul	Aug	Sep	Oct	Nov	Dec
1												
2												
3												
4												
5											p	p
6									p	p	p	p
7							p	p	p	p	p	p
8				p	p	p	p	p	p	p	p	p
9		p	p	p	p	p	p	p	p	p	p	p
10	p	p	p	p	p	p	p	p	p	p		
11	p	p	p	p	p	p	p	p				
12	p	p	p	p	p	p						
13	p	p	p									
14	p											
15												
16												
17												
18												
19												
20												
21												
22												
23												
24												
25												
26												
27												
28												
29												
30												
31												
Total												

SUGGESTED READING

ANXIETY AND NEUROSIS Charles Rycroft (UK: Pelican, 1979. USA: Penguin, 1979).

BABY AND CHILD Penelope Leach (UK: Michael Joseph, 1977. USA: Alfred Knopf, 1977).

BIOFEEDBACK FASTING AND MEDITATION Gary Null (USA: Pyramid Books, 1974, distributed in UK by Thorson Publishers).

BIRTH AT HOME Sheila Kitzinger (UK & USA: Oxford University Press, 1979).

BIRTH WITHOUT VIOLENCE Frederick Leboyer (UK: Fontana, 1978. USA: Alfred Knopf, 1975).

BODY, THE Anthony Smith (UK: Penguin, 1978).

BOOK OF CHILD CARE, THE Hugh Jolly (UK & USA: George Allen & Unwin, 1976).

BOOK OF EST, THE Luke Rhinehart (UK & USA: Sphere Books, 1976).

CHEMICAL COMPOSITION OF FOODS, THE (McCance and Widdowson's) A. A. Paul and D. A. T. Southgate (UK: HMSO, 1978).

DEPRESSION Ross Mitchell (UK & USA: Pelican, 1979).

DON'T SAY YES WHEN YOU WANT TO SAY NO Herbert Fensterheim and Jean Baer (UK: Futura Publications, 1976. USA: Dell Publishing, 1975).

EAT WELL AND KEEP HEALTHY Merril Durrant (UK: Macdonald Guidelines, 1977. USA: Ideals Publishing Company, coming shortly).

EVERYWOMAN. A GYNAECO-LOGICAL GUIDE FOR LIFE Derek Llewellyn-Jones (UK & USA: Faber & Faber, 1978).

EXPERIENCE OF CHILDBIRTH, THE Sheila Kitzinger (UK & USA: Pelican, 1978).

FACT OF FOOD, THE Arnold Bender (UK & USA: Oxford University Press, 1975).

FAT IS A FEMINIST ISSUE Susie Orbach (UK: Paddington Press, 1978, Hamlyn Paperbacks, 1979. USA: Paddington Press, 1978, distributed by Grosset & Dunlap).

FROM WOMAN TO WOMAN Lucienne Lanson, MD, FACOG (UK: Cape, 1977. USA: Alfred Knopf, 1977).

GESTALT IS edited by John O. Stevens (UK & USA: Bantam, 1977).

GOOD AGE, A Alex Comfort (UK: Mitchell Beazley, 1977. USA: Crown, 1976, Simon & Schuster paperback, 1978).

HAIR Wendy Cooper (UK: Aldus Books, 1968. USA: Stein & Day, 1969).

HARD LABOUR: REALIST'S GUIDE TO HAVING A BABY Jean and John Lennane (UK: Victor Gollancz, 1977).

HEALTH OF WOMEN, THE Dr Wendy Greengross (UK: Family Doctor Publications, 1974).

HITE REPORT, THE Shere Hite (USA: Summit, 1978, distributed in UK by WHS Distributors).

LET'S EAT RIGHT TO KEEP FIT Adelle Davis (UK: Unwin, 1976. USA: Harcourt Brace Jovanovich, 1954).

LET'S GET WELL Adelle Davis (UK: Unwin, 1976. USA: Harcourt, Brace & World, 1965).

LIVING WELL, THE PEOPLE MAINTENANCE MANUAL (UK: Mitchell Beazley, 1977. USA: Rand McNally, 1977).

MEDICINES: A GUIDE FOR EVERY-BODY Peter Parish (UK: Penguin Books, 1979).

MENSTRUAL CYCLE, THE Katharina Dalton, MRCGP (UK: Pelican, 1970. USA: Pantheon, 1969).

MENSTRUAL TABOOS (The Matriarchy Study Group, London).

NATURAL BEAUTY BOOK, THE Clare Maxwell-Hudson (UK: Macdonald & Jane's, 1976).

NEW SEX THERAPY, THE Helen Singer Kaplan (UK: Ballière Tindall, 1975. USA: Brunner Mazel, 1974, distributed by Quadrangle).

NEW WOMEN'S HEALTH HAND-BOOK, THE edited by Nancy Mackeith (UK: Virago, 1978, distributed in USA by Academy Press and Women in Distribution).

NO CHANGE: BIOLOGICAL REVOLUTION FOR WOMEN Wendy Cooper (UK: Hutchinson, 1978).

NOT ALL IN THE MIND Richard Mackarness (UK: Pan, 1979).

ON BEING A WOMAN Fay Fransella and Kay Frost (UK: Tavistock Publications, 1977. USA: Methuen Inc, 1977).

OUR BODIES, OURSELVES Boston Women's Health Collective (UK: Penguin Books, 1978. USA: Simon & Schuster, 1976).

PERIODS WITHOUT PAIN Erna Wright (UK: Tandem, 1979. USA: Hart Publishing, 1979).

PLANNING OR PREVENTION? NEW FACE OF FAMILY PLANNING Peter Diggory and John McEwan (UK & USA: Marion Boyars Publishers, 1978).

PREGNANCY Gordon Bourne (UK: Pan Books, 1978. USA: Harper & Row, 1975).

PREMENSTRUAL SYNDROME AND PROGESTERONE THERAPY, THE Katharina Dalton, MRCGP (UK: William Heinemann Medical Books, 1977. USA: Year Book Medical Publications, 1977).

PSYCHOANALYSIS AND WOMEN edited by Jean Baker Miller (UK & USA: Pelican, 1973).

RELAXATION AND EXERCISE FOR NATURAL CHILDBIRTH the late Helen Heardman, revised and re-edited by Maria Ebner (UK & USA: Churchill Livingstone, 1975).

SELF-HELP AND HEALTH: MUTUAL AID FOR MODERN PROBLEMS David Robinson and Stuart Henry (UK: Martin Robertson, 1979, distributed in USA by Biblio-Distribution Center).

TEXTBOOK OF CONTRACEPTIVE PRACTICE John Peel and Malcolm Potts (UK & USA: Cambridge University Press, 1969).

THIS SLIMMING BUSINESS John Yudkin (UK: Penguin, 1977).

TREAT YOURSELF TO SEX Paul Brown and Carolyn Faulder (UK: J. M. Dent & Sons, 1977. USA: Universe Books, 1977).

WHEN I SAY NO, I FEEL GUILTY Manuel J. Smith (UK & USA: Bantam, 1975).

WOMAN'S BODY: AN OWNER'S MANUAL The Diagram Group (UK & USA: Paddington Press, 1977).

WORLD OF HAIR COLOUR, THE Daniel Galvin (UK: Macmillan, 1977. USA: Van Nostrand Reinhold, 1977).

WORLD'S LIVING RELIGIONS, THE Geoffrey Parrinder (UK: Pan Books, 1977. USA: Thomas Ray Crowell, 1964).

YEAR OF BEAUTY AND HEALTH, A Beverly and Vidal Sassoon (UK: Penguin Books, 1974. USA: Simon & Schuster, 1976).

YOUR BABY AND YOUR FIGURE Lois P. Burns (UK & USA: Churchill Livingstone, 1978).